Myology and Kinesiology for Massage Therapists

Enhanced Edition

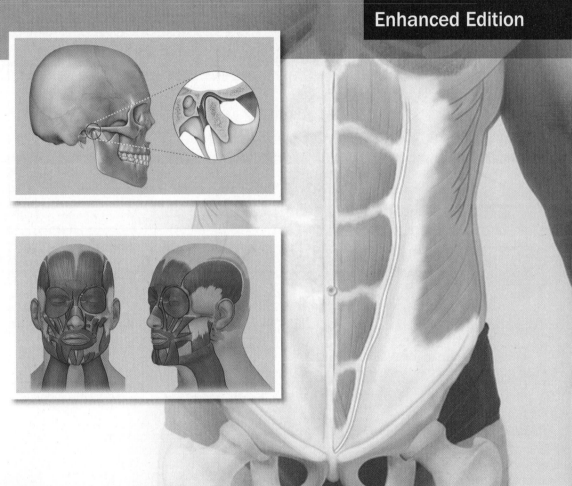

Myology and Kinesiology
for Massage Therapists

Enhanced Edition

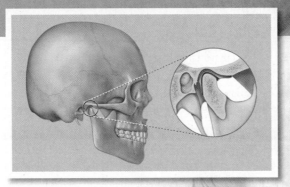

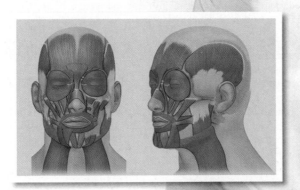

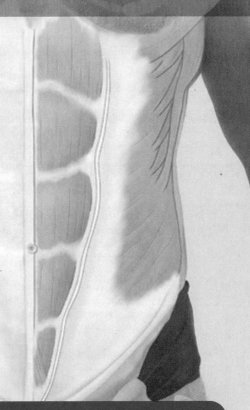

Cindy Moorcroft, BA, LMT
Center for Natural Wellness School of Massage Therapy
Albany, New York

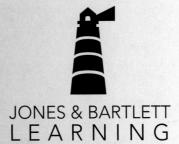

JONES & BARTLETT
LEARNING

World Headquarters
Jones & Bartlett Learning
5 Wall Street
Burlington, MA 01803
978-443-5000
info@jblearning.com
www.jblearning.com

Jones & Bartlett Learning books and products are available through most bookstores and online booksellers. To contact Jones & Bartlett Learning directly, call 800-832-0034, fax 978-443-8000, or visit our website, www.jblearning.com.

21841-1

Production Credits

VP, Product Management: Amanda Martin
Director of Product Management: Cathy Esperti
Product Manager: Sean Fabery
Product Specialist: Andrew LaBelle
Product Coordinator: Elena Sorrentino
Digital Project Specialist: Angela Dooley
Director of Marketing: Andrea DeFronzo
Marketing: Dani Burford

Production Services Manager: Colleen Lamy
VP, Manufacturing and Inventory Control: Therese Connell
Composition: S4Carlisle Publishing Services
Project Management: S4Carlisle Publishing Services
Cover Design: Kristin E. Parker
Senior Media Development Editor: Troy Liston
Rights Specialist: Rebecca Damon
Printing and Binding: LSC Communications

Library of Congress Cataloging-in-Publication Data
Library of Congress Cataloging-in-Publication Data unavailable at time of printing.

LCCN: 2020936107

6048

Printed in the United States of America
24 23 22 21 20   10 9 8 7 6 5 4 3 2 1

For my Family

Preface

This book is designed for massage therapy students taking a Myology (study of muscles) and/or Kinesiology (study of movement) course as part of their massage curriculum. Because muscles permit our body's movement, these topics complement each other. Massage therapy is frequently defined as the systematic manipulation of soft tissue of the body for therapeutic purposes. Muscles make up a significant portion of the body's soft tissue, so massage therapists address muscles in almost every massage technique they perform. In addition, therapeutic massage requires an understanding of both muscles and movement. Clients frequently complain of muscle pain and limited range of motion, and they often seek postural changes. For massage therapists to address limited movement and/or muscle pain, and address imbalances, the body's muscles, and the movements they perform need to be learned.

APPROACH

I began teaching myology and kinesiology at the Center for Natural Wellness School of Massage Therapy in 1999. At that time, although there were many wonderful atlases of human anatomy, there were very few texts written specifically for massage therapy students nor were there texts that explained how, when, and why massage may be necessary and beneficial to muscle health. I was looking for a text that contained all the information that massage therapy students would need about muscles but did not find one.

As I began to teach, I fine tuned my beliefs about what is needed in a myology text for massage therapy students. I realized that students benefit greatly from accurate and clear illustrations of muscles, with origins and insertions labeled. I saw that students learn and recall information about muscles much better when offered an understanding of why the muscles perform the actions they do. It remained clear to me that students must learn the relationship between each muscle and the common possible postural and functional issues with which massage therapy clients present. Further, I learned

that students need much repetition of the vast amount of material that makes up the study of myology and kinesiology, in order to recall and use the information in practical situations.

My observations led me to create various handouts and learning activities to help my students understand and retain the information about muscles relevant to massage therapy. I put these exercises together into a workbook which students complete as each muscle is covered in class. Students draw and record factual information about each muscle including origin, insertion, action(s), location, how to palpate, how to stretch, synergist and antagonist muscles, and potential postural and functional issues if the muscle is shortened and/or lengthened.

In addition, I created activities to assist visual and kinesthetic learners including cut and paste paper replications of the muscles, and worksheets to use with clay building of the muscles. Finally, I wrote up many case studies from my own practice of massage therapy, and I devised many review exercises and games to simply practice recall of the information.

The workbook and activities I use in the classroom have become the basis for this text. In addition, much research and feedback from colleagues has enabled this text to be expanded to its current state.

ORGANIZATION

Myology and Kinesiology for Massage Therapists, Enhanced Edition is divided into two distinct sections. Part I includes Chapters 1 and 2 and provides all the background information needed to begin the study of myology and kinesiology. The text assumes no prior knowledge; thus, the first chapter begins with an explanation of anatomical terms and movements. Chapter 2 provides basic information about the anatomy and physiology of bones and joints of the body, connective tissue, skeletal muscle cells as well as the physiology of muscle contraction. The physiology presented is necessary for a thorough understanding of the skeletal muscles. The remainder of Part I applies previously learned information to massage therapy.

The terms origin and insertion are defined, and an explanation of shortened and lengthened muscles is provided. In addition, synergists and antagonists are discussed.

Part II includes Chapters 3, 4, and 5, and is a detailed study of 119 skeletal muscles organized by body region. The presentation of each muscle includes a beautiful illustration with origin and insertion clearly labeled. At the end of each chapter, regional pictures are included so that students may view each muscle in the context of surrounding muscles. For each muscle, text is included that provides an explanation of the etiology of the name, pronunciation, location and how to palpate the muscle, origin and insertion, actions and an explanation of why each muscle performs each action, a list of synergists and opposing muscles, implications of the muscles shortening and lengthening, instructions about how to stretch the muscle, and finally, innervation and arterial supply for each muscle.

Each chapter also includes a workbook section. Students must "work" to learn myology and kinesiology and the work-book section provides a variety of activities for students to complete to reinforce the understanding and memorization of the above material. Art and writing activities, palpation exercises, review charts, and case studies are included.

VISION

I believe the process of becoming a massage therapist involves a unique combination of learning technical, scientific information and techniques, and developing the art of touch and connection to another. But perhaps most important, the process of becoming a massage therapist and the practice of massage therapy requires a willingness to connect to our own source of inner knowledge and peace. I frequently speak to my students about the need to center themselves, quiet the mind, and practice awareness of their bodies, feelings, and beliefs. Only by knowing and facing ourselves fully will we be able to be fully present and provide our best work for our clients. Good luck!

Acknowledgements

Writing this book has been a journey; an invitation to take the rich subject of myology and kinesiology and delve into it in a way I have never done so before. This process has allowed me to take time to reorganize my teaching materials, research the fascinating nuances of many muscles, and engage in give-and-take dialogue with colleagues. I am grateful for the opportunity and the assistance provided to create this book.

Many people have helped me along the way. I wish to thank John Goucher, who first proposed this project and helped to keep it on track. I wish to thank Jennifer Ajello for answering my many questions and ensuring that the project moved along as necessary. I wish to thank David Payne for his thoughtful feedback and amazing job of selecting artwork to accompany the text. And thank you to the many others who quietly worked behind the scenes to support and direct this project. It takes a collective effort to complete a textbook.

I also wish to thank my coworkers and fellow instructors at CNW Massage School. Dale Perry and Lisa Satalino, thank you for sharing your experience and insights about the content of this text. Lisa Kay, thank you for helping me to visualize the structure of the text. Laura Iacovone, thank you for being a walking thesaurus and grammar chief. Dan Cronin, thank you for the opportunities and support you have provided. I wish to thank all my coworkers for their encouragement, support, and commitment to academic excellence, and unwavering belief in the ability of massage therapy to change the world for the better.

Thanks to all the students who have graced my classrooms. I have been a teacher for 27 years and I still enjoy almost every day in the classroom. It is an honor to teach. Thank you for your continual inspiration and for teaching me so much.

I thank my massage therapy clients who have shared their stories and lives, and deepened my gratitude for health and community.

I thank my family and friends. My parents have shared their wisdom and their belief in working hard to reach the finish line. Thank you for that. I thank Lisa for her huge heart and bright light. Yes, it is the size of North America and may it shine forever. Thank you Laura and Liz for your endless support! And Fern, I thank you for all you have brought into my life. Parenting is so very rich! May you always believe in yourself and may you fly!

Reviewers

Tamara J. Erickson, BA
Director of Dental Assisting
Herzing College, Lakeland Academy Division
Crystal, Minnesota

Mari Frohn, AS, BS
Professor
Tri-County Regional Vocational Technical High School
Franklin, Massachusetts

Kristyn Hawkins, LDH, BGS
Clinical Instructor
Indiana University, South Bend
South Bend, Indiana

Toni Hoffa, BS
Instructor
Lakeland Academy Division of Herzing College
Crystal, Minnesota

Stella Lovato, CDA, MSHP, MA
Chair of Allied Health
San Antonio College
San Antonio, Texas

Martha McCaslin, BSBM
Dental Assisting Program Director
Dona Ana Branch Community College
Las Cruces, New Mexico

Rita Ohrdorf, MA
Instructor
University of Northern Colorado
Pueblo, Colorado

Sue Raffee, RDH, EFDA, MSA
Sinclair Community College
Dayton, Ohio

Sheila Semler, PhD
Instructor
Lansing Community College
Lansing, Michigan

Diana Sullivan, ME
Dental Department Chair
Dakota County Technical College
Rosemount, Minnesota

Jo Szabo, CDA, CDR, BEd
Coordinator
Niagara College
Welland, Ontario

Mary Clare Szabo, CDA, CDR
Professor
George Brown College
Toronto, Ontario

Mark Thoreson, DDS
The Academy of Dental Assisting
Redmond, Oregon

Contents

PART ONE

Foundational Concepts of Myology and Kinesiology

1

Anatomical Terminology and Body Movements

■ CHAPTER OUTLINE

KEY TERMS

Anatomical position: a standard body position that is used to provide consistent orientation to the body from which directional terms are referenced. Body is standing erect while head, feet, and palms face forward.

Cephalic region: region of the head

Cranium: includes top and back of the head

Thorax: region of the body between the neck and abdomen

Sagittal plane: plane that divides the body into left and right sections

Frontal (coronal) plane: plane that divides the body into front and back sections

Transverse plane: plane that divides the body into upper and lower sections

Anterior: front or toward the front

Posterior: back or toward the back

Superior: above

Inferior: below

Proximal: closer to the trunk, typically used in reference to an extremity

Distal: farther from the trunk, typically used in reference to an extremity

Medial: closer to the midline

Lateral: farther from the midline

Ipsilateral: pertaining to the same side

Contralateral: pertaining to the opposite side

Unilateral: one-sided, typically either right- or left-sided

Bilateral: two-sided, typically right- and left-sided

Superficial: closer to the surface

Deep: farther from the surface

Flexion: bending movement that occurs at a joint

Dorsiflexion: ankle movement, in which the top of the foot moves toward the front of the leg

Plantarflexion: ankle movement, in which the sole of the foot moves downward, toward the back of the leg, or causes us to rise up on our toes.

Lateral flexion: movement of neck, trunk, or lower spine that involves bending to the side

Extension: straightening movement that occurs at a joint

Hyperextension: the movement of extension beyond anatomical position

Rotation: a turning movement that occurs at a joint

Supination: a turning movement that occurs within the forearm, causing the forearm to rotate laterally

Pronation: a turning movement that occurs within the forearm, causing the forearm to rotate medially

Abduction: a movement bringing a body part away from the midline or out to the side of the body

Adduction: a movement bringing a body part closer to the midline or across the midline of the body

Circumduction: movement of a body part in a circular direction, combining flexion, extension, adduction, and abduction

Horizontal abduction: movement of a limb in a horizontal manner away from the midline of the body

Horizontal adduction: movement of a limb in a horizontal manner toward and/or across the midline of the body

Inversion of the foot: movement of the sole of the foot inward toward the midline

Eversion of the foot: movement of the sole of the foot outward toward the side

Elevation: upward movement

Depression: downward movement

Protraction: movement in an anterior or forward direction

Retraction: movement in a posterior or backward direction

Upward rotation: turning movement of the shoulder blade or scapula, such that the right scapula turns counterclockwise or the left scapula or shoulder blade turns clockwise

Downward rotation: turning movement of the shoulder blade or scapula, such that the right scapula turns clockwise or the left scapula or shoulder blade turns counterclockwise

This chapter is designed to provide you with the terminology needed to study the muscles and movements of the body. We begin with a study of anatomical language. Massage therapists frequently communicate with each other and with other health care professionals, as well as with clients. Anatomical language allows you to communicate with precision and clarity about anatomical structures and locations, and the health issues that your clients may be facing. In addition, you will need to understand anatomical language as you look at the many illustrations included in this text. The pictures are shown from different perspectives and angles and are labeled with anatomical terms to help you understand the orientation of the picture. For many students, the study of anatomical language is like learning a foreign language. Give yourself enough study time to grasp the terms we will use.

After we cover anatomical language, we will explore the names of the movements we can perform. Understanding the terms that describe our body's movements will be essential for studying the muscles and their actions.

ANATOMICAL TERMINOLOGY

Because of the complexity of the body, a whole system of terminology has been developed to help accurately describe the orientation of each part of the body to the other parts and to the whole. These terms may be grouped into four categories: anatomical position, body regions, planes of reference, and directions.

Anatomical Position

Anatomical position refers to a standard body position that is used to give us a consistent orientation to the body from which directional terms are referenced (determined). Western anatomical position includes the following characteristics:

1. Standing erect (upright)
2. Arms at the sides
3. Facing forward (both head and feet)
4. Palms facing forward

Body Regions

Anatomists have divided the body into several distinct regions and named them with specific anatomical language. The head or **cephalic region** is subdivided into the cranium and face. The **cranium** includes the top and back of the head, and the face includes the area from the eyebrows down to the chin. The neck region lies between the head and the chest. The **thorax** is the region between the neck and the abdomen. The front of the thorax is typically called the *chest*, and the back of the thorax is commonly called the *upper* and *mid back*. The abdominal region lies between the thorax and the pelvis, and the pelvic region is the area between the abdomen and the lower extremities. When combined, the thorax, abdomen, and pelvis make up the *trunk*. In addition, the armpit area is called the *axilla*, and the front of the elbow is the *antebrachial area*. The groin area is called the *inguinal area*.

The extremities are divided into distinct areas, as well. In anatomical language, the arm is defined as the body part between the shoulder and the elbow. The forearm is defined as the body part between the elbow and the wrist. In anatomical language, the thigh is defined as the body part between the hip and the knee, and the leg is defined as the body part between the knee and the ankle.

Figure 1-1 shows a person in anatomical position, with body regions labeled.

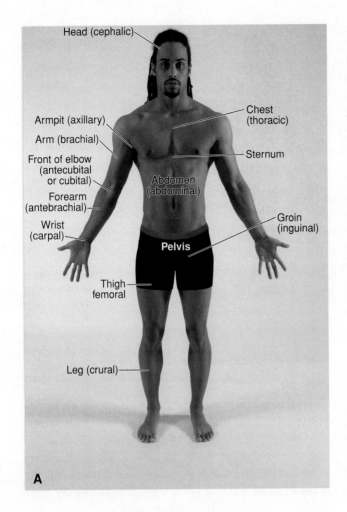
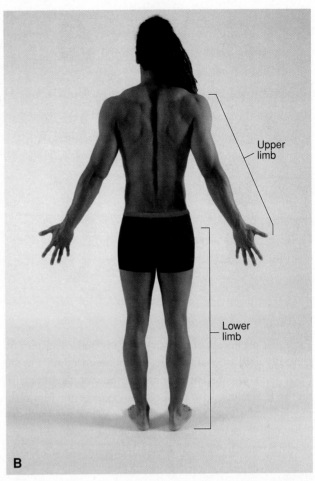

FIGURE 1-1 · Anatomical position showing the body regions.

Planes of Reference

The anatomical planes of reference are another tool useful for describing the body. Anatomical structures can be depicted from different perspectives to illustrate particular views. The plane that divides the body into right and left sections is called a **sagittal plane**. The plane that divides the body into front and back (*anterior* and *posterior*) sections is called a **frontal** or **coronal plane**. The plane that divides the body into upper and lower portions is called a **transverse plane**.

Figure 1-2 illustrates the planes of the body: A = sagittal, B = frontal or coronal, C = transverse.

Directional Terms

Directional terms allow us to communicate precisely about the locations of bodily structures. We will use these terms frequently to describe the locations of muscles and their attachment sites to bones.

Anterior

Anterior (or ventral) refers to the front of the body or the front of a body part, or closer to the front. (*Palmar* is a similar term, referring to the palm of the hand.) Examples of using the term

include the following: *The eyes and nose are on the anterior aspect of the face. A client complained of soreness in his anterior thighs.*

Posterior

Posterior (or dorsal) refers to the back of the body or the back of a body part, or closer to the back. Examples of using the term include the following: *The spine is most palpable on the posterior aspect of the body. A client has a sunburn on his posterior neck.*

Superior

Superior (or cephalad) means above or refers to a location closer to the top of the head. This term is generally applied to the head, neck, and trunk (and not the extremities). Examples of using the term include the following: *The chin is superior to the navel. A client's headache is felt directly superior to her eyes.*

Inferior

Inferior (or caudal) means below or closer to the feet. This term is generally used when referring to a location in the head, neck, and/or trunk. Examples of using the term include the following: *The chin is inferior to the nose. A client is experiencing back pain directly inferior to the 12th rib.*

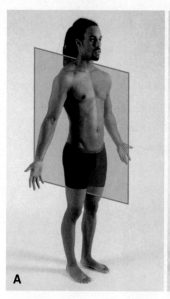
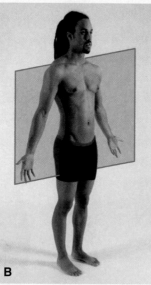
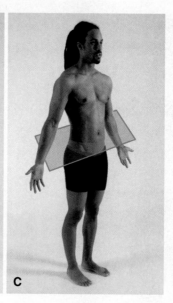

A   **B**   **C**

FIGURE 1-2 · Planes of the body.
A: Sagittal, **B:** Frontal or coronal, **C:** transverse

Proximal

Proximal means closer to the core of the body. This term is generally used when describing a location on a limb. On the upper limb, proximal means closer to the shoulder joint, and on the lower limb, proximal means closer to the hip joint. Examples of using the term include the following: *The elbow is proximal to the wrist. A client has a hairline fracture in her left, proximal femur (bone of the thigh).*

Distal

Distal means farther from the trunk of the body. Distal also means closer to the tips of the toes or fingers. This term is used when describing a location on a limb. On the upper limb, distal means farther from the shoulder joint and closer to the fingertips. On the lower limb, distal means farther from the hip joint and closer to the tips of the toes. Examples of using the term include the following: *The wrist is distal to the elbow. A client has osteoarthritis in the most distal joints of her fingers. Massage therapists' fingertips should be distal to their fingernails.*

Medial

Medial means closer to the midline or mid-sagittal plane. This term applies to all parts of the body. Examples of using the term include the following: *The nose is medial to the ears. A client complains of muscle tension in his right medial thigh.*

Lateral

Lateral means closer to the side or farther away from the midline. This term applies to all parts of the body. Examples of using the term include the following: *The hips are lateral to the navel. A client has a bruise on the lateral aspect of his right forearm.* **Note:** Without anatomical position, there would not be consistency in defining the lateral side the forearm. Why?

Ipsilateral

Ipsilateral means located on or pertaining to the same side of the body, either the right or left. An example of using this term is as follows: *A client has an ipsilateral shortening of the trapezius and levator scapula muscles on the right side.*

Contralateral

Contralateral means located on or pertaining to the opposite side of the body. Two examples of the use of this term include: *A lesion on the brain will commonly cause contralateral paralysis. A muscle, such as the right SCM, which is located on the right side of the neck, causes the neck to rotate to the left. This action is called contralateral rotation of the neck.*

Unilateral

Unilateral means one-sided, referring to the right side only or the left side only. Two examples of the use of this term follow: *One can experience a unilateral lung collapse. When a muscle, such as the SCM neck muscle, contracts unilaterally, it causes lateral flexion of the neck.*

Bilateral

Bilateral means two-sided. An example of using the term is as follows: *When the SCM muscles contract bilaterally—meaning that both right and left SCM muscles contract simultaneously—the result is flexion of the neck.*

Superficial

Superficial means closer to the surface of the body. Examples of using the term include the following: *The sternum (breast bone) is superficial to the heart. A client has a strain in his biceps brachii, the most superficial muscle in the anterior arm.*

Deep

Deep means farther away from the surface. Examples of using the term include the following: *The stomach is deep to the abdominal muscles. A client has shin splints because she tore a muscle in the deep posterior leg compartment.*

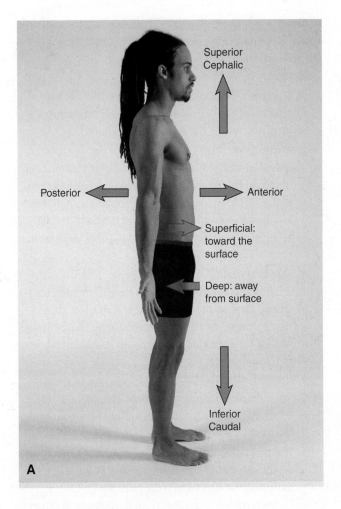

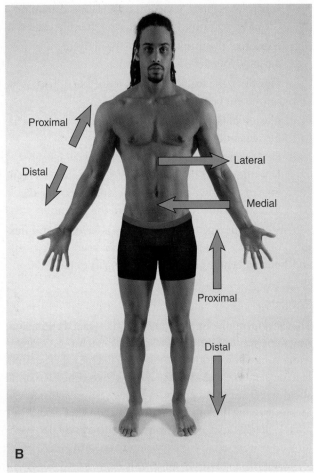

FIGURE 1-3 · Directional terms.

Figure 1-3 uses arrows to illustrate directional terms.

MOVEMENTS

Movement happens at joints. We will discuss the significance of joints in Chapter 2. The goal of this section is to help you become familiar with the language used to describe the names of the particular movements we perform. Movements are named in terms of the body parts that move, or in terms of the joint at which movement occurs, or both.

Flexion

The movement involved in bending is called **flexion**. Any joint you can bend can perform flexion. For example, when you bend your elbow, you are flexing it. When you bend your knee, you are flexing it. When you bend your fingers, you are flexing them.

Flexion is usually a forward movement (except for the knee and toes). When you move your arm forward, you are flexing it. When you move your thigh forward, you are flexing it. When you move your fingers forward, you are flexing

them. Of course, use of the word "forward" is from the perspective of anatomical position.

Flexion can also be seen as decreasing the angle between bones or body parts. Elbow flexion involves decreasing the angle between the forearm and the arm, and flexion of the knee involves decreasing the angle between the thigh and leg.

Examples of flexion are listed below:

1. Flexion of the forearm, elbow, or forearm at the elbow (these are all equivalent). This movement bends the elbow.
2. Flexion of the arm, humerus, shoulder, or arm at the shoulder (these are all equivalent). This movement brings the arm forward.
3. Flexion of the hand, wrist, or hand at the wrist. This movement brings the palmar surface of the hand closer to the anterior forearm.
4. Flexion of the head or neck. Technically, these can be different, depending on where specific movement occurs. That is, flexion of the head can mean a forward movement at the atlanto-occipital joint only, or it can mean a forward movement of the joints between the

cervical vertebrae. Sometimes, we have to determine the meaning through the context in which it is used.

5. Flexion of the trunk or spine. This movement bends a person forward.
6. Flexion of the leg, knee, or leg at the knee. This movement bends the knee.
7. Flexion of thigh (or femur), hip, or femur at hip. This movement brings the thigh forward.
8. Flexion of the foot at the ankle has special names. **Dorsiflexion** is moving the foot so that the toes point toward the nose, and **plantarflexion** is moving the foot so that the toes point toward the ground.

Flexion to the side, or side bending, is called **lateral flexion**. We can perform lateral flexion of the head, neck, trunk, and spine by bending the named body part to one side.

Extension

The movement involved in straightening is called **extension**. Any joint you can "straighten" permits extension. Straightening your elbow or knee is extending it. One can also think of extension as increasing the angle between bones. Think about relevance to the elbow and knee again. Extension can involve moving back to anatomical position after flexing any joint. Generally, extension involves moving a body part back. Moving your arm back is extension of the arm.

Examples of extension are as follows:

1. Extension of the forearm, elbow, or forearm at the elbow. This movement straightens the elbow.
2. Extension of the arm (or humerus), shoulder, or arm at the shoulder. This movement moves the arm posteriorly.
3. Extension of the hand, wrist, or hand at wrist. This movement involves bringing the dorsal side of the hand toward the posterior forearm.
4. Extension of the head or neck. These movements involve bringing the head or neck posteriorly.
5. Extension of the trunk or spine. This movement brings the spine backward, or straightens the spine from a flexed position.
6. Extension of the leg, knee, or leg at the knee. This movement straightens the knee.
7. Extension of the thigh (or femur), hip, or femur at the hip. This movement involves moving the thigh posteriorly.

Note: In the field of massage therapy, **hyperextension** typically refers to the position of a joint being extended past anatomical position.

Rotation

Any movement that involves turning is **rotation**. Think of rotation around an axis, if that is helpful. At the shoulder and hip joints, rotation is specified as medial (turning toward the midline) or lateral (turning toward the side). Anywhere in the spine, rotation is simply described as rotation to the left or rotation to the right.

Examples of rotation are as follows:

1. Rotation of the head (sometimes included as part of rotation of the neck; left or right). This movement involves turning the head to the right or left.
2. Medial (sometimes called internal) or lateral (sometimes called external) rotation of the arm, which is equivalent to medial (or internal) or lateral (or external) rotation of the shoulder. Medial rotation involves turning the arm inward toward the midline of the body, and lateral rotation involves turning the arm outward away from the midline of the body.
3. Medial (internal) or lateral (external) rotation of the thigh is also called medial (or internal) or lateral (external) rotation of the hip or lateral rotation of the femur. Medial rotation involves turning the thigh inward toward the midline of the body, and lateral rotation involves turning the thigh outward away from the midline of the body.
4. Rotation of the trunk to the right or rotation of the spine to the left. This movement turns the trunk to the right or left.
5. Rotation of the forearm has special names: **supination** is movement of the hand and forearm laterally, generally toward a position in which the palm faces up.
   Pronation is a movement of the forearm and hand medially, generally toward a position in which the palm faces down.

Abduction

Abduction is a movement away from the midline of the body, or a movement out to the side of the body. This definition suits abduction of the hip/thigh or shoulder/arm. In addition, abduction of the digits (fingers and toes) involves moving the fingers away from the midline of the hand (third digit or middle finger) or moving the toes away from the midline of the foot (second digit of foot). In other words, spreading the fingers or toes is abducting them.

Examples of abduction include the following:

1. Abduction of the arm, which is equivalent to abduction of the shoulder. This movement moves the arm out to the side of the body.
2. Abduction of the hip, which is equivalent to abduction of the thigh. This movement moves the thigh out to the side of the body.

Adduction

A movement toward the midline of the body, and/or across the midline of the body is known as **adduction**. This definition suits adduction of the hip/thigh or shoulder/arm. In addition, adduction of the digits (fingers and toes) involves moving the fingers toward the midline of the hand (third digit or middle finger) or moving the toes toward the midline of the foot (second digit of foot). In other words, bringing the fingers or toes closer together is adducting them.

Examples of adduction include the following:

1. Adduction of the arm or shoulder. This is a movement of the arm toward and across the body from a position of arm abduction.

2. Adduction of the hip or thigh. This is a movement of the thigh toward and across the body from a position of hip abduction.

Circumduction

Circumduction is a combination of four movements: abduction, adduction, extension, and flexion, all done continuously, so that the distal end of the moving body part traces a circle. Circumduction can occur only at joints that permit flexion, extension, adduction, and abduction.

Examples of circumduction include the following:

1. Circumduction of the arm or shoulder. This movement combines flexion, extension, abduction, and adduction of the shoulder joint.

2. Circumduction of the thigh or hip. This movement combines flexion, extension, abduction, and adduction of the hip joint.

3. Circumduction of the fingers at the metacarpophalangeal joints (knuckles). This movement combines flexion, extension, and radial and ulnar deviation of each digit at the metacarpophalangeal joint. Radial deviation moves a single digit or the whole hand toward the lateral forearm. Ulnar deviation is the movement of a single digit or of the whole hand toward the medial side of the forearm.

4. Circumduction of the head and trunk is debatable, because the joints between the individual vertebrae that make up the neck (between C2 and T1) do not perform adduction or abduction. However, the joints of the neck can perform lateral flexion, and the combined neck movements of flexion, extension, and lateral flexion to both the right and left mimic circumduction.

Horizontal Abduction

Horizontal abduction of the arm or shoulder is a movement of the arm along the transverse (horizontal) plane away from the body.

Horizontal Adduction

Horizontal adduction is a movement of the arm or shoulder in a horizontal or transverse plane toward and across the midline of the body.

Inversion of the Foot

Inversion is a movement in which the soles of the foot move toward the midline of the body (soles point in). (In some references, inversion may be referred to as supination. Technically, supination is a term indicating a combination of inversion, ankle dorsiflexion, and adduction of the ankle.)

Eversion of the Foot

Eversion is a movement in which the soles of the foot move away from the midline (soles point out). (In some references, eversion may be referred to as pronation of the foot. Technically, the term pronation of the foot means a combination of eversion of the foot, combined with abduction and plantarflexion of the ankle.)

Elevation

Elevation is an upward or superior movement. Elevation applies to the scapula (shoulder blade) and mandible (lower jaw bone).

Depression

Depression is a downward or inferior movement. Depression applies to the scapula (shoulder blade) and mandible (lower jaw bone).

Protraction

Protraction is an anterior or forward movement of the scapula or mandible.

Retraction

Retraction is a posterior movement of the scapula or mandible.

Upward Rotation

Upward rotation is a scapular movement, in which the scapula turns so that the glenoid fossa, a bone marking on the lateral, superior aspect of the scapula, turns upward. The glenoid fossa is the socket into which the humerus (arm bone) fits to form the shoulder joint. This rotation of the scapula is necessary for our arm to abduct beyond 90 degrees.

Downward Rotation

Downward rotation is a movement in which the scapula turns so that the glenoid fossa turns down. This scapular movement permits a greater range of arm movement when reaching down and back behind our body.

Figure 1-4 demonstrates these movements of the body.

Arm and Elbow movement

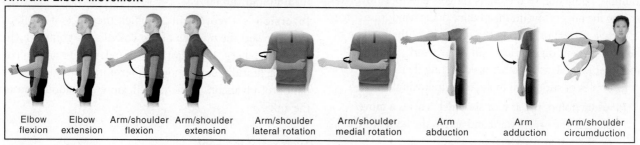

Elbow flexion | Elbow extension | Arm/shoulder flexion | Arm/shoulder extension | Arm/shoulder lateral rotation | Arm/shoulder medial rotation | Arm abduction | Arm adduction | Arm/shoulder circumduction

Leg movement

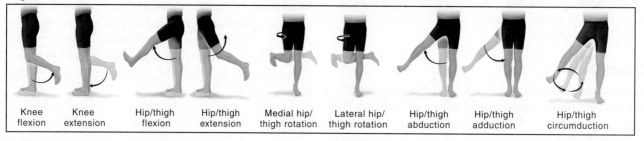

Knee flexion | Knee extension | Hip/thigh flexion | Hip/thigh extension | Medial hip/thigh rotation | Lateral hip/thigh rotation | Hip/thigh abduction | Hip/thigh adduction | Hip/thigh circumduction

Lower Arm and Hand movement

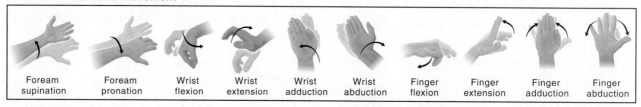

Foream supination | Foream pronation | Wrist flexion | Wrist extension | Wrist adduction | Wrist abduction | Finger flexion | Finger extension | Finger adduction | Finger abduction

Ankle and Foot movement

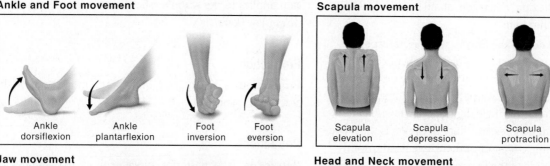

Ankle dorsiflexion | Ankle plantarflexion | Foot inversion | Foot eversion

Scapula movement

Scapula elevation | Scapula depression | Scapula protraction | Scapula retraction

Jaw movement

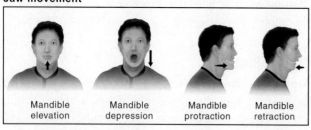

Mandible elevation | Mandible depression | Mandible protraction | Mandible retraction

Head and Neck movement

Neck flexion | Neck extension | Neck rotation | Lateral neck flexion

Trunk and Spine movement

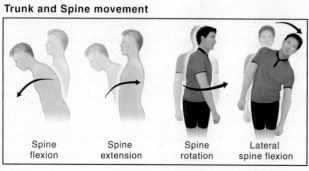

Spine flexion | Spine extension | Spine rotation | Lateral spine flexion

FIGURE 1-4 · Body movements.

■ CHAPTER SUMMARY

A thorough knowledge of anatomical language is necessary for the study of myology and the practice of massage therapy. We will use the terminology covered in this chapter throughout the text. In addition, this language is commonly used in communication between health care practitioners and in documentation by health care practitioners of all kinds, including massage therapists.

■ WORKBOOK

Palpation Exercises

Palpate or locate the following areas on your body:

1. Palpate the scapula (shoulder blade). Trace this triangular bone, located in the lateral upper back. Find the border or edge of the scapula that is closest to the spine. It is easier to locate this border of the scapula when the elbow is flexed and the arm is placed behind the body. Find the lateral border as well.

2. Palpate your anterior sternum (breast bone). Find the superior aspect of the sternum and gently find the pointy inferior aspect, which is called the xiphoid process.

3. Trace the superior border of your clavicle (collar bone) from medial to lateral.

4. Palpate your anterior leg (remember, the leg does not include the thigh). Notice where you can feel soft tissue and where you feel bone.

5. Palpate your medial forearm. Remind yourself of the difference between medial and lateral and the importance of anatomical position when distinguishing medial and lateral.

6. Palpate your posterior arm (remember, the arm does not include the forearm). Why do you suppose it feels fleshy?

7. Palpate your proximal, anterior forearm. Distinguish this from your distal anterior forearm. Which half of the anterior forearm is more muscular, the proximal half or the distal half?

8. Palpate your lateral thigh. Compare it to the medial thigh in terms of sensitivity.

9. Can you find the most distal bone in your thumb?

10. Find the lateral edges of the sternum (breast bone) and trace your ribs medially to laterally.

Review Exercises

Write the appropriate terms in the spaces below:

1. List four characteristics of anatomical position:

   a. _____

   b. _____

   c. _____

   d. _____

2. Which plane divides the body into right and left sections?

   _____

3. Which plane divides the body into anterior and posterior sections?_____

   _____

4. The chin is inferior to _____

   _____

5. Name a body part superior to the navel: _____

   _____

6. Name a structure medial to the shoulders: _____

   _____

7. Name a structure on the anterior aspect of the body: _____

   _____

8. Name something distal to your knees: _____

9. What side of your head is covered when you wear a hood?

   _____

10. Which joint is directly proximal to the hand? _____

    _____

2

Body Tissues and Basic Physiology

■ CHAPTER OUTLINE

KEY TERMS

Epithelial tissue: tissue that covers surfaces, and lines cavities and hollow organs.

Connective tissue: abundant and continuous tissue that supports, binds, and protects the body and structures within the body

Compact bone tissue: the dense type of bone tissue that comprises the entire outer surface of bones

Spongy bone tissue: the lighter type of bone tissue, formed by thin slivers of bone arranged in an irregular pattern and located deep to compact bone tissue

Axial skeleton: includes the bones that generally run along the vertical axis of the body, including the bones of the skull and spine, as well as the ribs, sternum (breast bone), and hyoid bone, which is a small curved bone in the anterior neck

Appendicular skeleton: includes all the bones of the upper and lower limbs, as well as the bones that hold the limbs to the axial skeleton, including the clavicle (collar bone) scapula (shoulder blade), and hip bones

Bone markings: special projections, shapes, and textures on bones that serve varied anatomical functions

Synarthrotic: immovable

Amphiarthrotic: slightly movable

Diarthrotic: freely movable

Synovial joint: a freely movable, diarthrotic joint in which the ends of the joining bones are covered with cartilage and held together by a synovial joint capsule containing synovial fluid

Endomysium: sheet-like connective tissue structure that surrounds each muscle

Perimysium: sheet-like connective tissue structure that surrounds each fascicle or group of muscle cells

Epimysium: sheet-like connective tissue structure that surrounds each individual muscle cell

Sarcolemma: cell membrane of a skeletal muscle cell

Myofibril: a basic structure that forms skeletal muscle cells and that contains multilayered rows of alternating protein fibers called myofilaments

Myosin: thicker myofilament or protein fibers that overlap with actin when a muscle shortens

Actin: thinner myofilament or protein fibers that overlap with myosin when a muscle shortens

Sarcoplasmic reticulum: a network of sacs and tubules that surround each myofibril

Sliding filament mechanism: the process by which myosin and actin are pulled closer together, resulting in muscle shortening

Motor units: a single motor neuron (nerve cell designed to allow movement) and the set of skeletal muscle cells innervated by that single neuron

Motor unit recruitment: the use of additional motor units to accomplish a muscle contraction or movement

Muscle tone: continuous contraction of alternating motor units, which causes muscles to have tension or firmness during rest

Muscle fatigue: exhaustion of muscle cells, so that they can no longer contract

Origin: muscles typically connect to two or more locations on at least two different bones; the stable or less movable location is called the origin

Insertion: muscles typically connect to two or more locations on at least two different bones; the more movable, less stable location is called the insertion

Action: movement that occurs at a joint when a muscle's insertion moves closer to the muscle's origin

Concentric contraction: a muscle contraction resulting in shortening of the muscle

Eccentric contraction: a muscle contraction resulting in lengthening of the muscle

Isometric contraction: a muscle contraction in which the length of the muscle does not change, yet muscle tension occurs

Synergists: muscles that perform one or more of the same actions

Antagonists: muscles that perform one or more opposite actions

Shortened muscle: a muscle that remains in a shortened position, with origin and insertion closer together than typical

Lengthened muscle: a muscle that remains in a lengthened position, with origin and insertion farther apart than typical

---

This chapter provides an introduction to the physiology of bones, joints, and muscles, and a brief overview of nerve and arterial supply to muscles. This information provides a framework for the understanding of myology and kinesiology, as these studies relate to massage therapy. We begin this chapter by discussing the types of tissue and the particular categories and functions of connective tissue. Within this discussion, we explore the bones and bone markings of the body, many of which serve as muscle attachment sites. Next, we explore joints of the body, including the different categorizations of joints and the movement permitted at each. Then, we move on to muscles, including their structure and functions and how they contract to allow us to move. We conclude this chapter with a look at shortened and lengthened muscles, how they impact posture and function, as well as the importance of muscles' innervation and arterial supply. Understanding these concepts prepares you for the study of myology and assists you in designing treatment plans for your clients.

TYPES OF TISSUE

A brief description of tissues can help create a context for learning about muscles, bones, and joints. *Tissue* is a mass of the same type of cells that form a particular kind of structure, for a particular purpose. There are four types of tissue in the body. **Epithelial tissue** lines the cavities, vessels, and hollow organs of the body and forms the outer covering of the body. It also comprises various glands. **Nervous system tissue** forms the brain, spinal cord, peripheral nervous system, and all supporting nerve tissue. Nervous system tissue is designed to sense stimuli and respond to it by generating nerve impulses. **Muscle tissue** is designed to contract, which enables it to shorten and lengthen and thus allow movement. **Connective tissue** includes all other tissue in the body and is the most abundant type of tissue we have. Connective tissue protects, supports, and binds together other tissue. Of these four types, this chapter will focus primarily on connective tissue and muscle tissue.

CONNECTIVE TISSUE

It is just as important for massage therapists to understand and address connective tissue as it is to address muscles. In fact, it is impossible to differentiate the massage of muscle from the massage of connective tissue. As we will see later in this chapter, muscles are infused with and surrounded by connective tissue. Restrictions in a client's connective tissue can cause pain, limited range of motion, and postural abnormalities, all of which can be addressed with massage therapy.

Connective tissue is made up of cells and matrix. The matrix, which is secreted by the cells, gives connective tissue its unique properties. The matrix is made of ground substance and fibers, and depending upon its composition, may be fluid, gel-like, fibrous and flexible, or solid.

Connective tissue includes bone, cartilage, fascia (dense and loose connective tissue), blood, and lymph. Each of these is described below.

Bones

It is important for you, as a massage therapist, to understand bones and bony landmarks, as they are attachment sites for muscles. In addition, an understanding of the exact location of muscles and their position relative to bones and joints is needed to understand the movements muscles allow us to perform. You will also benefit from understanding the exact location of a muscle's connection to bone, as it is often helpful to massage this area to enhance muscle relaxation, or to treat or prevent tendonitis.

Bones are a rigid form of connective tissue that provide the overall structure of the body. They have several important functions, including protecting organs, producing blood cells, and storing fats and minerals. In addition, bones provide attachment sites for muscles and act as levers, or solid structures that move when muscles contract.

Bone Tissue

There are two types of bone tissue: compact and spongy (Fig. 2-1). **Compact bone tissue** forms the outer layer of bones and is more solid in structure. **Spongy bone tissue** is deep to compact bone and is porous. Spongy bone tissue is composed of thin beams of bone, called *trabeculae*, which are patterned in a criss-cross or latticelike structure. The space between the beams of bone are filled with red bone marrow, which produces blood cells.

Shapes of Bones

Bones are classified by shape: long, short, flat, irregular, or sesamoid. Long bones are longer than they are wide. The bones of the arm, forearm, fingers, thigh, leg, and toes are all long bones. Typical adult long bones contain spongy bone only on the proximal and distal ends of the bone and a hollow space called the *medullary canal* in the shaft of the bone. The medullary canal is filled with yellow marrow and contains fat cells.

Short bones are small and somewhat square-shaped and contain an outer layer of compact bone and an inner layer of spongy bones. Most of the carpal bones (most proximal bones in the hand) and the tarsal bones of the foot are short bones. Flat bones are as named: They are flat. Flat bones consist of two outer layers of compact bone with an inner layer of spongy bone between them. Examples include the ribs, sternum, scapula, and many bones of the skull. Irregular-shaped bones have unusual shapes. They include the vertebrae and some facial bones. Sesamoid bones are shaped like sesame seeds. The patella is the most famous. Other sesamoid bones are present in varying numbers and are generally imbedded in tendons.

Axial vs. Appendicular Skeleton

The human skeleton contains 206 bones and is divided into the axial and appendicular skeletons (Fig. 2-2). The bones of the axial skeleton form somewhat of a vertical axis through the center of the body. The **axial skeleton** includes the 22 bones of the skull, six auditory ossicles, 26 bones that make up the vertebral column, the hyoid bone, 24 ribs, and the sternum. The **appendicular skeleton** consists of the bones of the appendages or limbs and the girdles that hold the limbs to the axial skeleton.

The bones of the appendicular skeleton include the shoulder girdle bones: two clavicles and two scapulae. The appendicular skeleton also contains the bones of the upper limb: two humerus, two ulna, and two radius bones, 16 carpal bones (which include two each of the following bones: scaphoid, lunate, triquetrum, pisiform, trapezium, trapezoid, capitate, and hamate), ten metacarpals, and 28 phalanges in the hands. The appendicular skeleton also contains the pelvic girdle, or two coxal or hip bones, and the bones of the lower limb, which include two femurs, two patellae, two tibia, two fibula bones, 14 tarsals (which include two each of the following bones: calcaneus, talus, navicular, medial cuneiform, intermediate cuneiform, lateral cuneiform, and cuboid), ten metatarsals, and 28 phalanges in the feet.

Bone Markings

Bone markings are specific markings and textures on the surface of bones that serve many purposes. Most relevant to myology is the fact that bone makings serve as muscle attachment sites and provide the particular shapes that allow the bones to articulate (join) with other bones, thus creating joints. The list below describes the common markings that are relevant to the joints and muscles covered later in this book (Fig. 2-3).

1. The *head* of a bone is generally rounded and appears at either the distal or the proximal end of many bones. Just distal or proximal to the head is a narrow portion of bone called a *neck*. A head may fit nicely into a socket to form a ball-and-socket joint. Other heads articulate with curved bone markings at joints that permit less movement. Note the heads of the humerus and radius in Figure 2-3, the ulna in Figure 5-2B, and the fibula in Figure 5-3A.

2. A *condyle* (which means knuckle) is also a rounded bone marking at the distal or proximal end of a bone. (The condyles of the occiput, a skull bone, are on the inferior aspect of the bone.) Condyles come in pairs.

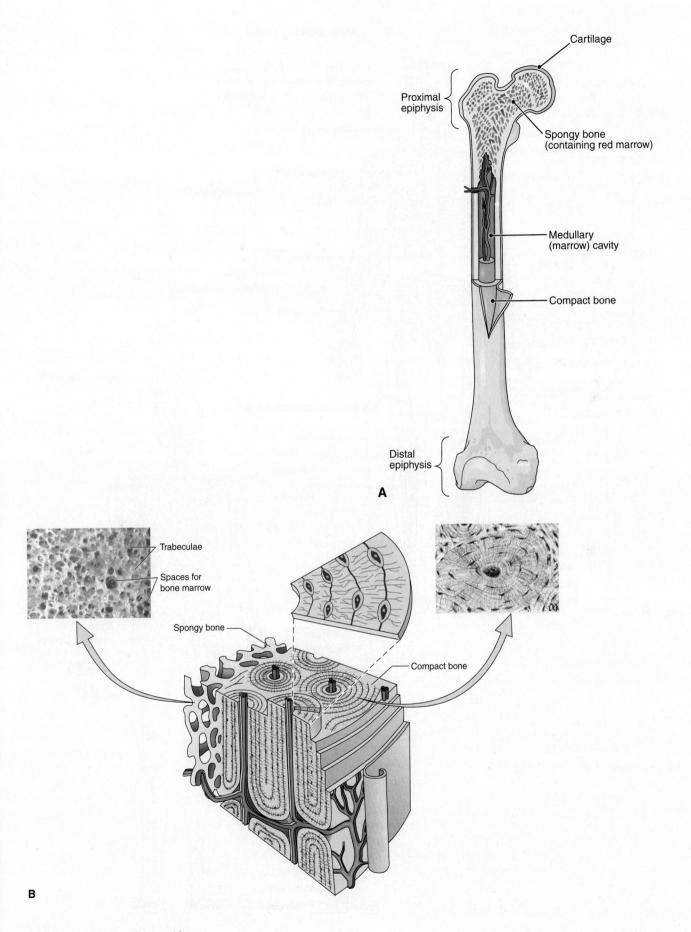

FIGURE 2-1 · Spongy and compact bone.

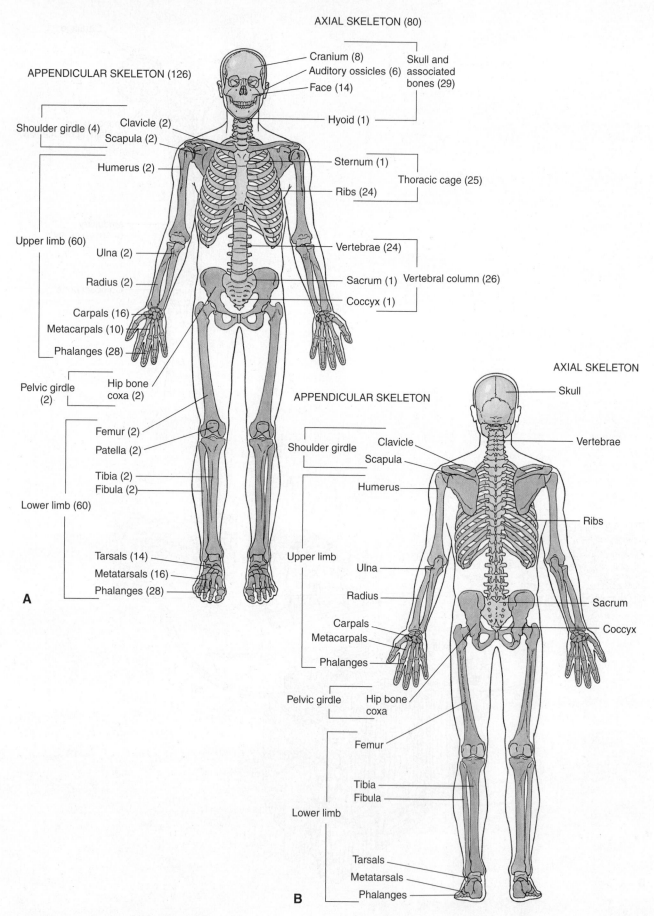

FIGURE 2-2 · Axial and appendicular skeleton.

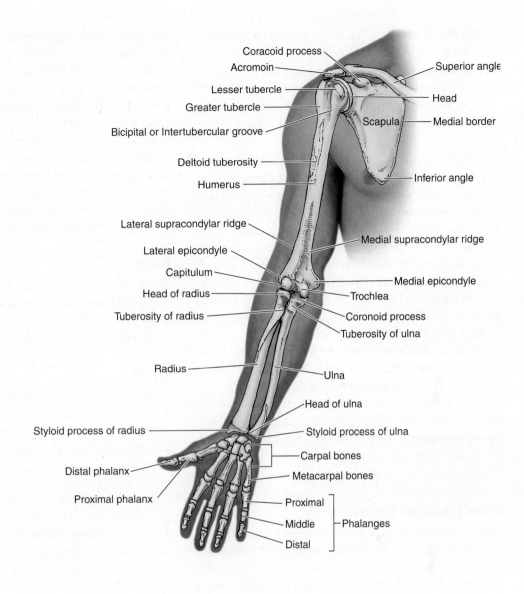

Coracoid process
Acromoin
Lesser tubercle
Greater tubercle
Bicipital or Intertubercular groove
Deltoid tuberosity
Humerus
Lateral supracondylar ridge
Lateral epicondyle
Capitulum
Head of radius
Tuberosity of radius
Radius
Styloid process of radius
Distal phalanx
Proximal phalanx

Superior angle
Head
Scapula — Medial border
Inferior angle
Medial supracondylar ridge
Medial epicondyle
Trochlea
Coronoid process
Tuberosity of ulna
Ulna
Head of ulna
Styloid process of ulna
Carpal bones
Metacarpal bones
Proximal
Middle — Phalanges
Distal

FIGURE 2-3 · Bone markings.   Anterior view

Note the condyles of the femur and tibia in Figure 5-2B. Note also that the distal end of the humerus has bone markings named *trochlea* (which means pulley) and *capitulum* (which means little head), rather than condyles.

3. *Epicondyles* ("epi" means upon) are raised areas on or near condyles. In Figure 2-3, note the medial and lateral epicondyles of the humerus.

4. A *tubercle* is a small, rounded projection. Note the tubercles on the humerus and scapula in Figure 2-3.

5. A *tuberosity* is a rounded, roughened area on a bone. Tuberosities tend to be larger than tubercles. Note the deltoid tuberosity on the humerus and the radial tuberosity in Figure 2-3.

6. A *trochanter* is a large projection on the femur. There are two trochanters on each femur, the greater

trochanter and the lesser trochanter. See Figure 5-2A.

7. Many bone markings are called *processes*, each with a descriptive name, such as the acromion process, the coracoid process, and the coronoid process. In Figure 2-3, look for these three processes.

8. A *crest* is a prominent, narrow ridge of bone. An example of a crest is the iliac crest. See iliac crest in Figure 5-1A.

9. A *spine* is a thin, sharp projection. The spine of the scapula can be seen in Figure 2-3.

10. A *fossa* is a shallow indentation in a bone. See Figure 5-1A to see the iliac fossa.

11. A *groove* is a narrow, linear indentation in a bone. Locate the bicipital groove, also called the intertubercular groove, in the proximal, anterior humerus in Figure 2-3.

12. A *facet* is a smooth, flat, articular surface on a bone. Facets are located on the ribs and vertebrae.

13. A *foramen* is a rounded opening in a bone. Typically, nerves or vessels pass through a foramen. Examples include the foramen magnum in the occiput and the obturator foramen in the hip or coxal bones.

Cartilage

Cartilage is made of a dense arrangement of collagen and elastic fibers within a rubbery ground substance that contains chondroitin sulfate. Cartilage has no blood or nerve supply. There are several types of cartilage, distinguished by the arrangement and composition of fibers and ground substance. *Hyaline* is the most common type of cartilage and covers the articular surfaces of most bones, providing them with smooth surfaces where they form joints. Hyaline cartilage forms the nose and parts of larynx. The function of hyaline cartilage is to provide flexibility and support.

Elastic cartilage has a matrix containing thin elastic fibers. The external ear is elastic cartilage. The function of elastic cartilage is to provide support and shape.

Fibrous cartilage has a matrix with abundant collagen fibers, making it the strongest type of cartilage. Fibrous cartilage is located in the intervertebral discs and at the pubic symphysis and is the cartilage of the knee joint. The function of fibrous cartilage is to provide support and attach structures.

Dense Connective Tissue

Dense connective tissue contains numerous, thick, densely packed fibers. There are several types of dense connective tissue. Dense regular connective tissue contains many collagen fibers organized in parallel groupings. Its function is attachment. Examples include *tendons*, which attach muscle to bone; *ligaments*, which attach bone to bone; and *aponeuroses,* which are flat, sheet-like tendons.

Dense irregular connective tissue also contains primarily collagen fibers, randomly arranged. Its function is to add strength. Examples include fascial membranes that cover, support, and separate muscles, deep layers of dermis of skin, membrane capsules around organs, and joint capsules.

Elastic connective tissue is made of elastic fibers that contain the protein elastin, and have the function of allowing elasticity (stretching). Examples of elastic connective tissue include lung tissue and the walls of arteries.

Loose Connective Tissue

Loose connective tissue contains fewer fibers and more cells than dense connective tissue, thus there is more space between fibers. There are several types of loose connective tissue. *Areolar* is soft, flexible tissue made of many types of fibers in semifluid ground substance. Its function is to cushion, protect, and give strength and elasticity. Areolar tissue also absorbs extra fluid when edema is present. An example of areolar tissue is the tissue surrounding organs.

Adipose tissue is dominated by fat cells. It functions as a temperature insulator and protector. Examples of adipose tissue include the tissue that protects and holds the eyeballs in their sockets, provides padding around the kidneys and heart, and makes up fat deposits.

Reticular connective tissue is composed of a fine, fibrous network, providing the framework of some organs such as the liver and spleen. An additional function of reticular connective tissue is to bind smooth muscle cells together. Examples include the framework of the liver, spleen, and lymph nodes.

Blood

Blood comprises blood cells and platelets in plasma. The function of blood is to transport oxygen, carbon dioxide, white blood cells, platelets, and many other substances needed for our body's health and homeostasis.

Lymph

Lymph is interstitial fluid that has passed into lymphatic vessels. Lymph assists in our body's immune response by transporting lymphocytes to areas where they are needed. Lymph also transports lipids and vitamins from the digestive tract to the blood.

The portion of connective tissue most relevant to massage therapists is the body's dense and loose connective tissue, which is collectively termed *fascia*. Fascia creates a continuous three-dimensional web around and within every structure of the human body, right down to the cellular level. Fascia is made of collagen and elastin fibers in a gel-like ground substance. Again, this web surrounds and connects every cell of the body, creating space between our cells while nourishing and protecting them.

Tears, adhesions, or other disruptions in the fascia are called *restrictions*, and these have a major impact on our health. Such restrictions can be caused by trauma, infection, or posture imbalances. In turn, fascial restrictions cause pain and limits in movement. Certain bodywork techniques directly impact the fascia, thus reducing pain and improving mobility. These techniques may lengthen the elastic components of fascia, leading to greater mobility, and/or they may change the viscosity of the ground substance, enhancing the overall health and function of the fascia.

JOINTS

It is important for massage therapists to have an understanding of joints and how different joints permit different movements. Massage therapy clients frequently have treatment goals related to the functioning of their joints. For many people, their sense of health is directly related to their ability to move, and movement occurs at joints. A common reason for clients to seek massage therapy is to improve their range of motion or reduce pain that occurs during movement. Many clients present with joint injuries and joint problems they would like addressed. To satisfy these clients, we need to understand the structure and function of the joints we have in our bodies.

An *articulation*, or a joint, is a point where bones come together. Joints are necessary to allow our bodies to move. The surfaces of bones that contact other bones are called *articular surfaces*, and bones are said to *articulate* with each other at joints. Joints are classified in two ways, functionally and structurally.

Functional Classification

Classifying joints functionally means placing joints into categories based on the amount of movement they allow. The three functional categories are listed below.

Synarthrotic

Synarthrotic joints are considered "immovable" joints. The joints between the skull bones are classified as synarthrotic joints. Many bodywork practitioners, however, recognize that movement is possible between the skull bones, and this movement is one of the cornerstone beliefs of craniosacral therapy. Other examples include the joints between the roots of the teeth and their sockets in the mandible and maxillae.

Amphiarthrotic

Amphiarthrotic joints are considered "slightly movable" joints. The joints between the bodies of the vertebrae are examples of amphiarthrotic joints. The bodies make up the anterior aspects of the vertebrae and are joined together by fibrocartilaginous discs. Other examples include the pubic symphysis, which is the joint between the two pubic bones, and the joint between the ribs and the sternum.

Diarthrotic

Diarthrotic joints are considered "freely movable" joints. Freely movable may appear to be a misnomer in some instances, as in the case of the intercarpal joints, which are located in the very proximal aspect of the hand. The joints between the eight tiny carpal bones do not permit a wide range of motion, but they are classified as diarthrotic. More obvious diarthrotic joints include the elbow, the shoulder or glenohumeral joint, the hip and the knee.

Structural Classification

The second way to categorize joints is structurally. Structural classification is based on whether joints have a synovial cavity and the type of connective tissue that holds the bones together. The three structural categories are listed below.

Fibrous

Fibrous joints are connected by fibrous tissue with plentiful collagen fibers and can be synarthrotic or amphiarthrotic. They do not have a synovial cavity. *Sutures*, the joints between our skull bones and *gomphoses*, which are joints between our teeth and their sockets, are classified as fibrous joints. Another type of fibrous joint is a *syndesmosis*, such as the distal tibiofibular joint of the leg. This joint is classified as amphiarthrotic.

Cartilaginous

Cartilaginous joints have no synovial cavity and are united either by hyaline cartilage, fibrous cartilage, or both. They allow little or no movement. The two types of cartilaginous joints are synchondroses and symphyses. *Synchondroses* are synarthrotic joints that are joined by hyaline cartilage. An example is the joint between the rib 1 and the sternum. *Symphyses*, such as the pubic symphysis, are amphiarthrotic joints in which hyaline cartilage covers the surfaces of the articulating bones, and the bones are united by strong fibrous tissue. The joints between the bodies of the vertebrae are also symphyses, as they are united by fibrocartilaginous discs. The joints between the ribs and the sternum are also symphyses.

Synovial

Synovial joints have four basic components. Articular cartilage (generally hyaline cartilage, although sometimes fibrocartilage) covers the ends of both bones forming the joint. An articular capsule or sleeve encloses the joint surfaces. This sleeve contains an outer layer of fibrous connective tissue and an inner layer called the *synovial membrane*. Inside the sleeve is a joint cavity filled with synovial fluid. In addition, most synovial joints contain reinforcing ligaments (either inside or outside of the joint capsule), which add strength to the fibrous capsule. Some synovial joints also contain discs or *menisci* (pads of fibrocartilage) to support and cushion the joint.

There are six types of synovial joints, described below (Fig. 2-4). It is important to understand the movement permitted at each type of synovial joint. This allows us to properly assess range of motion. The movement permitted at each joint is determined by the shapes of the articulating surfaces of the bones that come together to form the joint. The movement permitted at each joint is also influenced by the ligaments that stabilize the joints and the soft tissue located in the area.

Plane or Gliding

Plane or gliding joints permit the least movement of all the types of synovial joints. Usually, they are joints between two flat surfaces of bone and permit only a small amount of back-and-forth or gliding movement. Examples include the intercarpal joints, the joint between the sternum and clavicle, and the joint between the acromion of the scapula and the clavicle (AC joint).

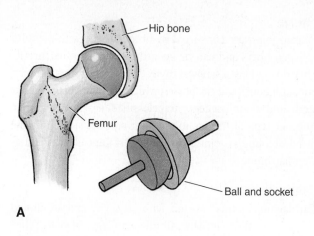

A

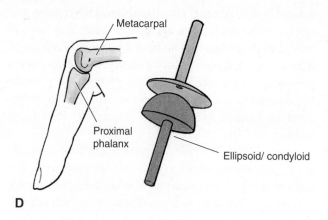

D

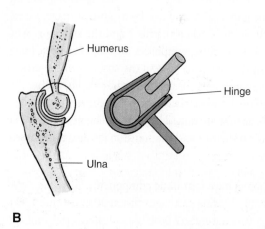

B

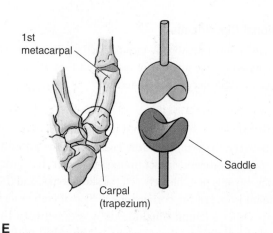

E

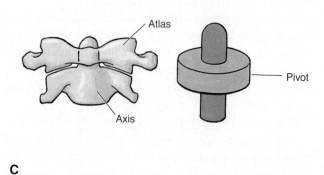

C

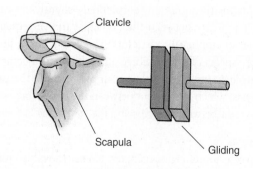

F

FIGURE 2-4 · Types of synovial joints.

Condyloid or Ellipsoidal

Condyloid or ellipsoidal joints permit flexion, extension, abduction, and adduction, or in other words, circumduction. Condyloid joints bring together convex and concave surfaces. You could perhaps picture an egg in an oval bowl. The egg can roll in two directions but cannot turn or spin. Examples of condyloid joints include the wrist, the joint between the occiput and C1 (atlanto-occipital joint), and the metacarpophalangeal joints.

Saddle

The saddle joint brings together the trapezium bone in the proximal hand with the metacarpal of the thumb. Saddle joints permit a greater range of circumduction than do condyloid joints.

Pivot

Pivot joints allow rotation only. They are formed by the articulation between a rounded surface on a bone and a concave surface on a bone. They may also be formed by a ring of bone articulating with an axis of bone. Examples of pivot joints include the joints between the radius and ulna within the forearm and the atlantoaxial joint between C1 and C2.

Hinge

Hinge joints permit flexion and extension only and mimic a door opening and closing. Examples of hinge joints in the body include the elbow, the knee, and the ankle.

Ball-and-Socket

Ball-and-socket joints permit the most movement of any synovial joint. There are only two ball-and-socket joints in the body, the shoulder and the hip. The articulating surfaces of this type of joint are shaped like a ball and a socket.

MUSCLES

As massage therapists, we must know and understand the muscles we touch so we can provide the most effective massage and achieve the goals our clients seek. In addition, educating our clients about their bodies and potential postural or functional imbalances requires an understanding of and ability to communicate about our muscles.

Muscles are organs, composed of fiber-like cells, which are specialized to contract and thus allow movement. Muscles move not only our bones, but also food, fluids, and other substances through the body. In addition, muscle contraction generates 85% of our body's heat and allows us to maintain our body's internal temperature, despite a colder external environment. Muscles also help us to maintain our posture, such as standing up or holding our head up. Finally, muscles cross our joints and thus help to stabilize them. Muscles make up 40% to 50% of our body's weight.

Muscle Tissue

There are three types of muscle tissue: skeletal, smooth, and cardiac. Skeletal muscle attaches to our bones and moves them. It contracts voluntarily, meaning it is generally under our conscious control. Skeletal muscles also appear striated or striped when viewed under an electron microscope. The stripes are caused by alternating bands of thin and thick myofilaments, as will be discussed later.

Smooth muscle lines many of our body's organs and vessels and contracts to move food, fluids, and other substances along their pathways. Smooth muscle is considered involuntary, as it is not generally under conscious control. Cardiac muscle is the muscle of the heart. It contracts to push blood throughout our body. Cardiac muscle is also considered involuntary, although we have some capacity to control our heart rate through breathing and imagery.

Structure of a Skeletal Muscle

A typical skeletal muscle contains hundreds to thousands of long, thin muscle cells called muscle fibers. The gastrocnemius muscle contains roughly one million muscle fibers, whereas the first dorsal interosseus muscle contains roughly 80,000. Muscle cells line up next to each other. Each muscle fiber is encased in a thin, areolar connective tissue covering called an **endomysium**. Within each muscle, fibers are grouped together into bundles called *fascicles*. Each fascicle is wrapped in a dense regular connective sheet covering called a **perimysium**. Many fascicles are bundled together to make a muscle. The most superficial connective tissue wrapping around each muscle is called an **epimysium**. Epimysium is also made of dense regular connective tissue.

Skeletal Muscle Cell Components

Each muscle fiber or cell contains many components that are necessary for muscle contraction. The **sarcolemma** is the cell membrane, surrounding the muscle cell. The sarcolemma is responsible for controlling what enters and exits the cell. **Myofibrils** are the structural components of the muscle cell, which actually contract and shorten. Myofibrils are cylindrical in shape and contain thousands of thread-like protein structures beautifully positioned in organized rows and segments. These thread-like protein structures are called *myofilaments*.

Myofilaments are classified as thick or thin. There are alternating rows of thick and thin myofilaments, lying next to each other within each myofibril. Thick myofilaments appear darker on an electron micrograph and are primarily composed of the protein **myosin**. Thin myofilaments appear lighter on an electron micrograph and are composed primarily of the protein **actin**. Although myofibrils run the full length of each muscle fiber, the myofilaments do not. The shorter myofilaments of myosin and actin line up end to end along the length of a muscle cell, as well as next to each other. The lineup of myosin and actin is such that an actin myofilament extends beyond each end of the myosin. This lineup permits the actin myofilaments to slide toward the center of each myofibril segment. Each segment of a myofibril, which includes the myosin and the actin myofilaments that extend beyond the myosin, is called a *sarcomere*. Figure 2-5 illustrates the lineup of actin and myosin and the length of a sarcomere.

Myosin myofilaments have projections called *crossbridges*, which connect to the actin. During concentric contraction, myosin's crossbridges swivel and pull or slide the actin myofilaments toward the center of the sarcomere. Bringing the actin myofilaments toward the center of the sarcomere literally shortens the muscle. Myosin uses adenosine triphosphate (ATP) (energy) to do the work of pulling the actin.

The thin actin myofilaments have two regulatory proteins, tropomyosin and troponin, which can prevent myosin's crossbridges from pulling the actin myofilaments toward the center

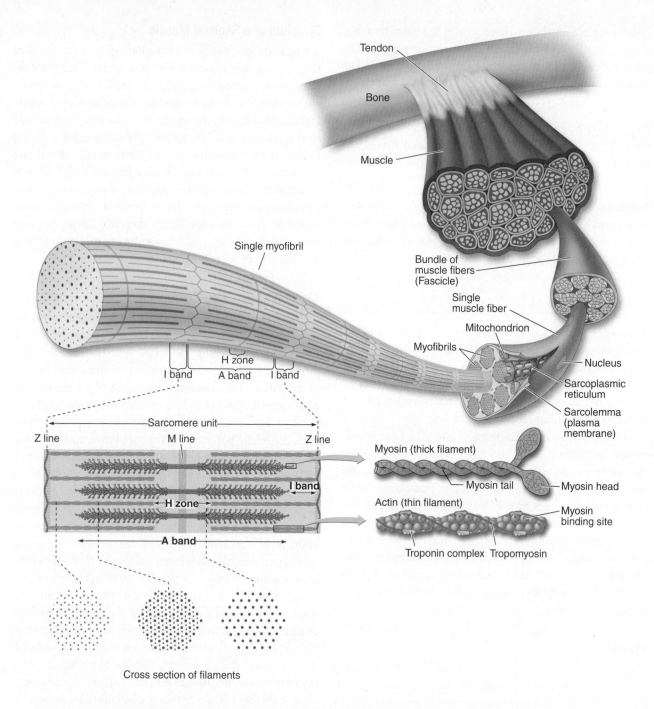

FIGURE 2-5 · **Skeletal muscle and the myofilaments within a skeletal muscle cell.**

of the sarcomere. When troponin and tropomyosin cover the myosin binding sites on the actin, contraction is impossible. However, as soon as the troponin and tropomyosin are removed from the actin, the myosin crossbridges are free to swivel and pull the actin toward the center of the sarcomere.

The **sarcoplasmic reticulum** is a specialized network of smooth tubules and sacs that surround each and every myofibril like a loosely knit sweater. The sacs in the sarcoplasmic reticulum store calcium ions, which are essential for contraction. Figure 2-5 illustrates a skeletal muscle and the myofilaments within a skeletal muscle cell.

Skeletal Muscle Contraction

The contraction of skeletal muscle is complex and involves many components and factors. These are discussed below.

Sliding Filament Mechanism

The concept of the **sliding filament mechanism** was first introduced in 1954 and was called *sliding filament theory.* Since that time, researchers have refined their knowledge of muscle contraction, allowing us to have a more detailed understanding of the process. As time passes, it is likely that our understanding of how muscles contract and allow us to move will be developed even further.

The sliding filament mechanism is the means by which muscles contract or shorten. For a muscle to contract, a nerve impulse or electrical signal is required. As an illustration, we will follow the path of a nerve impulse toward the biceps brachii muscle, located in the superficial anterior arm. Biceps brachii helps us to flex our elbow. For biceps brachii to contract and for us to flex our elbow, a nerve impulse must be sent from the brain, travel down the spinal cord, and move out a spinal nerve heading toward the anterior arm. The nerve cell that carries the impulse required for muscle contraction is called a *motor neuron*. The particular fiber within the motor neuron that carries the nerve impulse toward a muscle is called a *motor axon*. At the end of the motor axon, the axon branches into axon terminals. At the end of each axon terminal, there are synaptic end bulbs, which house acetylcholine (ACh).

When a nerve impulse travels down a motor axon, then down the axon terminals, it reaches the synaptic end bulbs. The synaptic end bulbs do not touch the muscle; there is a space between the axon terminal and the muscle cell called a *synaptic cleft*. The nerve impulse must reach the skeletal muscle cell to cause contraction. If the impulse is strong enough, it will stimulate the release of ACh from the synaptic end bulbs. Acetylcholine is a neurotransmitter that carries the nerve impulse across the synaptic cleft and attaches to particular receptor sites on the sarcolemma. These receptor sites on the sarcolemma are called *motor end plates.*

Once the ACh has carried the nerve impulse and attached to its receptor sites on the sarcolemma, the sarcolemma becomes temporarily permeable to sodium ions. The interstitial fluid surrounding muscle cells contains a high concentration of positively charged sodium ions. When the sarcolemma becomes permeable to sodium, sodium ions rush into the cell. The entry of positive sodium ions alters the electrical charge within the cell and causes an electrical signal (called an *action potential*) to travel along the sarcoplasmic reticulum. The action potential causes the sarcoplasmic reticulum to release calcium from its storage sacs. The calcium travels to the troponin and tropomyosin, which is resting on actin, the thin myofilament. Calcium and the troponin–

tropomyosin unit react chemically, causing the troponin–tropomyosin units to move away from the actin, thus revealing the myosin binding sites. With the myosin binding site exposed, the myosin crossbridges automatically attach to the actin and pull the actin myofilaments from both ends of the muscle toward the center of the sarcomere, thus shortening the muscle. As the muscle shortens, the muscle's tendons pull the bones, causing them to move closer to each other. In the case of elbow flexion, the forearm is pulled closer to the anterior arm. As additional action potentials are produced, and enough ATP energy and calcium are available, myosin continues to pull the actin over and over to sustain the contraction. This type of muscle contraction, in which the muscle shortens, is called a *concentric contraction.*

Relaxation of a muscle fiber happens when the nerve impulse ends and ACh is no longer released. Acetylcholinesterase is released to break down the acetylcholine in the synaptic cleft. Without the continuation of nerve impulses reaching the sarcolemma, the chain of events needed for muscle contraction stops. Energy is used to return calcium to the sarcoplasmic reticulum and remove sodium from the cell. Troponin and tropomyosin also return to cover the myosin binding sites on the actin. At this point, the myosin no longer can pull the actin. Contraction stops, and the muscle relaxes and returns to its original length. Figures 2-6 and 2-7 illustrate the position of actin and myosin during muscle contraction and relaxation.

Motor Units

Some types of motor axons each carry nerve impulses to just a few muscle cells, as is the case with motor axons that serve the muscles that move our eyes. Other motor axons can carry impulses that reach roughly 750 muscle cells, as do the motor axons that bring impulses to the biceps brachii muscle. Some motor axons carry impulses to thousands of skeletal muscle cells. The single motor axon and all the skeletal muscle cells it stimulates are together called a **motor unit**. The number of motor units that comprise and serve each muscle varies greatly. Some small muscles contain just a few motor units, whereas others have hundreds.

Because we have motor units, our bodies can move in many ways and in varying degrees. For instance, we can flex our elbow

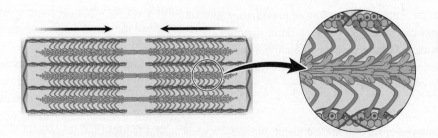

FIGURE 2-6 · Position of actin and myosin during muscle contraction.

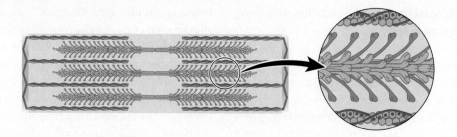

FIGURE 2-7 · Position of actin and myosin during muscle relaxation.

a little or a lot. We can flex our elbow when we have nothing in our hand, or we can flex it while carrying a 5-pound weight. A small movement with little force applied requires a smaller number of motor units. A larger movement with greater force applied requires the contraction of a greater number of motor units. Thus, the size and number of motor units contracting at any one time determines the amount of movement possible and the strength of the movement. In addition, motor units take turns contracting; some are engaged while others rest. This enables us to maintain contraction for a longer period of time.

All-or-Nothing Principle

When a motor unit does contract, every muscle cell within the motor unit contracts fully. This means that the entire set of actin and myosin myofilaments within each cell shorten to their full extent. In other words, there is no partial contraction within a muscle cell. This concept is called the *all-or-nothing principle*.

Motor Unit Recruitment

When we perform repetitive movements or use our muscles for a long time, we require more motor units to be activated. The generation of more nerve impulses to more skeletal muscle fibers to assist in muscle contraction is known as **motor unit recruitment**. When additional motor units are recruited, the ones in use initially can rest and get ready to contract again.

Muscle Tone

A small number of motor units are involuntarily activated to produce **muscle tone**. The motor units take turns being active to sustain these contractions, which create tone or firmness in our muscles.

Muscle Fatigue

When muscle fibers can contract for a prolonged period, they eventually fatigue and can no longer contract. Some factors that contribute to **muscle fatigue** are lack of calcium, insufficient oxygen, depletion of glycogen and other nutrients, and possibly the buildup of lactic acid.

Types of Skeletal Muscle Fibers

There are three main types of skeletal muscle fibers. *Slow oxidative* (SO) fibers are small in diameter and appear red because they have large amounts of myoglobin, a red protein that binds oxygen in muscle fibers. SO fibers have many large mitochon-

dria, which generate ATP slowly. They contract slowly but are resistant to fatigue and can maintain sustained contraction for many hours. Muscles used in distance running and other endurance activities have higher concentrations of SO fibers.

A second type of skeletal muscle fiber is *fast oxidative glycolytic* (FOG). They are intermediate in diameter, are red because they contain much myoglobin, and can generate ATP by aerobic cellular respiration and glycolysis. Aerobic cellular respiration involves a series of oxygen-requiring mitochondrial reactions that produce ATP. Glycolysis is a series of ten reactions that break glucose into pyruvic acid and form ATP. The muscles in our lower limbs that we use for walking have a high concentration of FOG fibers.

Fast glycolytic (FG) fibers, the third type, are largest in diameter, and are white because they contain little myoglobin, and generate ATP by glycolysis. Muscles we use for weight lifting have a high concentration of FG fibers. They fatigue quickly. Most skeletal muscles have mixtures of these three types of fibers. Amazingly, we seem able to change the concentrations of these three types of fibers within our individual muscles to adapt to the type and level of activity we perform.

Origin, Insertion, and Action

Now that we have discussed muscle contraction in some depth, we can begin to prepare for the study of individual muscles. There are some terms we will need to understand to help us study the muscles. Recall that concentric skeletal muscle contraction involves a shortening of a muscle due to the sliding of myofilaments toward the center of the muscle's sarcomere. As a muscle shortens, a pull occurs on both ends of the muscle, and thus a pull, via the muscle's tendons, on both of the sites where the muscle connects to bones. The shortening of a muscle occurs when the more movable attachment site moves toward the more stable attachment site. The more stable attachment site of a muscle is called the **origin**. The more movable attachment site of a muscle is called the **insertion**.

For each muscle we will discuss in this text, we will name the origin and insertion. It is important for massage therapists to know and remember many origin and attachment sites, as this helps us know the exact location of a muscle. It is also helpful to remember the origin and insertion sites of muscles because these sites are useful places to provide massage, particularly friction, as we seek to help muscles relax.

Practice will make it easier to determine origin and insertion sites of the muscles and to remember them. If we consider how our bodies typically move, we can determine which body parts are more movable (and thus contain insertion sites) and which are more stable (and contain origin sites). For example, the forearm is more movable that the arm. It is certainly easier to bring the forearm closer to the arm than it is to bring the arm closer to the forearm. Consider a muscle that flexes the elbow and that attaches to both the arm and forearm. The attachment on the humerus will be the origin and the attachment on the forearm will be the insertion.

Likewise, the hand is more movable than the forearm. It is easier to bring the fingers closer to the forearm than it is to bring the forearm closer to the fingers. A finger flexor's attachment on the forearm will be the origin and the attachment on the fingers will be the insertion.

We could consider another muscle that attaches to the ribs and also to the humerus. The ribs are more stable than the humerus: it is easier to move the humerus toward the ribs than it is to move the ribs toward the humerus. Therefore, the origin of such a muscle would be on the ribs and the insertion would be on the humerus. The bone that moves when performing an action will be the bone that contains the insertion site. Muscles that are located in the extremities will have origin sites more proximal than their insertion sites, as the more proximal body parts in an extremity are more stable.

The **action** that a muscle performs is simply the name of the movement that occurs when insertion moves toward origin. Note that it is possible for muscles to contract and pull origin toward insertion. This is true if both muscle attachments are relatively equal in their mobility or if we fix the insertion, making it more stable. For instance, if we are hanging onto a chin-up bar, we have fixed our forearm, and when an elbow flexor contracts, the arm will actually move toward the forearm. It is essential for you to learn and remember the actions of muscles as the muscle's actions determine postural and functional problems. When a client presents with a postural or functional problem that he or she wishes to have addressed, you must determine the action he or she is having trouble with, or the action he or she is performing too much, so you can determine which muscle to address in your massage session. For this purpose, the actions of each muscle covered in this book are listed under that muscle as a reference for you.

Concentric, Eccentric, and Isometric Contractions

It is important to note that the above description of muscle contraction refers only to concentric contractions. **Concentric contractions** involve shortening of muscles. However, muscles may contract while lengthening or without any movement at all. A muscle contraction that occurs when a muscle lengthens is called an **eccentric contraction**. Eccentric contractions often occur when one moves to resist a force such as gravity. An example of eccentric contraction occurs when you slowly set a heavy stack of books down in front of

you. Let us assume that you set the books down by slowly extending your elbows. In this instance, your elbow extensors are relaxing, and your elbow flexors are working or contracting. The elbow flexors contract to control the rate at which you set the books down, preventing gravity from pulling the books down quickly. Thus, the elbow flexors contract eccentrically. Another example to describe the difference between concentric and eccentric contractions can be illustrated as follows. Suppose you abduct your arm with a 5-pound weight in your hand. This action requires your arm abductors to contract concentrically. If you slowly lower the weight by adducting your arm, you are using your arm abductors eccentrically. Every muscle can be used concentrically and eccentrically, depending on the circumstances.

In addition, one can contract a muscle with no movement at all. This type of muscle contraction is described as an **isometric contraction**. Literally, isometric means "same length." A muscle contracting isometrically does not shorten or lengthen, so it remains the same length. An example of an isometric use of arm flexors is to hold your arms out in front of you in a position of flexion. If you hold your arms in a flexed position, you can notice that the arm flexors are working to allow you to maintain this position. Gravity would pull your arms back to your sides if you did not use muscles to hold your position. Another example of an isometric use of muscles is how the neck extensors contract to simply hold the head up. All muscle can be used isometrically, when they tighten, but do not cause movement.

Synergists and Antagonists

Synergists are muscles that work together to perform an action at a given joint. In the following chapters of the book, synergists will be listed for each muscle presented. Reviewing synergists helps you to remember the actions of muscles.

Antagonist or **opposing** muscles are ones that perform the opposite action from each other. Antagonist muscles must operate at the same joint. Antagonists will also be listed for each muscle presented in the following chapters. To have optimal health and posture, we need a balance between opposing muscle groups. If opposing muscle groups are in balance, we can have both strength and flexibility in all muscles. However, most of us have some imbalance between opposing muscles. We tend to have certain groups of muscles that are shortened and opposing muscle groups that are lengthened. For example, it is common for medial rotators of the arm to be shortened and lateral rotators of the arm to be lengthened. Typically, a lack of balance occurs because one group of muscles becomes shortened, resulting in the lengthening of the opposing muscles.

Shortened and Lengthened Muscles

Muscles frequently become shortened due to overuse. If your job requires continuous or frequent elbow flexion, your elbow flexors become shortened. If you perform elbow curls, flexing your elbows repetitively with weights in your hands, you will likely cause your elbow flexors to shorten. Muscles also become shortened by being held in a position in which insertion has been moved toward origin. Wearing a sling that holds your elbow in a bent or flexed position for several weeks can cause shortened elbow flexors.

When muscles shorten, there are postural as well as functional implications. A **shortened muscle** causes one to hold the muscle in a contracted, shortened position. Perhaps you have noticed people who have slightly bent elbows, without intention to bend them. It is likely that such people have shortened elbow flexors.

In addition, shortened elbow flexors limit the ability to extend the elbow fully. In other words, a shortened muscle limits the range of motion of the opposite action. Shortened hip adductors result in limited hip abduction. Shortened knee extensors limit the ability to perform knee flexion fully. For many of the individual muscles covered in this text, we will explore the postural and functional implications of the muscle's shortening.

Muscles can also become weak and/or lengthened. Whenever a muscle shortens, its opposing muscle lengthens. Thus, muscles that remain in a shortened state cause their antagonists to remain in a lengthened state. Because shortened muscles receive continuous impulses to contract, the impulses to contract the opposing lengthened muscles may be inhibited, causing them to seem weak. These **lengthened muscles** that seem weak may be overworked, as they may need to contract eccentrically or isometrically to counteract the pull of a shortened muscle. For example, a muscle like the pectoralis minor, that pulls our scapulae (shoulder blades) forward and causes a posture of rounded shoulders, is commonly shortened and feels tight. Thus, the rhomboid muscles, which pull our scapulae back toward the spine, remain lengthened. A client with this particular muscular imbalance may experience pain in the area of the lengthened rhomboids. These rhomboids may feel tight and ropy to the massage practitioner. But the fact of the matter is that they are lengthened, so they will not benefit from lengthening massage strokes. The solution lies in lengthening the shortened muscles to restore balance. This solution is likely to restore strength to the weak muscles.

Muscles can also become weak when their nerve innervation is interrupted or when they have been injured. For many of the muscles covered in this text, we will discuss the implications of individual lengthened muscles.

Massage therapy techniques such as deep effleurage, friction, and range-of-motion work can literally lengthen muscles. Such massage applied to shortened muscles can help to restore the balance between opposing shortened and lengthened muscles. Circulatory massage to lengthened muscles can also assist their overall health. When approaching imbalances between muscle groups, it is commonly recommended to massage the shortened muscles first and with techniques designed to break adhesions and lengthen fibers. Afterward, it may appropriate to address the weaker, lengthened muscles with techniques that strengthen them. However, as mentioned in the example above, lengthening the shortened muscles can be enough to restore the strength of the lengthened muscles.

Palpation and Massage of Muscles

For each muscle discussed in this text, a suggestion for how to palpate the muscle and a list of appropriate massage strokes for the muscle are provided. Although the list of strokes is certainly not exhaustive, it gives you a sense of appropriate and helpful strokes to use to reduce muscle tension and adhesions in this muscle. Keep in mind that knowledge of each muscle's action keep allows you to use *reciprocal inhibition* to assist in muscle relaxation Reciprocal inhibition requires that you engage the opposing muscle isometrically. By causing the opposing muscle to contract, you limit the nerve impulse to contract to your target muscle and create an opportunity for lengthening the muscle. For example, if you wish to use reciprocal inhibition to relax the plantarflexors of the ankle, simply dorsiflex the ankle isometrically. Continued research and exploration allows our understanding of the nervous system to grow and change. We now know that reciprocal inhibition is much more complicated than the simple concept that our nervous system cannot simultaneously innervate opposing muscles. In fact, there are many instances when nerve impulses are sent to opposing muscles simultaneously, particularly muscles that cross more than one joint. However, it does seem that impulses to contract sent to a muscle can, at times, inhibit impulses to the antagonist. This is why reciprocal inhibition is such an effective cramp reduction technique.

For most muscles discussed, directions to stretch the muscle are offered. To stretch a muscle is to move the origin and insertion away from each other. This means that you can stretch muscles by performing the opposite action(s) of the muscle you wish to stretch. Sometimes you have to experiment with various combinations of opposite actions you perform when seeking a stretch. Remember that stretching should never hurt, and if you wish to stretch a client's muscles, you must give him or her a clear explanation of what you are doing before you begin a stretch. You must also tell your client to let you know as soon as he or she feels a good stretch and if any pain is experienced. Stretching is an excellent technique for lengthening a muscle and increasing range of motion at a joint.

NERVE SUPPLY TO MUSCLES

As described above in the section on the sliding filament mechanism, nerves are needed to carry impulses for contraction to all muscles. Any disruption in the process of bringing a nerve impulse to a muscle can cause mobility problems. Massage therapy clients may present with mobility problems, and thus it is important to have as full an understanding as possible of the physiology of movement. A brief overview of the nervous system, as well as information about which nerves innervate which muscles, is given below.

The nervous system is divided into the *central nervous system,* which consists of the brain and the spinal cord, and the *peripheral nervous system,* which includes the nerves that extend from the brain and spinal cord and carry impulses to all parts of the body. There are two sets of nerves in the peripheral nervous system, the cranial nerves, which carry impulses to and from the brain, and the spinal nerves, which carry impulses to and from the spinal cord. There are 12 pairs of cranial nerves and 31 pairs of spinal nerves. The 31 pairs of spinal nerves are named according to the area of the spine from which they emerge (cervical, thoracic, lumbar, sacral, or coccygeal) and the level of the spine from which they emerge. The first pair of spinal nerves emerges between the occiput and C1 (C1 is the first vertebra and is also called the *atlas*). Each of the remaining spinal nerves emerges from a space between the vertebrae that is called the *intervertebral foramen.* The spinal nerves include eight pairs of cervical nerves, twelve pairs of thoracic nerves, five pairs of lumbar nerves, five pairs of sacral nerves, and one pair of coccygeal nerves.

The structure of spinal nerves is quite elaborate. Each spinal nerve has an anterior and a posterior root, which emerge directly from the spinal cord. These roots join together, pass through the intervertebral foramen, and divide immediately into two branches called rami (*rami* is the plural of *ramus*). The roots split into a ventral ramus, which innervates muscles of the extremities and the lateral and anterior trunk, and a dorsal ramus, which innervates deep muscles and the skin of the back. Most of the ventral rami form plexuses (Latin for *braid*), or networks of adjacent spinal nerves. The main plexuses are the cervical, brachial, lumbar, and sacral. The plexuses consist of spinal nerves that divide, join with other nerves, divide again, and rejoin other nerves to create a complex configuration of nerve pathways. The plexuses eventually become individual nerves that innervate particular body areas and muscle groups.

The cervical plexus comprises the ventral rami of spinal nerves C1 to C4, and a portion of C5. The cervical plexus innervates some muscles of the head, neck, and the diaphragm.

The brachial plexus primarily innervates muscles of the upper extremity (Fig. 2-8). The brachial plexus begins as the ventral rami of spinal nerves C5 to C8 and T1. The rami of spinal nerves C5 and C6 unite to form the superior (or upper)

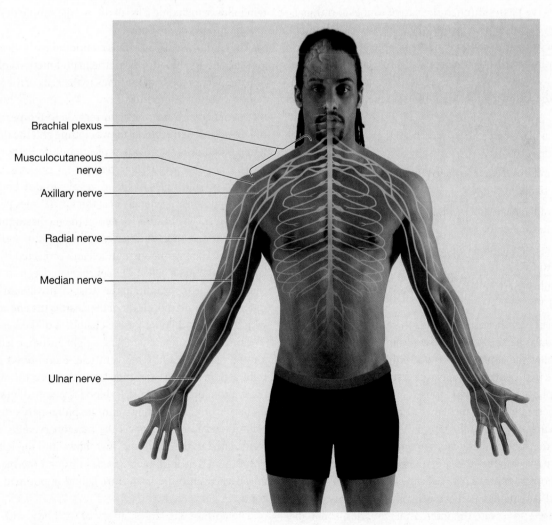

Brachial plexus

Musculocutaneous nerve

Axillary nerve

Radial nerve

Median nerve

Ulnar nerve

FIGURE 2-8 · Brachial plexus.

trunk of the brachial plexus. The ventral ramus of C7 becomes the middle trunk. The ventral rami of C8 and T1 unite to form the inferior (or lower) trunk. The three trunks divide into anterior and posterior divisions. The anterior divisions from the superior and middle trunks unite to form the lateral cord. The anterior division of the inferior trunk continues on its own to become the medial cord. The posterior divisions from all three trunks unite to form the posterior cord. (The lateral cord runs more laterally, the posterior cord more posteriorly, and the medial cord more medially.) The cords branch into many specifically named nerves that innervate muscles of the upper extremity.

There are five major nerves that arise from the cords of the brachial plexus. They include the axillary nerve, which supplies the deltoid and teres minor muscles and thus is necessary for arm abduction. The musculocutaneus nerve supplies the coracobrachialis, biceps brachii, and brachialis and thus is largely responsible for elbow flexion. The radial nerve supplies muscles of the posterior arm and forearm and is thus responsible for elbow, wrist, and finger extension. The median nerve supplies most of the anterior forearm compartment and some muscles in the hand. The median nerve passes through the carpal tunnel and thus is the nerve that becomes irritated when one has carpal tunnel syndrome. Finally, the ulnar nerve supplies some anteromedial muscles of the forearm and most muscles of the hand.

Note the following regarding the source of certain nerve fibers:

- All axillary nerve fibers arise from the ventral rami of C5 and C6.
- All musculocutaneous nerve fibers arise from the ventral rami of C5 to C7.
- All radial nerve fibers arise from the ventral rami of C5 to C8 and T1.
- All median nerve fibers arise from the ventral rami of C5 to C7.
- All ulnar nerve fibers arise from the ventral rami of C8 and T1.

Other nerves that emerge from this plexus include the suprascapular nerve, which emerges from the superior trunk and supplies the supraspinatus and infraspinatus muscles. The nerve to the subclavius emerges from the superior trunk and supplies the subclavius muscle. The medial pectoral nerve emerges from the medial cord and supplies the pectoralis major and pectoralis minor. The subscapular nerve supplies the subscapularis and teres major. And the thoracodorsal nerve supplies the latissimus dorsi.

The thoracic nerves T2 to T12 are simply numbered and organized as singular nerves rather than a plexus. These spinal nerves innervate the intercostals muscles, some abdominal muscles, and some deep back muscles.

The nerves of the lumbar plexus, L1 to L4, innervate some abdominal muscles, some thigh flexors, all knee extensors, and all hip adductors.

The nerves of the sacral plexus, L4, L5, and S1 to S4, serve the gluteal muscles, hamstrings, and many muscles of the leg and foot.

ARTERIAL SUPPLY TO MUSCLES

Each muscle requires a blood supply to function. Blood is delivered to the muscles via arteries, which branch and narrow to arterioles. Massage therapy has long been credited with the enhancement of blood flow. While the exact effect of Swedish massage on the overall circulatory system is the subject of ongoing research and debate, it is commonly believed that massage enhances local circulation, reduces edema, and alters the interstitial fluid to enhance removal of metabolic waste and delivery of nutrients to the body's cells.

An understanding of the circulatory system enables massage therapists to better understand the effects of our work. A basic explanation of the structure and function of the system follows, including a list of the arterial supply to the major muscle groups of the body.

The cardiovascular system is comprised of the heart, blood vessels, and the blood. One of the main functions of the system includes delivery of nutrients to the cells of the body and removal of waste products from cells. Another function is maintenance of homeostasis in regards to temperature and pH. In addition, the blood allows clotting and the delivery of white blood cells to provide protection from pathogens.

The heart is a muscular pump that pushes our blood through 60,000 miles of blood vessels in our bodies. The healthy adult heart generally beats about 70 times per minute while at rest. The heart is located in the mediastinum, which is between our lungs and between the sternum and thoracic vertebrae. The heart is surrounded and protected by a three-layered membrane called the *pericardium*. Deep to the pericardium is the myocardium, the striated, involuntary cardiac muscle. The innermost layer of the heart is the endocardium, which provides a lining for the chambers of the heart.

The heart has four chambers, a right atrium, a left atrium, a right ventricle, and a left ventricle. Blood flows from the right atrium through the tricuspid valve into the right ventricle. From the right ventricle, blood is pumped into the pulmonary trunk, which splits into the pulmonary arteries that bring blood to the lungs via the pulmonary veins. Blood is oxygenated in the lungs and then flows into the left atrium. From the left atrium, blood passes through the bicuspid or mitral valve into the left ventricle and is pumped into the aorta.

The aorta is the largest artery of the body, with a width of close to 1 inch. The aorta contains four sections. The

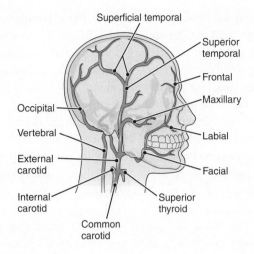

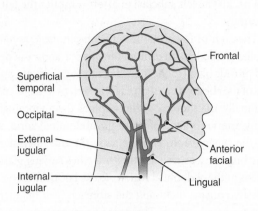

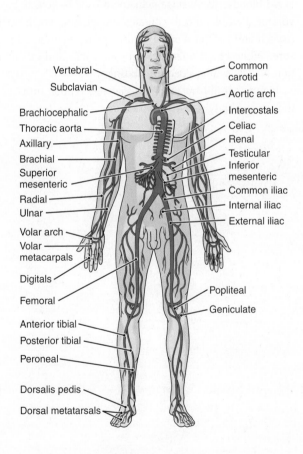

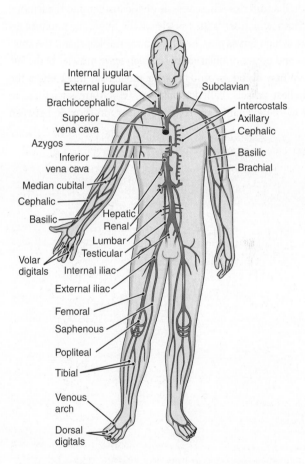

FIGURE 2-9 · Arterial supply and venous return to various body areas.

ascending aorta carries blood directly from the left ventricle of the heart. The right and left coronary arteries branch from the ascending aorta and bring blood to nourish the heart muscle. The ascending aorta becomes the *arch* of the aorta, which is aptly named for its curved shape. Three major arteries branch off of the arch of the aorta: the brachiocephalic trunk, the left common carotid artery, and the left subcla-

vian artery. The brachiocephalic trunk divides into the right subclavian artery and the right common carotid artery. The right subclavian artery carries blood to the brain and spinal cord, as well as to muscles of the neck, shoulder, and scapula regions. The right common carotid artery carries blood to the right side of the head and neck. The left common carotid artery carries blood to the left side of the head and neck. The left subclavian artery supplies the left upper extremity.

The arch of the aorta becomes the thoracic aorta. Many smaller vessels branch off from the thoracic aorta as it descends and provide blood to the bronchial tubes, esophagus, and muscles of the chest wall and rib cage, as well as to the diaphragm.

Finally, the thoracic aorta becomes the abdominal aorta. Many arteries branch off from the abdominal aorta, including the celiac trunk, and the superior and inferior mesenteric branches, as well as other branches serving glands and organs in the abdominal region. The celiac trunk serves some digestive organs including the stomach, gall bladder, liver, pancreas, and spleen. The superior mesenteric trunk supplies the small and large intestines. The inferior mesenteric branch delivers blood to portions of the colon and rectum.

The abdominal aorta branches into the right and left common iliac arteries. These vessels divide further into the femoral arteries, which serve the muscles of the thigh; the popliteal artery, which serves muscles of the posterior knee; and the anterior and posterior tibial arteries, which serve muscles of the leg.

When blood is brought to a muscle, it must enter the smallest vessels, called *capillaries*, which are structures to allow the exchange of oxygen and carbon dioxide between blood and muscle cells. Oxygen is diffused through capillary walls, into the interstitial fluid, where it can be accessed by our cells. Carbon dioxide is diffused into the capillaries, and the blood carries it into venules (small veins), then veins, and then back into the right atrium.

We have two types of circulation: systemic and pulmonary. Systemic circulation refers to the delivery of oxygenated blood from the left ventricle to the body's tissues and organs. Pulmonary circulation is the delivery of deoxygenated blood to the lungs, where it gains oxygen, and delivery of this oxygenated blood from the lungs to the heart.

The blood is a liquid connective tissue that contains plasma (about 91% water and some dissolved substances) and formed elements (red blood cells, white blood cells, and platelets). *Hematocrit* is the percentage of blood volume that is red blood cells. Average hematocrit is 38%–46% of blood volume. Red blood cells contain hemoglobin, which carries oxygen and carbon dioxide, and helps regulate blood pressure. White blood cells help fight infections and inflammation. Platelets are needed for clotting.

Figure 2-9 illustrates the arterial and venous supplies to the various body areas.

■ CHAPTER SUMMARY

Chapter 2 has provided a basic introduction to the physiology of connective tissue (including bones, cartilage, fascia, blood, and lymph), joints, and muscles, and an introduction to the nerve and blood supplies to muscles. This information should equip you to begin a comprehensive study of the muscles of the body.

■ WORKBOOK

Review Exercises

Connective Tissue

1. What are bones?

   _____

   _____

2. List five functions of bones:

   a. _____

   _____

   b. _____

   _____

   c. _____

   _____

   d. _____

   _____

   e. _____

   _____

3. Two main types of bone tissue are:

   a. _____

   _____

   b. _____

   _____

4. List the five shapes of bones:

   a. _____

   b. _____

   c. _____

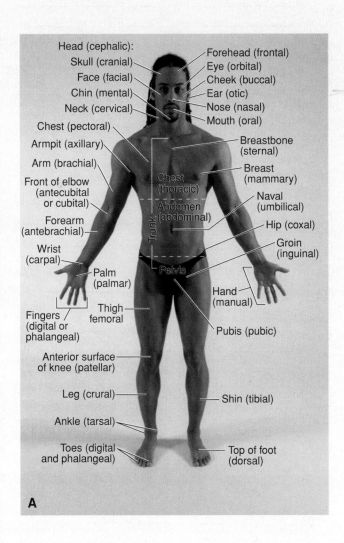

A

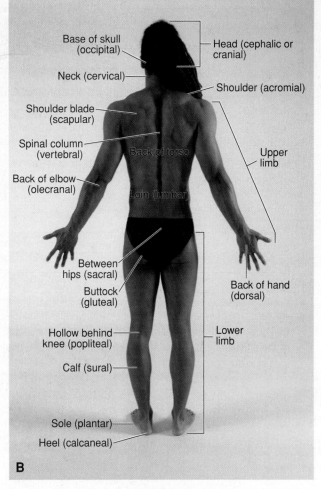

B

d. _____

e. _____

5. Skeleton is divided into axial and appendicular segments.

  a. The axial skeleton consists of:

_____

_____

_____

  b. The appendicular skeleton consists of:

_____

_____

_____

6. Define fascia, and give four examples of connective tissue structures that are called fascia:

_____

  a. _____

  b. _____

  c. _____

  d. _____

Joints

1. Fill in the appropriate functional classifications of joints:

  a. _____ = immovable joint

  b. _____ = slightly movable joint

  c. _____ = freely movable joint

2. Structural classifications of joint use the following terms:

  a. _____ joints are held together by fiber.

  b. _____ joints are held together by cartilage.

  c. _____ joints contain all the components of synovial joints.

3. List the four components of a synovial joint:

  a. _____

  b. _____

  c. _____

  d. _____

4. For each type of synovial joint listed below, please fill in the following: a., the movement permitted at this joint; b., the shape of the articulating surfaces; and c., an example of where this joint is in the body.

1. Plane or gliding

  a. _____

  b. _____

  c. _____

2. Condyloid or ellipsoidal

  a. _____

  b. _____

  c. _____

3. Saddle

  a. _____

  b. _____

  c. _____

4. Pivot

  a. _____

  b. _____

  c. _____

5. Hinge

  a. _____

  b. _____

  c _____

6. Ball-and-socket

  a. _____

  b. _____

  c. _____

Muscles

1. What are muscles?

_____

_____

_____

2. Three types of muscle tissue include:

  a. _____, which is _____, _____, and

_____

  b. _____, which is _____, _____, and

_____

  c. _____, which is _____, _____, and

_____

3. Functions of muscles include:

  a. _____

  b. _____

  c. _____

d. _____

e. _____

4. Structure of a skeletal muscle:

   a. Each individual muscle cell is enclosed in a connective tissue sheath called an

   _____ .

   b. Each fascicle, or group of muscle cells, is wrapped in a connective tissue sheath called a

   _____ .

   c. Many fascicles, bound together to form a muscle, are wrapped in a covering called a

   _____ .

   d. The epimysium blends into a tendon or aponeurosis, attaching muscles to bone.

5. List and define the components of a skeletal muscle cell:

   _____

   _____

   _____

6. Write out the steps involved in the sliding filament mechanism:

   _____

   _____

_____

_____

_____

_____

_____

_____

_____

_____

7. Define a motor unit, and explain the relationship between motor units and the all-or-nothing principle.

   _____

   _____

   _____

8. What is the difference between origin and insertion?

   _____

   _____

9. Give an example of a concentric contraction and an example of an eccentric contraction:

   _____

   _____

   _____

   _____

PART TWO

Individual Muscles by Body Region

3
Upper Limb

■ CHAPTER OUTLINE

(Continued)

OVERVIEW OF THE REGION

The upper limb includes the shoulder girdle, shoulder joint, arm, elbow, forearm, wrist, and hand. This limb is designed for great mobility and is used to complete many activities of daily living. Lifting, eating, reaching, gesturing, pushing, pulling, shaking, waving, and grasping are just a few of the many tasks performed by our upper limbs. Most of us take for granted the vast mobility of the upper limb and its joints, which are constructed to allow a wide range of motion in multiple directions. The structure of these joints prioritizes mobility over stability, and thus several of the joints in the upper extremity are less stable than corresponding joints in the lower extremity. In a later chapter, we will look at the structure of the lower limb, which is designed for weight bearing and thus requires greater stability than the upper limb.

BONES AND BONE MARKINGS OF THE REGION

As we prepare to study the muscles of the upper limb, we will look at the relevant bones and joints first. We will begin with the bones of the thorax (the region between the neck and the abdomen) and spine. Many muscles that move the upper limb attach to the spine, sternum, or ribs, thus we must understand these bones prior to studying the muscles of the upper limb. Next, we will discuss the bones of the shoulder girdle and the bones of each upper limb, including the humerus, radius, ulna, carpals, metacarpals, and phalanges of the hand Figure 3-1 illustrates the bones of the upper extremity.

Sternum

The sternum is part of the axial skeleton. It is a flat bone that is somewhat shaped like a sword. It is divided into three parts. The manubrium (handle) is the superior portion of the sternum. The body (gladiolus) is directly inferior to the manubrium and is the longest part of the sternum. The most inferior aspect is called the xiphoid process, which is composed of cartilage at birth and does not fully ossify until approximately age 40 years. Figure 3-2 shows the sternum, clavicle, and ribs.

Spine

The spine or vertebral column consists of a stack of vertebrae, which connects superiorly to the occipital bone of the skull and inferiorly to the ilium of the pelvis. The spine is constructed so that little muscular energy is necessary to keep one upright. The column has discs between the vertebrae, which serve to absorb shock and allow movement between adjacent vertebrae. Functions of the vertebral column include supporting the head, upper limbs, and trunk; protecting the spinal cord; and providing attachment sites for muscles.

A normal, developed vertebral column has four curves. At birth, the spine has just one curve, keeping one in the fetal position. When an infant begins to hold her or his head up to look around, the cervical curve, running in the opposite direction from the original spinal curve, is created. With more development (sitting up), the lumbar curve, or lordotic curve, is also created. The term "lordosis" is used to indicate a typical lumbar curve, and it is also used to indicate an exaggerated lumbar curve. Additionally, the term *lordosis* is sometimes used to refer

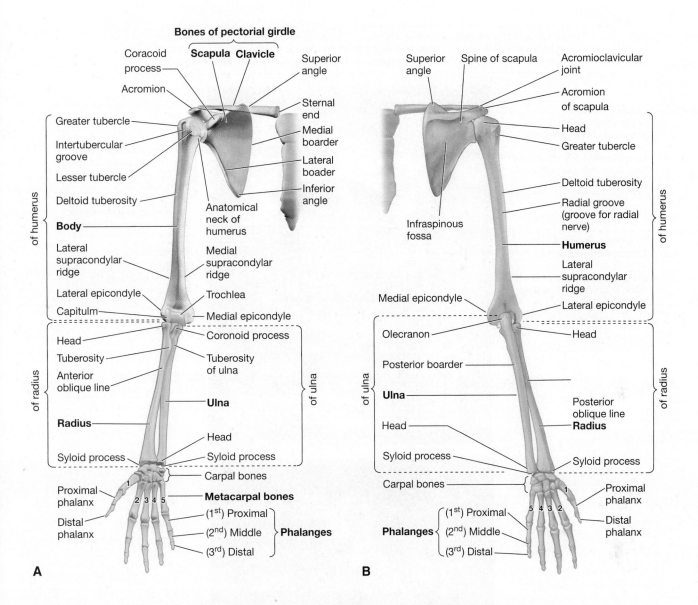

Bones of pectoral girdle

A — Anterior view labels:
Coracoid process — Scapula — Clavicle — Superior angle
Acromion — Sternal end
Greater tubercle — Medial boarder
Intertubercular groove — Lateral boader
Lesser tubercle — Inferior angle
Deltoid tuberosity — Anatomical neck of humerus
Body
Lateral supracondylar ridge — Medial supracondylar ridge
Lateral epicondyle — Trochlea
Capitulm — Medial epicondyle
Head — Coronoid process
Tuberosity — Tuberosity of ulna
Anterior oblique line
Radius — **Ulna**
Syloid process — Head
— Syloid process
Proximal phalanx — Carpal bones
Distal phalanx — **Metacarpal bones**
(1st) Proximal
(2nd) Middle — **Phalanges**
(3rd) Distal

of humerus / of radius / of ulna

B — Posterior view labels:
Superior angle — Spine of scapula — Acromioclavicular joint
Acromion of scapula
Head
Greater tubercle
Infraspinous fossa — Deltoid tuberosity
Radial groove (groove for radial nerve)
Humerus
Lateral supracondylar ridge
Medial epicondyle — Lateral epicondyle
Olecranon — Head
Posterior boarder
Ulna — Posterior oblique line
Head — **Radius**
Syloid process — Syloid process
Carpal bones — Proximal phalanx
Phalanges (1st) Proximal — Distal phalanx
(2nd) Middle
(3rd) Distal

FIGURE 3-1 · Anterior and posterior views of the bones and bone markings of the upper extremity, including sternum, clavicle, humerus, radius ulna, carpals, metacarpals, phalanges of the hand

to the cervical curve, which follows the same direction as the lumbar curve. *Hyperlordosis* is a term that is used to indicate an exaggeration of the lumbar curve. The thoracic and sacral-coccygeal are retained from the original position at birth. (The condition of having an extreme thoracic curve, is called *kyphosis* or *hyperkyphosis*.) Each curve compensates for others and allows the body to be balanced. Figure 3-3 shows a lateral view of the vertebral column, with the sections of the spine and curves labeled.

A typical vertebra consists of a body, a vertebral arch (also called a *neural arch*), and three projections. Each body is comprised of an outer circle of compact bone surrounding spongy bone tissue. The body is cylindrical in shape, and flat on both superior and inferior aspects. A fibrocartilaginous disc connects each vertebral body to the vertebral body above it and below it. The vertebral arch has sections called *laminae* and *pedicles*. There are two pedicles, each joining to a side of the

posterior body, and two laminae, each joining to a pedicle. The vertebral arch extends posteriorly from the vertebral body. The arch surrounds a foramen (a hole and bony landmark), through which passes the spinal cord. Three processes emerge from the vertebral arch. Two are *transverse processes,* which project out from each side of the vertebrae, right where the pedicle and lamina join. Vertebrae have a single *spinous process,* which projects posteriorly at the junction of the two laminae. In addition, each vertebra has four articulation sites called *facets.* Facets are smooth articular surfaces on bones. Each vertebra has two superior articulating facets and two inferior articulating facets, which allow each vertebra to join to the vertebra above and the vertebra below. The thoracic vertebrae have additional facets that serve as articulation sites for the ribs. Figure 3-4 shows a typical vertebra with body, lamina, pedicle, transverse processes, spinous process, and the vertebral foramen labeled.

The **acromioclavicular (AC) joint** is formed by the articulation of the acromion process of the superior scapula with the lateral clavicle.

Two bones comprise the **shoulder girdle**: the clavicle and the scapula. The shoulder girdle is also called the **pectoral girdle**.

The **coracoid process** of the scapula protrudes anteriorly and inferior to the clavicle, to form a strong bony attachment for several muscles of the shoulder.

The **sternoclavicular joint** is the articulation of the medial clavicle with the manubrium of the sternum.

The **manubrium** is the most superior portion of the sternum.

This shallow depression is the **glenoid fossa** of the scapula. It forms the socket of the **glenohumeral joint** which is the articulation of the glenoid fossa with the head of the humerus. The glenohumeral joint is commonly called the **shoulder joint**.

The **sternum** articulates with the ribs via costo-cartilage to form the anterior of the slightly moveable ribcage.

Body of Sternum

Xiphoid process

Humerus

A

Spine of scapula

Clavicle

Manubrium

Acromion process

Body of sternum

The anterior surface (undersurface) of the scapula is somewhat concave, forming the subscapular fossa. This depression is the origin of the subscapularis muscle of the rotator cuff.

Xiphoid process

The **epicondyles of the humerus** form prominent attachment sites for muscles of the elbow and forearm.

Shaft of humerus

B

FIGURE 3-2 · **Sternum (manubrium, body, and xiphoid process), clavicle, and ribs;** includes sternoclavicular joint and acromioclavicular joint. **A:** Anterior view of thorax; **B:** Lateral view of thorax. (*continued*)

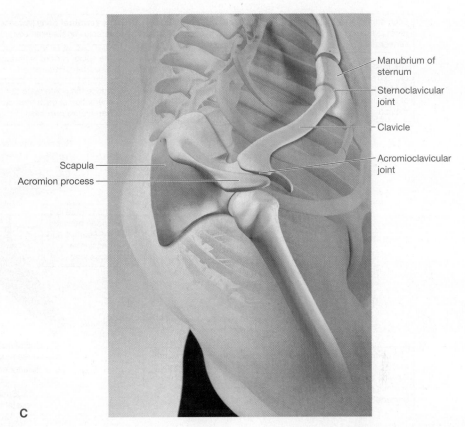

FIGURE 3-2 · *(Continued)*
C: Superior-lateral view of
clavicle and scapula.   **C**

Cervical Vertebrae

There are seven cervical vertebrae. The bodies of cervical vertebrae are small, and the pedicles are short. The transverse processes of the upper six cervical vertebrae have transverse foramina (plural of foramen), through which pass arteries and veins to the vertebrae. The transverse processes also have grooves for spinal nerves to pass through. Most spinous processes are short and forked or *bifid*. C1 and C2 are very different from the other cervical vertebrae. C1 is called the *atlas*. It has no body, but is shaped like a circular ring of bone. C2 is called the *axis*. It has a special, vertically oriented projection called a *dens*, which projects upward into the opening of the atlas. The joint between C1 and C2 allows much rotation. C7 has a large spinous process, which you can palpate on yourself and generally can see easily on others as a significant bump at the base of the back of the neck. Figure 3-5 shows C1 and C2.

Thoracic Vertebrae

There are 12 thoracic vertebrae. The bodies and transverse processes of the thoracic vertebrae have attachment sites for the ribs. The spinous processes of the thoracic vertebrae are long and descend to a level even with the body of the vertebra below. For example, the spinous process of T6 is even with the body of T7.

Lumbar Vertebrae

There are five lumbar vertebrae. The bodies of the lumbar vertebrae are large and strong to accommodate the physical demands placed on this area.

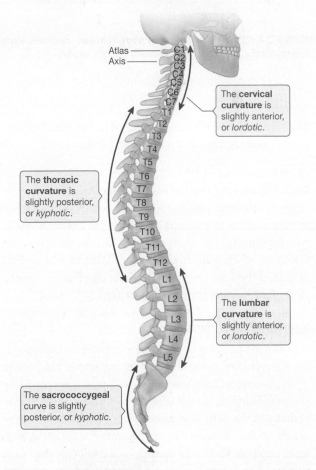

The **cervical curvature** is slightly anterior, or *lordotic*.

The **thoracic curvature** is slightly posterior, or *kyphotic*.

The **lumbar curvature** is slightly anterior, or *lordotic*.

The **sacrococcygeal** curve is slightly posterior, or *kyphotic*.

FIGURE 3-3 · **Lateral view of the vertebral column, with sections of spine labeled and curves of spine**

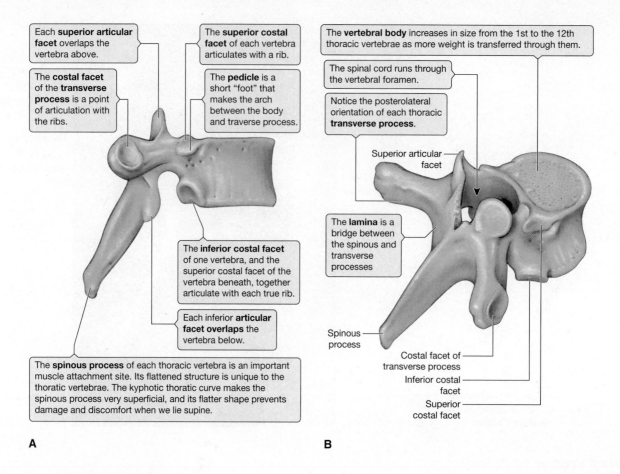

Each **superior articular facet** overlaps the vertebra above.

The **costal facet** of the **transverse process** is a point of articulation with the ribs.

The **superior costal facet** of each vertebra articulates with a rib.

The **pedicle** is a short "foot" that makes the arch between the body and traverse process.

The **inferior costal facet** of one vertebra, and the superior costal facet of the vertebra beneath, together articulate with each true rib.

Each inferior **articular facet overlaps** the vertebra below.

The **spinous process** of each thoracic vertebra is an important muscle attachment site. Its flattened structure is unique to the thoratic vertebrae. The kyphotic thoratic curve makes the spinous process very superficial, and its flatter shape prevents damage and discomfort when we lie supine.

The **vertebral body** increases in size from the 1st to the 12th thoracic vertebrae as more weight is transferred through them.

The spinal cord runs through the vertebral foramen.

Notice the posterolateral orientation of each thoracic **transverse process**.

Superior articular facet

The **lamina** is a bridge between the spinous and transverse processes

Spinous process

Costal facet of transverse process

Inferior costal facet

Superior costal facet

A

B

FIGURE 3-4 · Typical vertebra with body, laminae, pedicles, vertebral foramen, transverse processes, and spinous process labeled. A: Lateral view of a vertebra; **B:** Superior-lateral view of a vertebra

Sacrum

The sacrum is a single bone composed of five vertebral segments fused together. It is triangular in shape.

Coccyx

The coccyx is composed of four vertebrae fused into a single segment or as two bone segments. The coccyx is either fused to the sacrum or attached via ligaments. The sacrum is united with the ilium (a bone of the pelvis) at the sacroiliac joint. The iliac crest, which is an attachment site for the latissimus dorsi muscle, is the superior part of the ilium. See Figure 3-6 for a view of the sacrum, coccyx, and iliac crest.

Intervertebral Foramen

A final bone marking to note that is relevant to the spine is the intervertebral foramen. This opening permits the passage of spinal nerves. Each intervertebral foramen is created by the articulating surfaces of adjacent vertebrae, specifically the pedicles of the vertebrae above, joining the pedicles of the vertebra below. Because the pedicles are not as tall as the bodies of vertebrae, there is an opening on the sides between each vertebra. See Figure 3-7, which illustrates an intervertebral foramen.

Ribs

There are 12 pairs of ribs, which unite with the 12 thoracic vertebrae posteriorly. Rib 1 connects to the body and transverse process of vertebra T1. Rib 2 connects to the bodies of T1 and T2 and the transverse process of T2. Rib 3 connects to the bodies of T2 and T3 and the transverse processes of T3. Ribs 4 to 9 follow this same pattern, connecting to two adja-

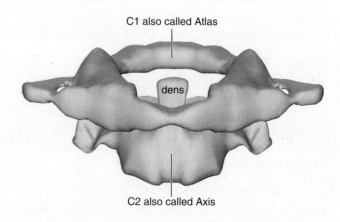

C1 also called Atlas

dens

C2 also called Axis

FIGURE 3-5 · Vertebrae C1 and C2 and the joint between them

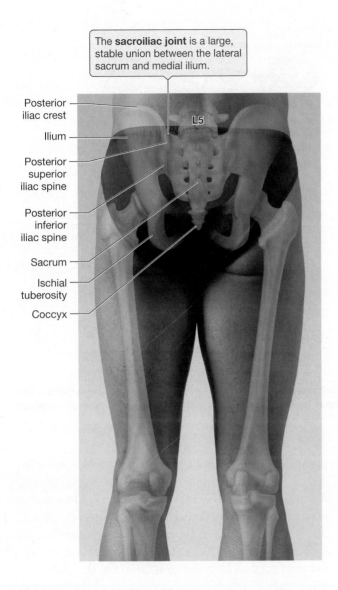

> The **sacroiliac joint** is a large, stable union between the lateral sacrum and medial ilium.

Posterior iliac crest

Ilium

Posterior superior iliac spine

Posterior inferior iliac spine

Sacrum

Ischial tuberosity

Coccyx

L5

FIGURE 3-6 · **Sacrum, coccyx, posterior iliac crest, and sacroiliac joint**

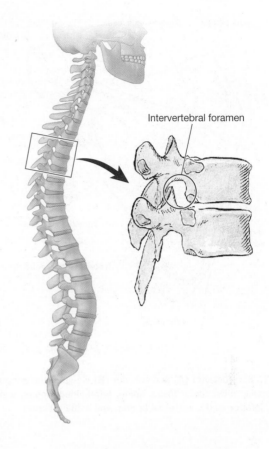

Intervertebral foramen

FIGURE 3-7 · **An intervertebral foramen**

cent vertebral bodies and one transverse process. Ribs 10 connects to the body and transverse process of T10 alone; rib 11 joins to the body and transverse process of T11 alone; and rib 12 connects to the body and transverse process of T12 alone.

The ribs form the protective circular structure of the *thorax*, enclosing the heart and lungs. The anterior, medial aspect or each of the upper seven pairs of ribs attach to the sternum via a slip of costal cartilage, earning them the title of "true ribs." Ribs 8–10 join to the sternum via the costal cartilage of rib 7, and thus they are called "false ribs." Ribs 11 and 12 do not articulate with the sternum at all, and thus they are called "floating" ribs, as well as "false" ribs. See Figure 3-2 for an anterior view of the ribs.

Shoulder Girdle: Clavicle and Scapula

The shoulder girdle or pectoral girdle is made of the clavicle and scapula. The clavicle is an S-shaped bone positioned horizontally inferior and lateral to the neck. The medial aspect of the clavicle articulates or joins with the manubrium of the sternum at the sternoclavicular joint (see Fig. 3-2). The lateral aspect of the clavicle articulates with the scapula at the acromioclavicular (AC) joint, which is between the acromion process of the scapula and the lateral aspect of the clavicle. Figure 3-2 illustrates the sternoclavicular and acromioclavicular joints.

The scapulae are two flat, triangular-shaped bones in the upper-mid back. As already mentioned, each scapula articulates with a clavicle at an AC joint. The acromion is a flat bone marking on the lateral, superior part of the scapula. Each scapula contains a bone marking called the *glenoid fossa*, also located on the lateral aspect of the bone. This is the shallow socket that accepts the head of the humerus to form the shoulder joint. In addition to the acromion and the glenoid fossa, there are several other important bone markings on the scapula. Just above and just below the glenoid fossa are two tubercles (small rounded projections) called the *supraglenoid tubercle* and the *infraglenoid tubercle*. There are two named borders of the scapula, simply called the vertebral and axillary borders. There are two named angles as well, the superior angle and the inferior angle. The scapula has a process that projects anteriorly on the lateral, superior aspect of the bone called the *coracoid* (crow's beak) *process*. The scapula has a prominent projection on the posterior part of the bone called the *spine* of the scapula. The root of the spine of the scapula is a bone marking located on the spine of the scapula where the

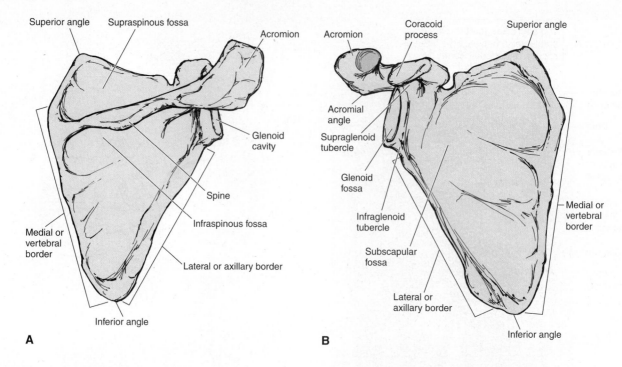

FIGURE 3-8 · Posterior (A) and anterior (B) views of the scapula with the following bony landmarks: coracoid process, acromion, glenoid fossa, subscapular fossa, spine, infraspinous fossa, supraspinous fossa, supraglenoid tubercle, infraglenoid tubercle, superior angle, inferior angle, vertebral border, and axillary border

spine meets the vertebral border. In addition to the glenoid fossa, the scapula has three additional fossas. One is the subscapular fossa, and it makes up the entire anterior aspect of the bone. Two other fossa are located on the posterior aspect of the bone: the supraspinous fossa and the infraspinous fossa. The supraspinous fossa is located above the spine of the scapula, and the infraspinous fossa is located below the spine of the scapula. Figure 3-8 provides anterior, posterior, and lateral views of the scapula with the bone markings noted above.

Humerus

The humerus is the bone of the arm. It is a long bone that is wider at the proximal and distal ends but narrower and rather cylindrical between the ends. The narrow and more cylindrical portion of the bone is called the *shaft* or *body* of the bone. The head of the humerus is a rounded bone marking on the proximal, medial aspect of the humerus. The head of the humerus articulates with the glenoid fossa to complete the shoulder joint. The humerus has two tubercles (small roundish projections), also on the proximal aspect of the bone. They are called the *greater tubercle* of the humerus and the *lesser tubercle* of the humerus. Between the greater and lesser tubercles of the humerus lies the intertubercular groove ("inter" means "between"). The intertubercular groove is also called the *bicipital groove* because the tendon of origin of the long head of the biceps brachii lies right in the groove.

The deltoid tuberosity (roughened area on a bone) is located on the lateral shaft of the humerus. The distal end of

the humerus contains two unique bone markings: on the lateral side, we have a capitulum (little head), and on the medial side, we have a trochlea (pulley). These two rounded bone markings replace the condyles of the humerus. The medial epicondyle of the humerus is a small projection on the medial side of the trochlea, and the lateral epicondyle of the humerus projects from the lateral aspect of the capitulum. Many muscles attach to the epicondyles of the humerus. Proximal to the medial and lateral epicondyles are two supracondylar ridges, medial and lateral. The distal aspect of the humerus is flatter than the rounded central part of the bone, thus resulting in these two bony ridges. Figure 3-9 provides both anterior and posterior views of the humerus.

The trochlea of the humerus articulates with the trochlear notch (see below) of the proximal ulna, and the capitulum of the humerus articulates with the head of the radius (see below) to form the elbow joint.

Radius and Ulna

The radius is the lateral forearm bone. It has three notable bone markings. The head of the radius is the rounded, proximal aspect of the bone. The head of the radius articulates with the capitulum of the humerus (as a cap sits on a head). The radial tuberosity is slightly distal and medial to the head of the radius. On the lateral, distal aspect of the bone lies the styloid process of the radius.

As already noted, the anterior, proximal end of the ulna has a sizable notch called the *trochlear notch*, which joins the

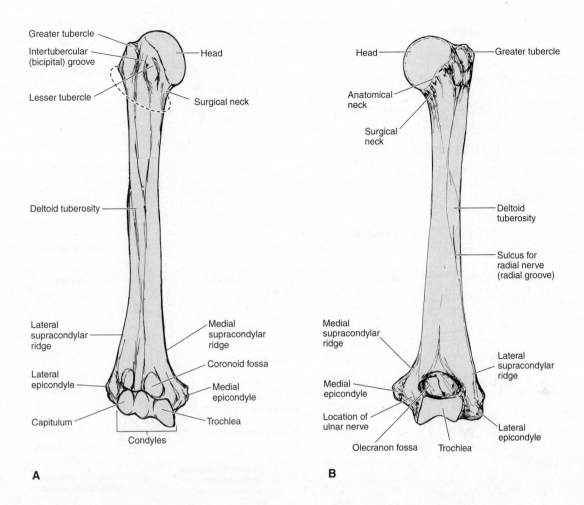

FIGURE 3-9 · Anterior and posterior views of the humerus with bone markings: greater tubercle, lesser tubercle, intertubercular sulcus (also called the bicipital groove), deltoid tuberosity, capitulum, trochlea, medial and lateral epicondyles, and the medial and lateral supracondylar ridges

trochlea of the humerus. The coronoid process of the ulna and the ulnar tuberosity are both located on the proximal anterior aspect of the ulna, just inferior to the trochlear notch. The olecranon process is a prominent projection on the posterior aspect of the proximal humerus. The olecranon process makes the "tip" of the elbow. The ulna has two bone markings on its distal aspect: the styloid process and the head of the ulna. The head is visible in most people when viewing the ulnar side of the distal, posterior forearm. The styloid process is a thin projection extending distally from the head of the ulna. Its small size and placement make is difficult to see and palpate. Figure 3-10 shows anterior and posterior views of the radius and ulna with bone markings labeled.

Bones of the Hand

Before discussing the bones of the hand, it is useful to note that the thumb and fingers are referred to as *digits*. The thumb is digit 1, the index finger is digit 2, the middle finger is digit 3, the "ring finger" is known as the fourth digit, and the smallest finger is called the fifth digit.

The most proximal set of bones within the hand are called the carpal bones. These eight tiny bones are commonly called the

bones of the "wrist," because they are so close to the wrist joint; however, they are actually located within the hand. The carpals are arranged roughly in two rows. The proximal row contains the scaphoid, lunate, triquetrum, and pisiform. The pisiform is the most palpable of the carpal bones and can be felt at the palmar side of the medial wrist crease. The distal row of carpals includes the trapezium, trapezoid, capitate, and hamate.

Distal to the carpals are five metacarpals, one for each digit. The metacarpals are located within the hand, and are quite palpable on the dorsal side of the hand. Distal to the metacarpals are the bones of the fingers and thumb, called the *phalanges*. The thumb, or the first digit, has two phalanges: a proximal phalanx and a distal phalanx. The fingers (digits 2 to 5) have three phalanges each, a proximal, middle, and distal phalanx per digit. Figure 3-11 shows a palmar view of the right hand.

JOINTS, LIGAMENTS, AND BURSAE OF THE REGION

As you know, our bones articulate with other bones to form joints and permit movement. The spine contains many joints between adjacent vertebrae. The sternum, clavicle, and

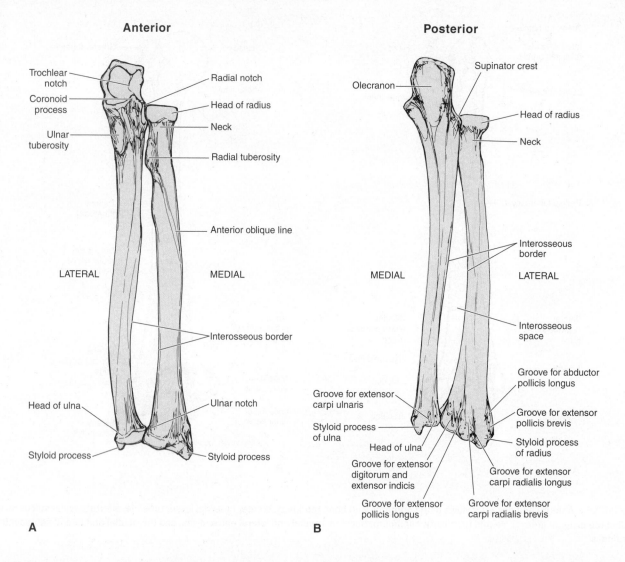

Anterior

Trochlear notch
Coronoid process
Ulnar tuberosity
Radial notch
Head of radius
Neck
Radial tuberosity
Anterior oblique line
LATERAL
MEDIAL
Interosseous border
Head of ulna
Ulnar notch
Styloid process
Styloid process

A

Posterior

Olecranon
Supinator crest
Head of radius
Neck
Interosseous border
MEDIAL
LATERAL
Interosseous space
Groove for abductor pollicis longus
Groove for extensor carpi ulnaris
Groove for extensor pollicis brevis
Styloid process of ulna
Styloid process of radius
Head of ulna
Groove for extensor digitorum and extensor indicis
Groove for extensor carpi radialis longus
Groove for extensor pollicis longus
Groove for extensor carpi radialis brevis

B

FIGURE 3-10 · **The radius and ulna with the bony landmarks: head of radius, radial tuberosity, styloid process of the radius, trochlear notch of the ulna, the olecranon process of the ulna, the coracoid process of the ulna, head of the ulna, styloid process of the ulna, and the interosseus membrane. A:** Anterior view of radius and ulna; **B:** Posterior view of radius and ulna.

scapula are all involved in joints. The upper limb contains a variety of synovial joints that allow the different movements within the upper extremity. Ligaments stabilize our joints, and *bursae*, which are synovial fluid–filled sacs, strategically placed to prevent friction between adjacent structures.

Joints Within the Spine

Movement of the vertebral column typically occurs when many joints move together. Remember that the anterior intervertebral joints are classified as slightly movable, fibrocartilaginous joints. So, the spine is composed of many slightly movable joints that together permit much movement, including flexion, extension, lateral flexion, and rotation of the spine. The thickness of intervertebral discs and the tightness of ligaments and muscles, which connect aspects of the spine, determine the amount of movement permitted at each area of the spine. Greatest movement is possible in the cervical (especially flexion) and lumbar regions (especially extension).

These two areas are also the most frequent sites of pain and serious injury. The thoracic vertebrae's connection to the ribs and indirect connection to the sternum adds stability to the thoracic vertebrae and limits the movement in the region.

Sternoclavicular Joint

The sternoclavicular joint links the entire upper limb to the axial skeleton. In other words, the sternoclavicular joint is the only bone-to-bone connection between the upper limb and the trunk. The medial end of the clavicle fits into a notch in the lateral aspect of the manubrium (proximal part of the sternum) and the costal cartilage of the first rib. A disc separates the two points of connection, providing cushioning and stabilization. The sternoclavicular ligaments provide additional stability to the joint. The medial aspect of the clavicle lies superior to the manubrium, making this joint easy to palpate. The sternoclavicular joint is typically categorized as a plane or gliding joint, although some sources categorize it

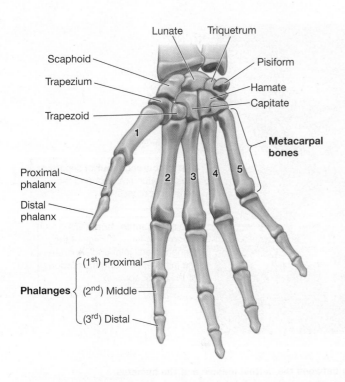

Lunate Triquetrum

Scaphoid

Pisiform

Trapezium

Hamate

Capitate

Trapezoid

Metacarpal bones

1

Proximal phalanx

2 3 4 5

Distal phalanx

(1st) Proximal

Phalanges (2nd) Middle

(3rd) Distal

FIGURE 3-11 · Palmar view of the right hand with all carpals, metacarpals, and phalanges labeled

as a saddle joint. A good degree of movement is possible at the sternoclavicular joint. Whenever one moves the scapula, the sternoclavicular joint moves as well. See Figure 3-2 for an illustration of the sternoclavicular joint.

Acromioclavicular Joint

The AC joint, between the acromion process of the scapula and the lateral aspect of the clavicle, is the junction of two flat bone markings. This joint is a plane type of synovial joint and allows minimal gliding movement. Movement of the scapula causes movement at the AC joint. The AC ligament supports this joint. See Figure 3-2 for an illustration of the AC joint.

The scapula does not articulate with the ribs via a bone-to-bone connection. However, the scapula can move along with the rib cage. The movements of the scapula include elevation and depression, protraction and retraction, and upward and downward rotation. Scapular movements allow for a much greater range of motion of the arms. For example, protracting the scapulae allows one to reach farther to the front. Upward rotation of the scapula allows a greater range of arm abduction.

The scapula is held against the chest wall by many muscles, most notably the serratus anterior muscle. The rhomboids assist in this task as well.

Shoulder Joint

The shoulder joint is a ball-and-socket joint that permits great mobility at the expense of stability. We have an extensive capacity to flex, extend, abduct, adduct, horizontally abduct,

horizontally adduct, medially rotate, and laterally rotate the shoulder joint. The socket of the shoulder joint (glenoid fossa) is shallow, permitting great movement of the humerus in almost all directions, but sacrificing stability. The shoulder joint is one of the most easily dislocated joints on the body. We rely on soft tissue, particularly the rotator cuff muscles, and ligaments to stabilize and help maintain the integrity of the joint.

Notable ligaments include the transverse humeral ligament, which joins the greater and lesser tubercles of the humerus; the coracohumeral ligament, which joins the coracoid process of the scapula to the neck of the humerus; and the coracoacromial ligament, which links the coracoid process of the scapula and the acromion process.

There are several bursae close to the shoulder joint. Bursae are sacs containing synovial fluid and are positioned to prevent friction between adjacent structures. The subscapular bursa is located between the scapula and the tendon of insertion of the subscapularis muscle. The subacromial bursa is located inferior to the acromion and deep to the deltoid muscle and superior to the tendon of insertion of the supraspinatus muscle. This bursa prevents rubbing of the supraspinatus tendon and the deltoid muscle when one abducts the arm. Figure 3-12 shows the subacromial bursa, in position to prevent friction between the deltoid muscle and the humerus.

Elbow Joint

The elbow can be a confusing joint, as it is considered a hinge joint, which allows the movements of flexion and extension only. Actually, the elbow joint capsule contains three different joints, the humeroulnar joint, the joint between the capitulum and head of the radius, and the proximal radioulnar joint. The humeroulnar joint in conjunction with the joint between the capitulum and head of the radius create the hinge joint. Meanwhile, the joint between the radius and ulna is a pivot joint, allowing supination and pronation of the forearm. In this text, the elbow joint will refer to the hinge joint between the arm and forearm.

The elbow joint is supported by the radial and ulnar collateral ligaments. The radial collateral ligament joins the lateral epicondyle of the humerus to the annular ligament, which attaches the proximal radius to the proximal ulna. The ulnar collateral ligament joins the medial epicondyle of the humerus to the coronoid process of the ulna and the olecranon process of the ulna. Figure 3-13 illustrates the elbow (humeroulnar) joint, and the proximal radioulnar joint.

Several bursae are located around the elbow joint. The subtendinous bursa prevents friction between the olecranon process of the ulna and the tendon of insertion of the triceps brachii. Another significant bursa is the radioulnar bursa, which creates space between the radiohumeral joint and the supinator muscle. A third bursa is the bicipitoradial bursa, which lies between the tendon of insertion of the biceps brachii and the radial tuberosity.

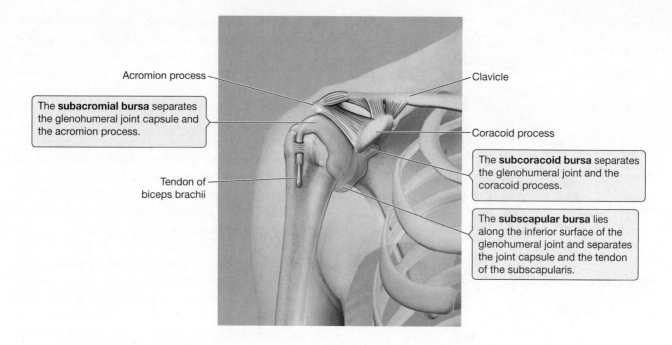

Acromion process

Clavicle

The **subacromial bursa** separates the glenohumeral joint capsule and the acromion process.

Coracoid process

Tendon of biceps brachii

The **subcoracoid bursa** separates the glenohumeral joint and the coracoid process.

The **subscapular bursa** lies along the inferior surface of the glenohumeral joint and separates the joint capsule and the tendon of the subscapularis.

FIGURE 3-12 · Subacromial bursa, in position to prevent friction between the deltoid muscle and the humerus

Radioulnar Joints

There are two pivot joints connecting the radius and ulna. Both the proximal and distal radioulnar joints allow supination and pronation to occur. In the proximal radioulnar joint, the head of the radius articulates with the radial notch in the proximal ulna. The distal radioulnar joint is between the head of the ulna and the ulnar notch of the radius.

When one performs the actions of supination and pronation, the radius rotates around the ulna. As already mentioned, the annular ligament stabilizes the proximal radial ulnar joint. In addition, a strong, thin, fibrous interosseous membrane connects the radius and ulna, providing greater stability to the forearm and serving as a muscle attachment site.

Wrist Joint

The wrist joint is a condyloid joint between the radius and the scaphoid and lunate. Wrist movements include flexion, extension, abduction (radial deviation), and adduction (ulnar deviation).

Joints Within the Hand

The joints between the carpals, or intercarpal joints, are plane joints, which permit only a small amount of gliding movement. This movement is not done in isolation, but rather to increase the range of motion of the fingers and wrist.

The joints between the carpal bones and the metacarpals (carpometacarpal or CMC joints) are also plane joints, with the exception of the joint between the trapezium and the first metacarpal. This joint is called a *saddle joint* because of the unique shape of the articulating surfaces of the joints, which

appear as a saddle and a rider. This joint permits flexion, extension, abduction, adduction, and a small amount of rotation. The joints between the metacarpals and the phalanges are called *metacarpophalangeal* (MP) joints. They are ellipsoidal joints and allow flexion, extension, abduction, and adduction. The joints between phalanges are called *interphalangeal* (IP) joints. Each finger has two IP joints, a proximal one (PIP) and a distal one (DIP). The thumb has only two phalanges and thus has a single IP joint. All IP joints are hinge joints. Figure 3-14 provides a dorsal view of the bones and joints of the hand.

CONNECTIVE TISSUE STRUCTURES OF THE REGION

Several connective tissue structures are relevant to muscles of the upper limb. The flexor retinaculum is a strap-like band of fascia that joins the scaphoid and trapezium to the hamate and pisiform. The flexor retinaculum forms the roof of the carpal tunnel. Many flexor tendons, along with the median nerve, pass deep to the flexor retinaculum and through the carpal tunnel. Flexor tendon sheaths are connective tissue structures on the palmar side of the fingers that contain pulleys for the flexor tendons to pass through. The sheaths helps keep these tendons in position for efficient flexion of the fingers. The extensor mechanism is a more complex connective tissue structure than the flexor tendon sheath, located on the dorsal side of the fingers. Its purpose is to guide extensor tendons (keep them in position) and serve as an attachment site for some hand muscles. The palmar aponeurosis/palmar fascia is a triangular-shaped fascia on the palm that provides

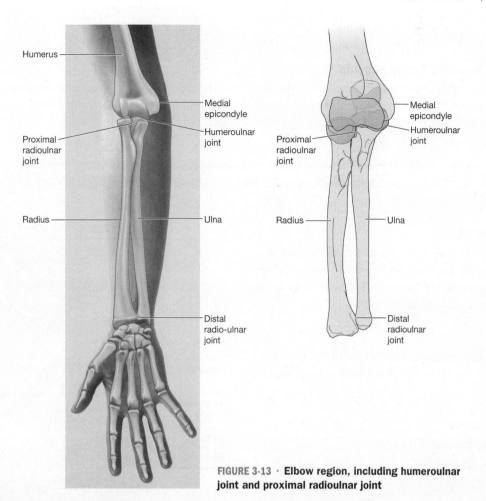

FIGURE 3-13 · Elbow region, including humeroulnar joint and proximal radioulnar joint

protection for nerves and vessels in the center of the palm and serves as a muscle attachment site for one of the wrist flexors. The extensor retinaculum is a connective tissue structure creating a tunnel on the dorsal side of the wrist. The tendons of insertion of the wrist and finger extensors pass through this tunnel.

The ligamentum nuchae is a line of connective tissue running from a bone marking on the posterior aspect of the head (the external occipital protuberance) to the spinous process of C7 and joining the spinous processes of C1 through C7. The bones and bone markings of the skull will be covered in a later chapter. The thoracolumbar aponeurosis is a wide sheet of fascia connecting to the sacrum and posterior iliac crest. This sheet-like fascia serves as the origin tendon of latissimus dorsi.

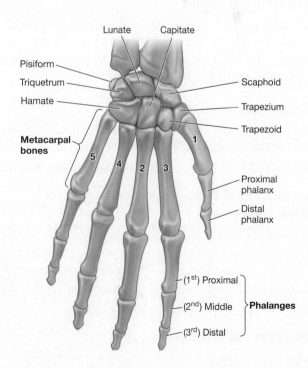

FIGURE 3-14 · Dorsal view of the bones and joints of the hand, with all carpals, metacarpals, and phalanges labeled

INDIVIDUAL MUSCLES

Muscles That Move the Arm or Scapula

We will begin our study of individual muscles by exploring the muscles that move the arm at the shoulder joint. These muscles insert on the humerus and can perform one or more of the following actions: flexion, extension, abduction, adduction, medial rotation, lateral rotation, horizontal abduction, and horizontal adduction.

CORACOBRACHIALIS (kor-a-ko-bra-ke-al-is)

Meaning of Name

The first part of this muscle's name, *coraco*, tells us that muscle connects to the coracoid (crow's beak) process of the scapula. The second part of the muscle's name tells us that the muscle connects to the arm or *brachium*.

Location

Medial arm. Coracobrachialis blends in with the short head of biceps brachii (an elbow flexor that we will cover later on in this text).

Origin and Insertion

Origin: coracoid process of the scapula
Insertion: medial humerus

Actions

Flexion and adduction of arm at the shoulder joint

Explanation of Actions

Because the origin is above the insertion and this muscle crosses the anterior aspect of the shoulder joint, it performs shoulder flexion. Because the origin is medial to the insertion, coracobrachialis also adducts the arm.

Notable Muscle Facts

Coracobrachialis is a small, relatively weak arm mover. Coracobrachialis can flex the arm to approximately 90 degrees. Arm flexion beyond 90 degrees lengthens this muscle.

Implications of Shortened and/or Lengthened/Weak Muscle

Shortened: Posture has arms in front of the body, and/or arms very close to the body. Limited ability to perform arm extension and arm abduction. (Note antagonists below.)
Lengthened: No significant postural or functional deficits are seen.

Palpation and Massage

When palpating this muscle, note that coracobrachialis is difficult to distinguish from the short head of biceps

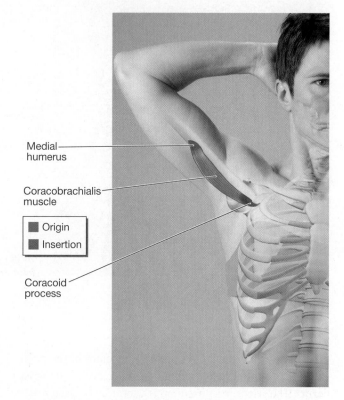

Medial humerus

Coracobrachialis muscle

■ Origin
■ Insertion

Coracoid process

FIGURE 3-15 · **Coracobrachialis**

brachii. However, because biceps brachii is an elbow flexor, you can ask the client to contract it isometrically by flexing the elbow against your resistance and feeling for the distinction between the firm, contracted biceps brachii and the relaxed coracobrachialis muscle, just medial to biceps brachii.

One way to massage coracobrachialis is to have your client supine and trace between the coracoid process and the medial humerus. One can provide gentle effleurage and pétrissage to the medial arm, taking care not to put pressure on the median nerve, brachial artery, medial antebrachial nerve, or the basilic vein, which are all located in the medial arm. Circular friction around the coracoid process will also address coracobrachialis.

How to Stretch This Muscle

Extend and laterally rotate the arm.

Synergists

Arm adductors: pectoralis major, latissimus dorsi, and teres major
Arm flexors: pectoralis major, anterior deltoid, and biceps brachii

Antagonists

Arm abductors: supraspinatus and middle deltoid

Arm extensors: latissimus dorsi, teres major, infraspinatus, teres minor, posterior deltoid, pectoralis major (extension from a flexed position), and triceps brachii

Innervation and Arterial Supply

Innervation: musculocutaneous nerve, which passes right through the muscle
Arterial supply: brachial artery

PECTORALIS MAJOR (pek-tor-al-is ma-jor)

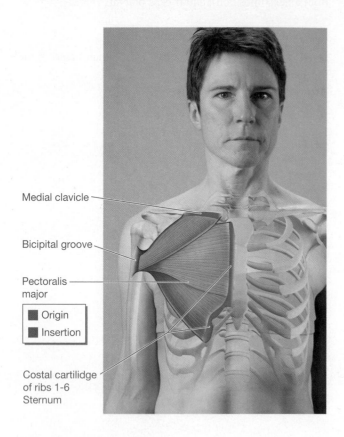

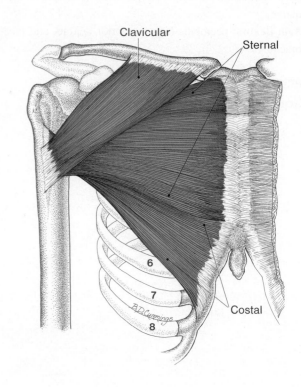

FIGURE 3-16 · Pectoralis major

Meaning of Name

Pectoralis means "chest." The word *major* means "larger," and distinguishes pectoralis major from pectoralis minor, a smaller muscle.

Location

Pectoralis major is located in the superficial, anterior chest. This muscle forms the contour of the anterior chest.

Origin and Insertion

Origin: medial clavicle, sternum, and costal cartilage of ribs 1 to 6

Insertion: lateral lip of the bicipital groove

Actions

Flexion, extension from a flexed position, medial rotation, adduction, and horizontal adduction of the arm at the shoulder joint

Explanation of Actions

This muscle has two distinct sections, or heads, called the *clavicular head* and the *sternal head*. (Some books list three parts/heads to the muscle: clavicular, sternal, and costal/ abdominal). The clavicular head can perform arm flexion, as the origin on the clavicle is above the insertion on the bicipital groove. The inferior portion of the sternocostal head performs extension of the arm from a flexed position. Pectoralis major can perform extension because the origin of sternocostal head is below the insertion on the bicipital groove. When both clavicular and sternocostal heads contract together, the muscle performs medial rotation, adduction, and horizontal adduction of the arm. These actions of adduction and horizontal adduction are possible because the origin is medial to the insertion. Medial rotation of the arm is possible because the insertion is lateral enough on the humerus to provide the leverage necessary to rotate the arm medially.

Notable Muscle Facts

Pectoralis major is a thick muscle that creates the shape or contour of the chest. It is a particularly strong medial rotator and adductor of the arm. The fibers of the clavicular head actually insert below the fibers of the sternal head, creating an overlap of fibers at the insertion and giving the muscle added density at the bicipital groove.

Implications of Shortened and/or Lengthened/ Weak Muscle

Shortened: Posture has dorsal side of hands facing forward, arms in front of the body, and/or arms very close to body. Limited ability to perform arm extension, arm flexion, lateral rotation of the arm, abduction of the arm, and/or horizontal abduction of the arm. (Note antagonists below.)

Lengthened: Significant loss of arm adduction, medial rotation, and flexion is seen.

Palpation and Massage

Pectoralis major can be palpated in the anterior chest and can be traced from the sternum to the bicipital groove. Effleurage across the anterior chest, compression into the anterior chest, and digital pétrissage of the lateral aspect of the muscle close to the anterior axillary area are all appropriate strokes for this muscle. Palpating and providing friction to the inferior aspect of the medial clavicle and lateral edge of the sternum allows us to access and massage much of the origin of pectoralis major. Friction to the lateral edge of the muscle, by pressing the tissue into the lateral ribs and humerus beneath, can also be helpful. Work with care in the anterior chest area, working into breast tissue only to the extent that it feels comfortable and appropriate for both the client and you.

How to Stretch This Muscle

Horizontally abduct and laterally rotate the arm.

Synergists

Arm medial rotators: subscapularis, anterior deltoid, latissimus dorsi, and teres major

Arm flexors: anterior deltoid, coracobrachialis, and biceps brachii

Arm horizontal adductor: anterior deltoid

Antagonists

Lateral rotators of the arm: posterior deltoid, infraspinatus, and teres minor

Arm extensors: latissimus dorsi, teres major, infraspinatus, teres minor, posterior deltoid, and triceps brachii

Arm horizontal abductor: posterior deltoid

Innervation and Arterial Supply

Innervation: medial and lateral pectoral nerves

Arterial supply: pectoral branches of the thoracoacromial trunk

DELTOID (del-toyd)

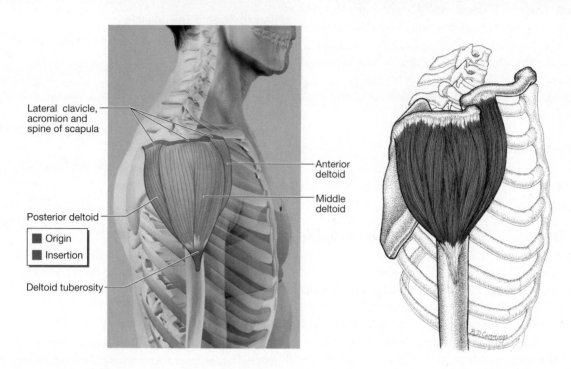

FIGURE 3-17 · **Deltoid**

Meaning of Name

The deltoid muscle is named for the Greek letter *delta*, which has a triangular shape.

Location

The superficial, strong, triangularly shaped deltoid muscle forms the contour of our shoulder. It is referred to as the *shoulder cap*, because its density and superficial location make it seem like a cap upon the shoulder. The deltoid is divided into three sections: anterior, middle, and posterior. We will look at the three sections of the deltoid muscle separately.

Anterior Deltoid

Origin and Insertion

Origin: lateral clavicle
Insertion: deltoid tuberosity

Actions

Medial rotation, flexion, and horizontal adduction of the arm

Explanation of Actions

Because the origin is located above insertion, and because anterior deltoid crosses the anterior aspect of the shoulder, anterior deltoid performs flexion. Medial rotation is possible because the lateral clavicle is more medial than the insertion, and because the insertion is on the lateral aspect of the proximal humerus, giving anterior deltoid the leverage to turn the

humerus medially. Horizontal adduction of the arm is possible because the origin is more medial than the insertion.

Middle Deltoid

Origin and Insertion

Origin: acromion
Insertion: deltoid tuberosity

Actions

Abduction of the humerus at the shoulder joint

Explanation of Actions

Middle deltoid crosses the lateral aspect of the shoulder joint, with its origin directly above the insertion. Moving the deltoid tuberosity toward the acromion causes abduction of the arm. However, when the arm is by the side of the body, an upward pull on the deltoid tuberosity toward the acromion would cause the proximal humerus to contact the acromion. The arm must be abducted a small amount in order for middle deltoid to have the leverage to abduct the arm without the humerus hitting the acromion. Another muscle, the supraspinatus, initiates arm abduction, to bring the arm into position for middle deltoid to perform its action.

Posterior Deltoid

Origin and Insertion

Origin: spine of the scapula
Insertion: deltoid tuberosity

Actions

The actions of posterior deltoid include lateral rotation, extension, and horizontal abduction of the arm at the shoulder joint.

Explanation of Actions

Posterior deltoid crosses the posterior aspect of the shoulder with origin above insertion. This location allows the muscle to perform arm extension. Because the origin is medial to the insertion, and the muscle crosses the posterior aspect of the shoulder joint, posterior deltoid can perform lateral rotation and horizontal abduction.

Notable Muscle Facts

The fibers of the deltoid muscle have a unique multipennate pattern, creating significant strength. In fact, the deltoid muscle is one of the strongest muscles in the body per unit of volume.

Implications of Shortened and/or Lengthened/ Weak Muscle

Shortened anterior deltoid: Posture has dorsal side of hand facing forward, and/or arms in front of the body. Limited ability to perform arm extension, lateral rotation of the arm, and/or horizontal abduction of the arm. (Note antagonists below.)

Lengthened anterior deltoid: Limited ability to perform arm flexion, medial rotation of the arm, and/or horizontal adduction of the arm is noted.

Shortened middle deltoid: Limited ability to perform arm adduction is seen. (Note antagonists below.)

Lengthened middle deltoid: Limited ability to perform arm abduction is present.

Shortened posterior deltoid: Posture has palmar side of hand facing forward. Limited ability to perform arm flexion, medial rotation of the arm, and/or horizontal adduction of the arm. (Note antagonists below.)

Lengthened posterior deltoid: Limited ability to perform arm extension, lateral rotation of the arm, and/or horizontal abduction of the arm is noted.

Palpation and Massage

The deltoid muscle can be palpated by contacting the superficial shoulder cap. One can trace from the lateral clavicle, to the acromion, and across the spine of the scapula to access the full origin. Isometrically contracting the deltoid, by abducting the arm against resistance, allows the muscle to tense, and one can follow the sides of this triangular muscle inferiorly to the deltoid tuberosity. Because of the bulky nature of this muscle, pétrissage is an appropriate massage stroke to apply to it. Effleurage and friction are also appropriate. Consider applying gentle friction across the full origin, pressing upward into the inferior aspect of the lateral clavicle, across the lateral acromion, and upward into the inferior aspect of the spine of the scapula. Consider applying gentle friction at the deltoid tuberosity on the anterolateral humerus. Consider using reciprocal inhibition by having your client contract his or her arm adductors isometrically.

How to Stretch This Muscle

Anterior deltoid: Fully extend, laterally rotate, and horizontally abduct the arm.

Posterior deltoid: Fully flex, medially rotate, and horizontally adduct the arm.

Anterior Deltoid

Synergists

Medial rotators of the arm: pectoralis major, subscapularis, latissimus dorsi, and teres major

Arm flexors: pectoralis major, coracobrachialis, and biceps brachii

Arm horizontal adductor: pectoralis major

Antagonists

Lateral rotators of the arm: posterior deltoid, infraspinatus, and teres minor

Arm extensors: latissimus dorsi, teres major, infraspinatus, teres minor, posterior deltoid, triceps brachii, and pectoralis major (extension from a flexed position)

Arm horizontal abductor: posterior deltoid

Middle Deltoid

Synergists

Arm abductor: supraspinatus

Antagonists

Arm adductors: pectoralis major, coracobrachialis, latissimus dorsi, and teres major

Posterior Deltoid

Synergists

Lateral rotators of the arm: infraspinatus, teres minor

Arm extensors: latissimus dorsi, teres major, infraspinatus, teres minor, triceps brachii, and pectoralis major (extension from a flexed position)

Antagonists

Medial rotators of the arm: pectoralis major, subscapularis, latissimus dorsi, teres major, and anterior deltoid

Arm flexors: pectoralis major, coracobrachialis, anterior deltoid, and biceps brachii

Arm horizontal adductors: pectoralis major and anterior deltoid

Innervation and Arterial Supply

Innervation: axillary nerve

Arterial supply: anterior and posterior circumflex humeral arteries

SUPRASPINATUS (su-pra-spin-a-tus)

Meaning of Name

The name *supraspinatus* tells us that this muscle is located above (superior to) the spine of the scapula. Supraspinatus is one of the four rotator cuff muscles, which form a "cuff" around the shoulder joint and help stabilize the joint.

Location

The supraspinatus muscle is a small muscle located on the posterior aspect of the scapula. The belly of the muscle fills the supraspinous fossa, and the tendon of insertion passes under the acromion on its way to the greater tubercle of the humerus.

Origin and Insertion

Origin: supraspinous fossa
Insertion: greater tubercle of the humerus

Actions

Initiates abduction of the arm at the shoulder joint

Explanation of Actions

Supraspinatus crosses the lateral aspect of the shoulder joint and is thus perfectly positioned for abducting the arm. Many sources claim that supraspinatus is important in initiating arm abduction, and once the arm is away from the body, the much stronger middle deltoid can take over and abduct the arm fully.

Notable Muscle Facts

Although supraspinatus is a relatively weak arm abductor, it plays an important role in stabilizing the shoulder joint. The tendon of insertion of supraspinatus crosses the glenohumeral joint just above the head of the humerus and attaches to the lateral aspect of the greater tubercle of the humerus. Thus, it is well positioned to hold the head of the humerus in the glenoid fossa and prevent the head of the humerus from moving inferiorly. However, the location of this tendon makes it susceptible to tendonitis, as it can rub between the acromion and head of humerus when the arm is abducted. Clients often refer to tendonitis of the tendon of insertion of supraspinatus as a *rotator cuff injury* or *tear*. This muscle's tendon is the most easily injured of the four rotator cuff tendons.

Implications of Shortened and/or Lengthened/ Weak Muscle

Shortened: Limited ability to perform arm adduction is noted.
Lengthened: Limited ability to perform arm abduction, and/or shoulder joint instability is present.

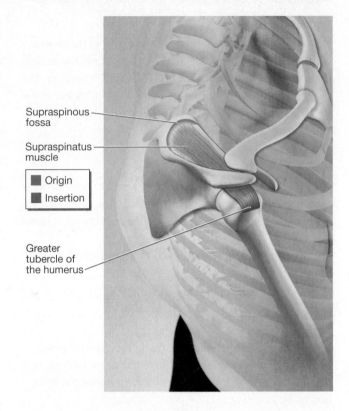

Supraspinous fossa

Supraspinatus muscle

■ Origin
■ Insertion

Greater tubercle of the humerus

FIGURE 3-18 · **Supraspinatus**

Palpation and Massage

To palpate and massage the supraspinatus, press into the tissue just above the spine of the scapula. You have to work through trapezius to access supraspinatus. Friction is an easy stroke to apply to this muscle, as it can be compressed into the scapula.

How to Stretch This Muscle

This is not an easy muscle to stretch, although one can adduct the arm as much as possible to get a stretch.

Synergists

Arm adductor: middle deltoid

Antagonists

Arm adductors: pectoralis major, coracobrachialis, latissimus dorsi, and teres major

Innervation and Arterial Supply

Innervation: suprascapular nerve
Arterial supply: suprascapular artery

INFRASPINATUS (in-fra-spin-a-tus)

Meaning of Name

Infraspinatus is named to convey its location just inferior to the spine of the scapula. It is a rotator cuff muscle and helps to stabilize the glenohumeral joint from a posterior perspective.

Location

Infraspinatus is a thick, flat muscle located in the infraspinatus fossa.

Origin and Insertion

Origin: infraspinous fossa
Insertion: greater tubercle of the humerus

Actions

Lateral rotation and extension of the humerus at the shoulder joint

Explanation of Actions

Infraspinatus crosses the posterior aspect of the shoulder joint, and its origin is medial to its insertion on the greater tubercle. When infraspinatus contracts, it pulls the greater tubercle, on the lateral aspect of the humerus, posteriorly, causing the humerus to turn laterally. By pulling the greater tubercle posteriorly, infraspinatus can assist with arm extension.

Notable Muscle Facts

Infraspinatus makes up a portion of the rotator cuff and helps to stabilize the glenohumeral joint from a posterior position. Infraspinatus is most active in its stabilization function when one is abducting or flexing the arm. Infraspinatus is a common site of *trigger points*, causing referral to the anterior and lateral shoulder and arm.

Implications of Shortened and/or Lengthened/ Weak Muscle

Shortened: Posture has palms facing forward and/or limited ability to medially rotate arm.
Lengthened: Limited ability to perform lateral rotation of the arm, and/or shoulder instability is noted.

Palpation and Massage

Infraspinatus can be palpated and massaged by putting pressure and friction inferior to the spine of the scapula. Locate the spine of the scapula and press in a superior direction into the spine's inferior border. One can also press directly into the posterior scapula, pressing the thumb at a 90-degree angle to the bone. Some of this muscle is deep to trapezius, yet the lateral aspect of infraspinatus is superficial. Infraspinatus is a

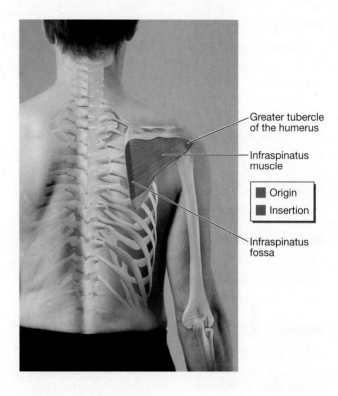

FIGURE 3-19 · Infraspinatus

frequent site of trigger points, so trigger point release work is often helpful. Friction to the tendon of insertion, around the greater tubercle of the humerus, although deep to the deltoid muscle, can also be helpful.

How to Stretch This Muscle

Fully flex the arm while medially rotating it.

Synergists

Lateral rotators of the arm: teres minor and posterior deltoid
Arm extensors: posterior deltoid, latissimus dorsi, teres major, teres minor, triceps brachii, and pectoralis major (extension from a flexed position)

Antagonists

Medial rotators of the arm: subscapularis, anterior deltoid, pectoralis major, latissimus dorsi, and teres major
Flexors of the arm: pectoralis major, anterior deltoid, coracobrachialis, and biceps brachii

Innervation and Arterial Supply

Innervation: suprascapular nerve
Arterial supply: suprascapular artery

TERES MINOR (ter-ez mi-nor)

Meaning of Name

Teres means "rounded" and *minor* means that this muscle is smaller than teres major. Although teres minor is not particular round in its overall shape, it is cylindrical. Teres minor is a rotator cuff muscle, and its tendon of insertion is part of the cuff that surrounds and stabilizes the shoulder joint. Teres minor provides stability to the shoulder joint from a posterior perspective.

Location

Teres minor lies along the axillary border of the scapula.

Origin and Insertion

Origin: midaxillary border of the scapula
Insertion: greater tubercle of the humerus, just inferior to the insertion of infraspinatus

Actions

Laterally rotates the arm and assists in arm extension

Explanation of Actions

Teres minor exhibits the same pull on the greater tubercle as infraspinatus does. By crossing the posterior aspect of the shoulder joint, with origin medial to insertion, the muscle pulls the greater tubercle posteriorly, causing lateral rotation of the arm. Because the axillary border of the scapula lies posterior to the humerus, this muscle pulls the greater tubercle back, causing arm extension.

Notable Muscle Facts

Teres minor makes up part of the posterior rotator cuff. Its tendon of insertion lies just inferior to the tendon of insertion of infraspinatus. Teres minor is also a common site of trigger points.

Implications of Shortened and/or Lengthened/ Weak Muscle

Shortened: Posture has palms facing forward and/or limited ability to medially rotate arm.
Lengthened: Limited ability to perform lateral rotation of the arm, and/or shoulder instability is noted.

Palpation and Massage

Find the lateral/axillary border of the scapula. Teres minor can be palpated and massaged by pressing directly into the middle third of the scapula's axillary border, applying friction as you press. You can also trace the tendon of insertion toward the greater tubercle of the humerus.

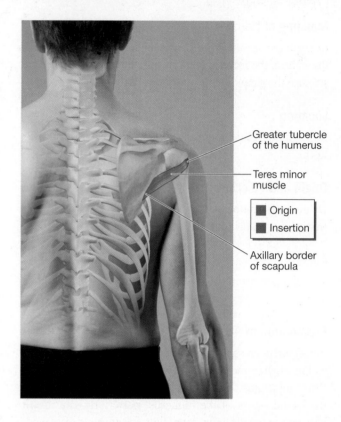

Greater tubercle of the humerus
Teres minor muscle
■ Origin
■ Insertion
Axillary border of scapula

FIGURE 3-20 · Teres minor

How to Stretch This Muscle

Flex, medially rotate, and abduct the arm.

Synergists

Lateral rotators of the arm: infraspinatus and posterior deltoid
Arm extensors: posterior deltoid, latissimus dorsi, teres major, teres minor, triceps brachii, and pectoralis major (extension from a flexed position)

Antagonists

Medial rotators of the arm: subscapularis, anterior deltoid, pectoralis major, latissimus dorsi, and teres major
Flexors of the arm: pectoralis major, anterior deltoid, coracobrachialis, and biceps brachii

Innervation and Arterial Supply

Innervation: axillary nerve
Arterial supply: circumflex scapular artery

SUBSCAPULARIS (sub-skap-yu-la-ris)

Meaning of Name
Subscapularis means "under the scapula," but the meaning of "under" is that the muscle is located on the anterior aspect of the scapula. Subscapularis is the fourth rotator cuff muscle.

Location
This muscle covers most of the anterior scapula, filling the subscapular fossa. The muscle's tendon of insertion passes in front of the shoulder joint and stabilizes the joint from the anterior perspective.

Origin and Insertion
Origin: subscapular fossa
Insertion: lesser tubercle of the humerus

Actions
Medial rotation of the arm at the shoulder joint

Explanation of Actions
Subscapularis crosses the anterior aspect of the shoulder joint. The origin is more medial and more posterior than the insertion, and thus when the lesser tubercle is pulled toward the anterior scapula, the humerus is turned medially.

Implications of Shortened and/or Lengthened/Weak Muscle
Shortened: Posture is one in which dorsal sides of hands face forward, and/or limited ability to perform lateral rotation of the arm.
Lengthened: Limited ability to perform medial rotation of the arm, and/or shoulder instability is present.

Notable Muscle Facts
Subscapularis forms the anterior portion of the rotator cuff, and thus assists in preventing an anterior dislocation of the humeral head from the glenoid fossa. This stabilization role of subscapularis is especially important when the shoulder is abducted. Some texts state that subscapularis is an arm adductor as well as a medial rotator.

Palpation and Massage
It is difficult to access much of subscapularis. The lateral aspect of the muscle is most accessible. With a client supine, carefully press your thumb or fingers into the side of your client's body, between the lateral aspect of the scapula and

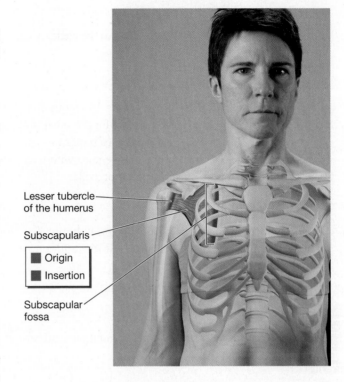

Lesser tubercle of the humerus
Subscapularis
■ Origin
■ Insertion
Subscapular fossa

FIGURE 3-21 · Subscapularis

the ribs, and press down toward the massage table to contact the anterior scapula. This same stroke can be done with the client in a side-lying position, as you press between the lateral scapula and ribs, into the lateral, anterior scapula. Subscapularis is a relatively thick muscle, so you will likely feel dense muscle between your fingers and the scapula.

How to Stretch This Muscle
Laterally rotate the arm.

Synergists
Other medial rotators: anterior deltoid, pectoralis major, latissimus dorsi, and teres major

Antagonists
Arm lateral rotators: infraspinatus, teres minor, and posterior deltoid

Innervation and Arterial Supply
Innervation: upper and lower subscapular nerves
Arterial supply: circumflex scapular artery

LATISSIMUS DORSI (la-tis-i-mus dor-si)

Meaning of Name

Latissimus means "widest," and *dorsi* refers to the back.

Location

Latissimus dorsi is the widest back muscle, covering much of the low and mid back. The thin, yet strong, latissimus dorsi muscle is almost entirely superficial except for the small, superior portion of the muscle that is deep to trapezius. The most superior, lateral portion of the muscle joins with teres major to form the soft tissue of the posterior axilla.

Origin and Insertion

Origin: thoracolumbar aponeurosis, sacrum, posterior iliac crest, spinous processes of T7–L5, lower few ribs, and sometimes the inferior angle of the scapula
Insertion: medial lip of the bicipital groove of the humerus

Actions

Extension (forcefully, if needed), medial rotation, and adduction of the arm at the shoulder joint

Explanation of Actions

The origin of latissimus dorsi is posterior and inferior to the insertion. Thus, the bicipital groove is pulled posterior, causing arm extension. Because the origin is more medial than the insertion, the bicipital groove is pulled medially, resulting in arm adduction. Finally, because the path taken by the latissimus dorsi muscle from the sacrum to the arm runs between the arm and the side of the body, the medial aspect of the bicipital groove is pulled back, causing the humerus to turn inward and perform medial rotation of the arm.

Notable Muscle Facts

Latissimus dorsi is a very strong muscle, despite its thin, flat shape. It is called the "crutch muscle," as it is needed to keep the arm extended when walking with crutches. It is also called the "wood chopping muscle," as it is the muscle we use in forceful extension actions, such as chopping wood. Latissimus dorsi has greater strength as an adductor when one brings the arm toward the midline behind the body. It is less strong when used to adduct the arm in front of the body.

Latissimus dorsi's multitude of attachments enables the muscle to influence posture and movement of several different body parts. In addition to arm movements, latissimus dorsi can depress the scapula. Because latissimus dorsi connects to the thoracolumbar fascia, spine, and ilium, it has the potential to affect the posture of the spine and pelvis.

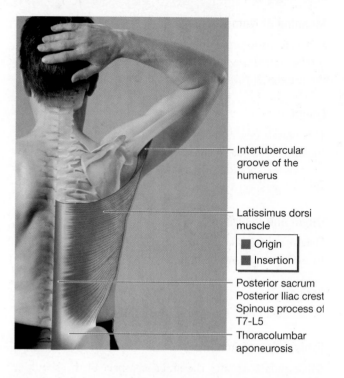

FIGURE 3-22 · Latissimus dorsi

Intertubercular groove of the humerus

Latissimus dorsi muscle

■ Origin
■ Insertion

Posterior sacrum
Posterior Iliac crest
Spinous process of T7-L5
Thoracolumbar aponeurosis

Implications of Shortened and/or Lengthened/Weak Muscle

Shortened: Posture is one in which dorsal sides of the hand faces forward, and/or arms are close to the body. Limited ability to perform lateral rotation, flexion, and/or abduction of the arm is noted.
Lengthened: Limited ability to perform arm extension, medial rotation of the arm, and/or arm adduction is seen.

Palpation and Massage

Latissimus dorsi is easy to find, as it is superficial and covers so much of the mid to low back. With the client prone, begin by locating the sacrum, and apply effleurage and friction superiorly and laterally across the mid to low back. Press inferiorly into the posterior iliac crest to address this portion of the origin. Locate the superior border of latissimus dorsi, just a few inches above the inferior angle of the scapula. Palpating laterally toward the axilla brings us to an area where latissimus dorsi is thicker and denser. In fact, palpating and pétrissaging the posterior axilla, lateral to the scapula, is a nice way to address the superior lateral aspect of this muscle. *Note:* The soft tissue of the posterior axilla is made primarily of latissimus dorsi and teres major.

How to Stretch This Muscle

Flex the arm while abducting and laterally rotating it.

Synergists

Arm adductors: coracobrachialis, pectoralis major, and teres major

Arm extensors: teres major, infraspinatus, teres minor, posterior deltoid, triceps brachii, and pectoralis major (from a flexed position)

Arm medial rotators: teres major, pectoralis major, subscapularis, and anterior deltoid

Antagonists

Arm abductors: supraspinatus and middle deltoid

Arm flexors: pectoralis major, anterior deltoid, coracobrachialis, and biceps brachii

Arm lateral rotators: infraspinatus, teres minor, and posterior deltoid

Innervation and Arterial Supply

Innervation: thoracodorsal nerve

Arterial supply: thoracodorsal artery

TERES MAJOR (ter-ez ma-jor)

Meaning of Name

Teres means "rounded," and *major* signifies that teres major is larger than teres minor.

Location

Teres major is located in the posterior axilla.

Origin and Insertion

Origin: inferior angle of the scapula
Insertion: lateral lip of the bicipital groove, just posterior to the insertion of latissimus dorsi

Actions

Extension, adduction, and medial rotation of the arm at the shoulder joint

Explanation of Actions

Teres major crosses the posterior aspect of the shoulder, and its origin is more posterior than its insertion. Thus, the insertion is pulled back, causing arm extension. Because its origin is more medial than its insertion, the bicipital groove is pulled toward the body, resulting in arm adduction. And, because teres major passes between the body and the arm and pulls the bicipital groove medially and posteriorly, it causes the humerus to turn inwardly, which is medial rotation of the arm.

Notable Muscle Facts

Teres major assists latissimus dorsi in all three actions, and is thus called "latt's little helper." Teres major's action of arm extension is most efficient when the arm moves from a flexed position to a position in which the arm is at the side.

Implications of Shortened and/or Lengthened/ Weak Muscle

Shortened: Posture is one in which back or hands face forward, with limited ability to flex and laterally rotate the arm.
Lengthened: Slight limit in ability to medially rotate, extend, and adduct the arm is noted.

Palpation and Massage

Palpating the soft tissue that forms the posterior axilla allows us to access teres major. With the client prone, find the axillary border of the scapula and search for the dense tissue between the axillary border of the scapula and the arm. Pétrissage is an appropriate stroke to apply to this muscle.

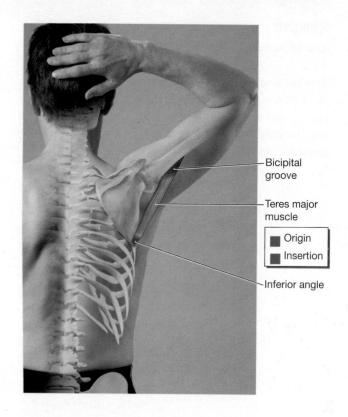

Bicipital groove

Teres major muscle

■ Origin
■ Insertion

Inferior angle

FIGURE 3-23 · Teres major

How to Stretch This Muscle

Flex the arm while abducting and laterally rotating it.

Synergists

Arm adductors: coracobrachialis, pectoralis major, and latissimus dorsi

Arm extensors: teres major, infraspinatus, teres minor, posterior deltoid, triceps brachii, and pectoralis major (from a flexed position)

Arm medial rotators: teres major, pectoralis major, subscapularis, and anterior deltoid

Antagonists

Arm abductors: supraspinatus and middle deltoid

Arm flexors: pectoralis major, anterior deltoid, coracobrachialis, and biceps brachii

Arm lateral rotators: infraspinatus, teres minor, and posterior deltoid

Innervation and Arterial Supply

Innervation: lower subscapular nerve

Arterial supply: circumflex scapular artery

Note: The next group of muscles moves the scapula. This means these muscles must insert on the scapula and perform one or more of the following actions: protraction, retraction, elevation, depression, upward rotation, and downward rotation of the scapula.

SERRATUS ANTERIOR (ser-at-tus an-ter-e-or)

Meaning of Name

Serratus means "jagged" and is so named due to its attachment on the ribs. *Anterior* signifies that serratus anterior is more anterior in its location than the serratus posterior muscles.

Location

Serratus anterior lies along the lateral trunk. It has a wide origin, as it joins to eight ribs, and narrows as it heads toward its origin on the scapula. Much of serratus anterior is deep to latissimus dorsi, scapula, and pectoralis major. However, there is a triangular-shaped area in which serratus anterior is superficial in the lateral mid rib area.

Origin and Insertion

Origin: lateral ribs 1 to 8
Insertion: anterior, vertebral border of the scapula

Actions

Serratus anterior is a strong protractor of the scapula, and the inferior fibers perform upward rotation of the scapula.

Explanation of Actions

Because the origin of serratus anterior is more anterior than the insertion on the scapula, this muscle pulls the scapula forward when contracting, thus producing protraction. Upon contraction, the inferior portion of the muscle pulls the inferior vertebral border of the scapula forward. This action tilts the scapula, so that the glenoid fossa moves upward, causing upward rotation of the scapula.

Notable Muscle Facts

Serratus anterior has the postural role of keeping the vertebral border of the scapula against the ribs. As there is no bone-to-bone joint between the scapula and ribs, we rely on muscles to hold the scapula in place. Serratus anterior has a major responsibility for maintaining the position of the scapula in relation to the thoracic wall.

Implications of Shortened and/or Lengthened/ Weak Muscle

Shortened: The shoulders are forward (protraction of the scapula more than is typical). Limited retraction and/or downward rotation of the scapula is noted.

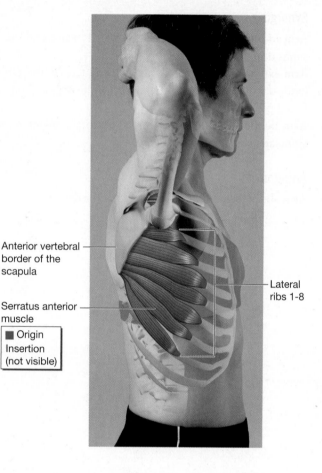

Anterior vertebral border of the scapula

Serratus anterior muscle

Lateral ribs 1-8

■ Origin
Insertion (not visible)

FIGURE 3-24 · **Serratus anterior**

Lengthened: The client likely exhibits the posture of "winged scapula," as the vertebral border of the scapula would not be held to the rib cage and would "wing out." In addition, scapula protraction is limited.

Palpation and Massage

Palpation and massage with direct pressure and friction along the lateral rib cage are a good way to access and massage serratus anterior. With the client supine, press directly (at 90-degree angle) into the lateral trunk, pressing into ribs as well as the space between the ribs. Because so many people protract the scapula repetitively, it can be quite helpful to massage this muscle in a full-body massage.

How to Stretch This Muscle

Downwardly rotate the scapula combined with retraction.

Synergists

Protractor of the scapula: pectoralis minor
Upward rotators of the scapula: upper trapezius and lower trapezius

Antagonists

Retractors of the scapula: rhomboids and middle trapezius
downward rotators of the scapula: levator scapula, rhomboids and pectoralis minor

Innervation and Arterial Supply

Innervation: long thoracic nerve
Arterial supply: dorsal scapular artery

PECTORALIS MINOR (pek-tor-al-is mi-nor)

Meaning of Name

Pectoralis means "chest," and *minor* signifies that pectoralis minor is smaller than pectoralis major.

Location

Pectoralis minor is located deep in the anterolateral chest area and is completely covered by the more superficial pectoralis muscle, pectoralis major.

Origin and Insertion

Origin: ribs 3, 4, and 5, close to the costal cartilage
Insertion: coracoid process of the scapula

Actions

Protraction, depression, and downward rotation of the scapula

Explanation of Actions

Pectoralis minor protracts the scapula because the origin is more anterior than the insertion, and by pulling the coracoid process anteriorly, one's scapula is protracted. Pectoralis minor performs both depression and downward rotation of the scapula because the insertion on the coracoid process is more superior than the origin on the ribs, and thus the coracoid process is pulled down. Downward rotation occurs when the coracoid process is pulled inferiorly. The coracoid process is just medial to the glenoid fossa, and when this area of the scapula is lowered, downward rotation results. To perform depression, pectoralis minor relies on another muscle to help. Pectoralis minor pulls the lateral aspect of the scapula downward, and when lower trapezius contracts simultaneously, the medial end of the scapula is also lowered. Together, these two synergists accomplish depression.

Notable Muscle Facts

Pectoralis minor helps to stabilize the lateral aspect of the scapula against the chest wall. In addition, pectoralis minor can serve as an accessory muscle of inhalation.

Implications of Shortened and/or Lengthened/ Weak Muscle

Shortened: If pectoralis minor is shortened, thoracic outlet syndrome may result. The brachial plexus, as well as the axillary artery and vein, passes directly deep to pectoralis minor and can become impinged by a short muscle.
Lengthened: If lengthened, pectoralis minor will not typically have any postural or functional implications, as it is a relatively weak muscle.

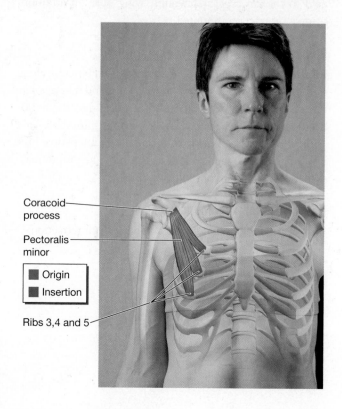

Coracoid process

Pectoralis minor

■ Origin
■ Insertion

Ribs 3,4 and 5

FIGURE 3-25 · Pectoralis minor

Palpation and Massage

Pectoralis minor can be palpated deep to pectoralis major in the anterolateral chest. Palpate with effleurage from the sternum to the lateral chest, feeling for a density increase as one's fingers press into pectoralis minor. Some therapists prefer to access pectoralis minor with their client supine, by applying pressure in a medial direction through the lateral axilla. Press deep to pectoralis major, feeling for the lateral edge of the dense pectoralis minor fibers. Friction of the muscle belly, as well as friction just inferior to the insertion site on the coracoid process, can be helpful to relax this muscle.

How to Stretch This Muscle

Perform upward rotation of the scapula in conjunction with retraction of the scapula. This is often done by leaning into a doorway with the arm abducted, scapula in a position of upward rotation, the elbow flexed, and pressing the anterior forearm into the side of the doorway while leaning through the doorway.

Synergists

Protractor of the scapula: serratus anterior
Depressor of the scapula: lower trapezius
Downward rotators of the scapula: levator scapula and rhomboids

Antagonists

Retractors of the scapula: rhomboids and middle trapezius
Elevators of the scapula: levator scapula and upper trapezius
Upward rotators of the scapula: upper trapezius, lower trapezius, and serratus anterior

Innervation and Arterial Supply

Innervation: medial and lateral pectoral nerves
Arterial supply: pectoral branches of the thoracoacromial trunk

LEVATOR SCAPULA (le-va-tor skap-yu-le)

Meaning of Name

The name indicates that this muscle performs elevation of the scapula.

Location

Levator scapula is located in the lateral neck region. The superior portion of the muscle is deep to sternocleidomastoid, and the inferior part of the muscle is deep to trapezius. The muscle twists between origin and insertion.

Origin and Insertion

Origin: transverse processes of cervical vertebrae 1 to 4
Insertion: superior angle of the scapula

Actions

Elevates the scapula and performs downward rotation of the scapula

Explanation of Actions

Because the origin of this muscle is superior to the insertion, levator scapula pulls the superior angle upward. An upward movement of the superior angle of the scapula results in a rotation of the scapula in which the glenoid fossa moves down. Thus levator scapula performs downward rotation of the scapula. In addition, when upper trapezius contracts simultaneously with levator scapula, the entire scapula is pulled superiorly. The result is elevation.

Notable Muscle Facts

Levator scapula has a postural role in stabilization of the cervical spine. In addition, when the scapula is fixed, levator scapula can cause neck rotation and neck extension.

Implications of Shortened and/or Lengthened/ Weak Muscle

Shortened: The shoulder or shoulders appear raised. Potential is present for limited rotation of the neck as well.
Lengthened: There are no significant postural or functional issues.

Palpation and Massage

Despite this muscle's lack of strength, it is easily overworked and causes much neck/upper back pain. Stress commonly causes a shortening of levator scapula and the raising of the

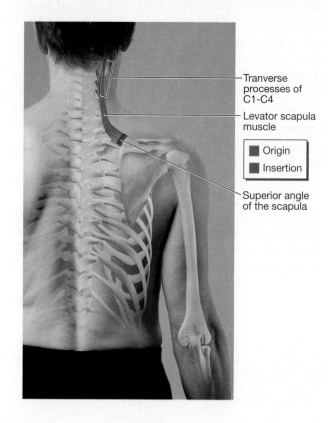

Tranverse processes of C1-C4

Levator scapula muscle

■ Origin
■ Insertion

Superior angle of the scapula

FIGURE 3-26 · Levator scapula

shoulders. When a client has difficulty turning the head to the right or left, a tight levator scapula can be the culprit. Find the root of the spine of the scapula, at the medial edge of the spine of the scapula. Move an inch or two above this root, and press down toward your client's feet. Friction to this area can be achieved by asking the client to turn his or her head slowly from side to side, as you press down into the superior angle. Circular friction around the transverse processes of C1–C4 is also a way to address this muscle.

How to Stretch This Muscle

Laterally flex to the right (for the left levator scapula) and laterally flex to the left (for the right levator scapula).

Synergists

Elevator of the scapula: upper trapezius
Downward rotators of the scapula: rhomboids and pectoralis minor

Antagonists

Depressors of the scapula: lower trapezius and pectoralis minor
Upward rotators of the scapula: upper trapezius, lower trapezius, and serratus anterior

Innervation and Arterial Supply

Innervation: dorsal scapular nerve
Arterial supply: dorsal scapular artery

RHOMBOID MAJOR AND RHOMBOID MINOR (rom-boyd ma-jor and rom-boyd mi-nor)

Meaning of Name
Rhomboids are named for their rhombus shape.

Location
The rhomboids are located between the spine and the scapula. The origin is superior to the insertion, causing an oblique direction of the muscle's fibers. The rhomboids are midlayer upper back muscles, superficial to the erectors yet deep to trapezius. Rhomboid minor is superior to rhomboid major, and of course minor is smaller than major.

Origin and Insertion
Origin: As a unit, the rhomboids originate on the spinous processes of C7–T5.
Insertion: the vertebral border of the scapula

Actions
Retraction and downward rotation of the scapula

Explanation of Actions
Because the origin of rhomboids is medial to the insertion, the vertebral border of the scapula is pulled toward the midline, which is retraction of the scapula. Because the origin is higher than the insertion, the vertebral border is pulled superiorly as well as medially, resulting in a downward tilt to the glenoid fossa and thus the action of downward rotation.

Notable Muscle Facts
Rhomboids help to stabilize the position of the scapula, preventing the scapula from protracting while the arm is being flexed or abducted. Rhomboids are frequently lengthened, due to the common shortening of the scapula protractors. Such an imbalance between protractors and retractors can result in a fairly constant isometric and/or eccentric contraction of the rhomboids, as we seek to balance our posture and keep the scapula closer to the spine. Such stretched and overworked rhomboids are common sites for trigger points.

Implications of Shortened and/or Lengthened/ Weak Muscle
Shortened: The shoulders appear pulled back (retracted more than is typical). Limited ability to protract and upwardly rotate the scapula is present.

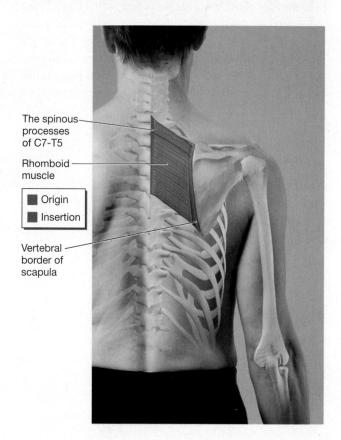

The spinous processes of C7-T5

Rhomboid muscle

■ Origin
■ Insertion

Vertebral border of scapula

FIGURE 3-27 · Rhomboid major and rhomboid minor

Lengthened: The client might have rounded shoulders, as well as difficulty retracting the scapula.

Palpation and Massage

To locate the rhomboids, find the spinous process of C7, which tends to be the largest posterior projection of the vertebrae in the area where the neck meets the back. After locating spinous process C7, count down five more spinous processes, so you reach T5. You have just outlined the origin of the muscle. Palpate the vertebral border of the scapula. Ask the client to place his or her forearm behind the back, as this shifts the angle of the vertebral border of the scapula and makes it easier to palpate. Providing effleurage and friction to the area between the spine and the scapula is a fine way to massage the rhomboids. One can also provide friction to the fibers of the insertion by pressing the muscle into the vertebral border of the scapula.

How to Stretch This Muscle

Protract the scapula and horizontally adduct the arm.

Synergists

Retractor of the scapula: middle trapezius
Downward rotators of the scapula: levator scapula and pectoralis minor

Antagonists

Protractor of the scapula: serratus anterior and pectoralis minor
Upward rotators of the scapula: upper trapezius, lower trapezius, and serratus anterior

Innervation and Arterial Supply

Innervation: dorsal scapular nerve
Arterial supply: dorsal scapular artery

TRAPEZIUS (trap-e-ze-us)

Meaning of Name

Trapezius means "little table" or "trapezoid-shaped."

Location

Trapezius covers much of the posterior neck and upper to mid back. It forms the contour between the shoulder and neck. Trapezius is commonly divided into three parts: upper trapezius, middle trapezius, and lower trapezius. The entire muscle is superficial

Origin and Insertion

Origin: external occipital protuberance, ligamentum nuchae, and spinous processes of C7–T12
Insertion: lateral clavicle and acromion (upper trapezius), spine of the scapula (middle trapezius), and root of the spine of the scapula (lower trapezius)

Actions

Elevation and upward rotation of the scapula (upper trapezius)
Retraction of the scapula (middle trapezius)
Depression and upward rotation of the scapula (lower trapezius)
Note: Trapezius can also extend the neck when insertion on the scapula is fixed and the attachment on the spine is more movable.

Explanation of Actions

Upper trapezius performs upward rotation because the origin is above the insertion, thus contraction causes an upward pull on the acromion. Because the acromion is on the lateral aspect of the scapula, pulling it upward results in upward rotation of the scapula. Upper trapezius is able to perform elevation of the scapula because the origin is above the insertion. Thus, shortening of the muscle provides an upward pull to the scapula. However, because upper trapezius generates an upward pull on the lateral aspect of the scapula only, levator scapula is a perfect complement to upper trapezius. When upper trapezius contracts simultaneously with levator scapula, the scapula experiences an upward pull on both the lateral and medial aspects of the bone, and thus elevation occurs.

Middle trapezius retracts the scapula because its origin is medial to its insertion. Thus, contraction draws the scapula closer to the spine, which is retraction.

The origin of lower trapezius is inferior to its insertion, and thus contraction pulls the root of the spine of the scapula downward, thus raising the glenoid fossa and resulting in upward rotation. Lower trapezius works simultaneously with pectoralis minor to cause depression. Because pectoralis

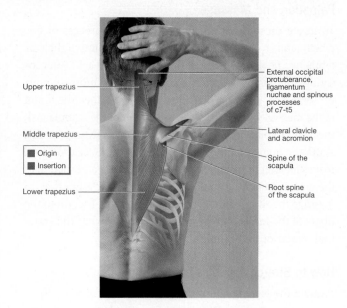

Upper trapezius

Middle trapezius

☐ Origin
☐ Insertion

Lower trapezius

External occipital protuberance, ligamentum nuchae and spinous processes of c7-t5

Lateral clavicle and acromion

Spine of the scapula

Root spine of the scapula

FIGURE 3-28 · Trapezius

minor contracts to pull the lateral aspect of the scapula down, and lower trapezius contracts to pull the medial part of the scapula down, depression of the scapula is possible.

Notable Muscle Facts

The trapezius muscle can play a role in stabilization of the scapula, as well as in stabilization of the cervical and thoracic spine. Such roles occur during movement of the upper extremity.

Implications of Shortened and/or Lengthened/ Weak Muscle

Shortened: If upper trapezius is shortened, a common posture is raised or shrugged shoulders (elevated more than is typical). Clients with short upper trapezius fibers likely experience limited ability to depress and/or downwardly rotate the scapula. Shortened middle trapezius fibers result in a posture in which the shoulders are pulled back (retracted more than is typical). Such clients have limited ability to protract the scapula. Clients with shortened fibers of lower trapezius likely experience limited ability to elevate and downwardly rotate the scapula.

Lengthened: Lengthened upper trapezius causes lowering of the contour between neck and shoulder and limited ability to fully elevate and upwardly rotate the scapula. Lengthened fibers of middle trapezius result in limited ability to retract the scapula fully. Lengthened fibers of lower trapezius cause limited ability to perform upward rotation of the scapula.

Palpation and Massage

Trapezius is one of the easiest muscles to palpate and massage, as it is entirely superficial. Find the external occipital protuberance by locating the prominent projection at the center of the posterior head. Apply friction just inferior to this bone marking. Palpate down the ligamentum nuchae, which is easier to feel if the client flexes his or her neck. Palpate the spinous processes of the cervical and thoracic regions and consider applying circular friction around them. You have thus outlined the origin of trapezius. Find the insertion of the muscle beginning with the lateral clavicle, keeping in mind that the muscle attaches to the posterior aspect of the lateral clavicle. Press into the posterior lateral clavicle. Find the entire spine of the scapula and apply pressure to the superior aspect of the spine. This enables you to address the remainder of the insertion of the muscle. The remainder of the muscle can be addressed by providing effleurage and pétrissage to the posterior neck, pétrissage to the area between neck and shoulder, friction to the high point of the upper trapezius right between neck and shoulders, effleurage to the upper and mid back, and friction to the upper and mid back. Trapezius is an extremely thin muscle and can be easily pressed into ribs and spine during friction.

How to Stretch This Muscle

Laterally flex the neck to the opposite side (upper trapezius).
Protract the scapula (middle trapezius).
Downwardly rotate the scapula (lower trapezius).

Synergists

Upper Trapezius
Elevator of the scapula: levator scapula
Upward rotators: lower trapezius and serratus anterior

Middle Trapezius
Retractor: rhomboids

Lower Trapezius
Depressor: pectoralis minor
Upward rotators: upper trapezius and serratus anterior

Antagonists

Upper Trapezius
Depressor of the scapula: pectoralis minor
Downward rotators: rhomboids, levator scapula, and pectoralis minor

Middle Trapezius
Protractors: serratus anterior and pectoralis minor

Lower Trapezius
Elevators: upper trapezius and levator scapula
Downward rotators: rhomboids, levator scapula, and pectoralis minor

Innervation and Arterial Supply

Innervation: cranial nerve XI and spinal accessory nerve
Arterial supply: transverse cervical artery and dorsal scapular artery

REGIONAL ILLUSTRATIONS OF MUSCLES

Figures 3-29 and 3-30 provide regional pictures of the muscles that move the shoulder and the muscles that move the scapula.

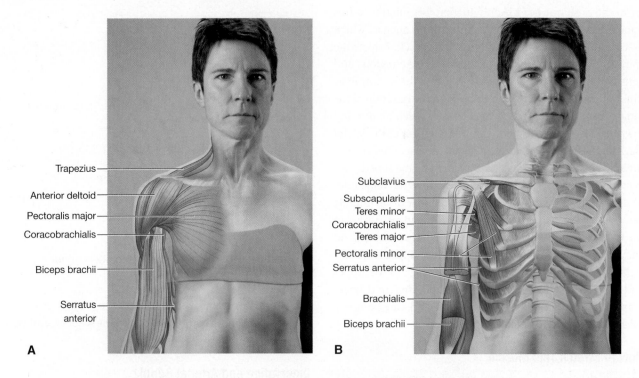

FIGURE 3-29 · **Anterior view: muscles that move the shoulder and scapula. A:** Superficial muscles; **B:** Deeper muscles.

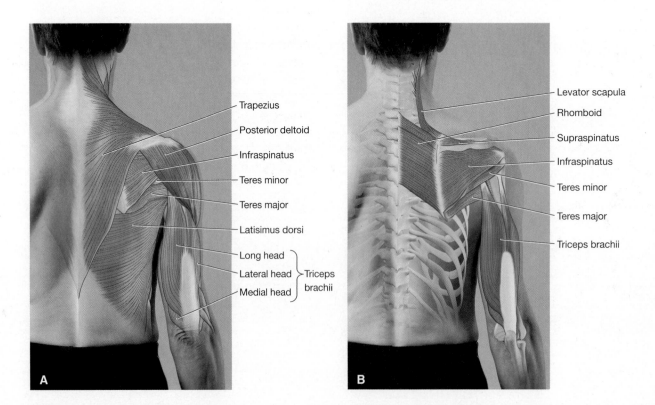

FIGURE 3-30 · **Posterior view: muscles that move the shoulder and scapula. A:** Superficial muscles; **B:** Midlayer muscles.

REGIONAL ILLUSTRATIONS OF ORIGIN AND INSERTION SITES

Figures 3-31 and 3-32 provide pictures of origin and insertion sites of these muscles.

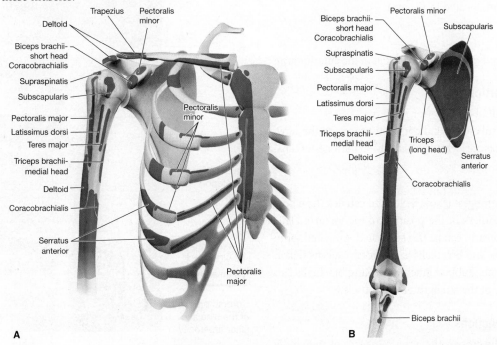

FIGURE 3-31 · Anterior view: origin and insertion sites of muscles that move the shoulder and scapula.
A: Anterior view of thorax; **B:** Anterior scapula and arm.

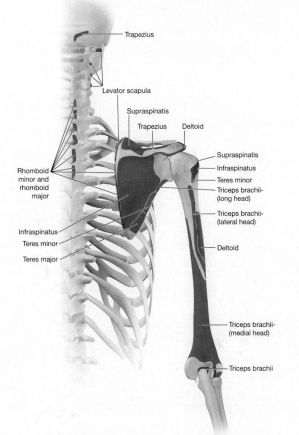

FIGURE 3-32 · Posterior view: origin and insertion sites of muscles that move the shoulder and scapula

Elbow Muscles

The next few muscles move the elbow joint and have the capacity to flex or extend the elbow. Some of the muscles perform additional actions, as well. Elbow movers must originate proximal to the elbow joint and insert distal to it. Flexors of the elbow must cross the anterior aspect of the joint, whereas extensors cross the back of the joint. There are three primary elbow flexors, and all contain the word part *brachi*, which means "arm." Two of the elbow flexors reside in the anterior arm, whereas one occupies the lateral forearm. There are two elbow extensors, one much larger and stronger than the other. We will begin by addressing the elbow flexors.

BRACHIALIS (bra-ke-a-lis)

Meaning of Name

Related to the arm, located in the arm

Location

Brachialis is located deep in the distal half of the anterior arm.

Origin and Insertion

Origin: distal half of the anterior humerus
Insertion: ulnar tuberosity and coronoid process of the ulna; both insertion spots are located proximally on the anterior ulna.

Actions

Brachialis is the strongest elbow flexor and can flex the elbow equally well regardless of the position of the forearm. This means that the forearm can be in a supinated, pronated, or in a neutral position, and brachialis is an effective elbow flexor. One of my students dubbed brachialis, "King brachialis," to remind everyone of the strength of this muscle.

Explanation of Actions

Because brachialis crosses the anterior aspect of the elbow and pulls the anterior ulna toward the anterior humerus, flexion is accomplished.

Notable Muscle Facts

Brachialis crosses only one joint and attaches to a significant amount of the humerus. These two factors contribute to the strength of the muscle.

Implications of Shortened and/or Lengthened/Weak Muscle

Shortened: The elbows are flexed more than is typical, and one would experience limited ability to fully extend the elbow.
Lengthened: A weakening of the action of elbow flexion is noted.

Palpation and Massage

Brachialis is easiest to massage when the client is supine, as it can be palpated deep to biceps brachii in the anterior arm. The distal portion of brachialis is wider than biceps brachii and thus can be palpated more easily than the proximal aspect of

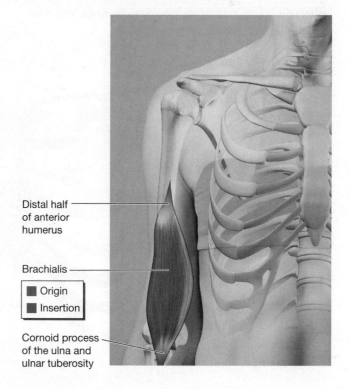

Distal half of anterior humerus

Brachialis

■ Origin
■ Insertion

Cornoid process of the ulna and ulnar tuberosity

FIGURE 3-33 · Brachialis

the muscle. Both effleurage and pétrissage to the anterior arm can effectively address both brachialis and biceps brachii.

How to Stretch This Muscle

Brachialis has limited ability to be stretched because the elbow can only be extended to 180 degrees; however, an extremely shortened brachialis can be stretched by extending the elbow fully. Using your fingertips to pin the muscle against the humerus beneath while the client extends his or her elbow can effectively stretch brachialis.

Synergists

Elbow flexors: biceps brachii, brachioradialis, and pronator teres

Antagonists

Elbow extensors: triceps brachii and anconeus

Innervation and Arterial Supply

Innervation: musculocutaneous nerve
Arterial supply: brachial artery

BICEPS BRACHII (bi-ceps bra-ke-i)

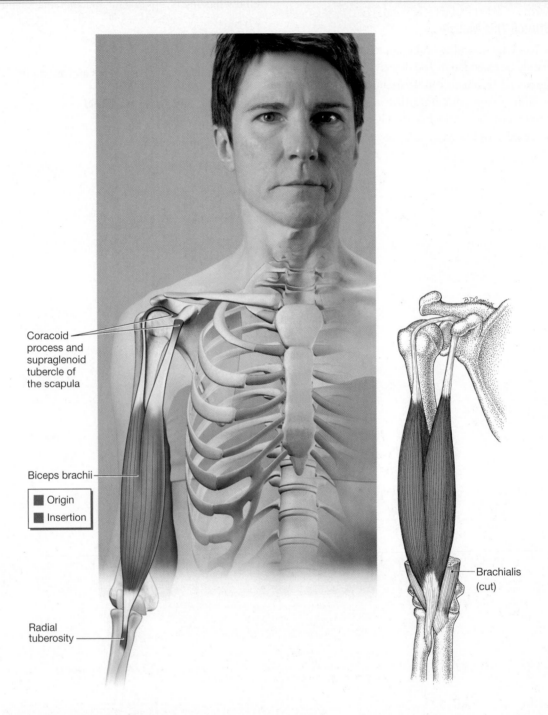

Coracoid process and supraglenoid tubercle of the scapula

Biceps brachii

Origin
Insertion

Radial tuberosity

Brachialis (cut)

FIGURE 3-34 · Biceps brachii

Meaning of Name

Biceps means "two heads," and *brachii* refers to the arm.

Location

Biceps brachii is located in the superficial, anterior arm.

Origin and Insertion

Origin: coracoid process of the scapula (short head) and supraglenoid tubercle of the scapula (long head); the long head passes through the intertubercular (or bicipital groove) on its way to the supraglenoid tubercle of the scapula.

Insertion (both heads): radial tuberosity and bicipital aponeurosis; the bicipital aponeurosis is a sheet of fascia, which joins the distal, medial portion of biceps brachii to the fascia of the anterior forearm.

Actions

Elbow flexion, supination of the forearm, and arm flexion

Explanation of Actions

Biceps brachii crosses the anterior aspect of both the elbow and shoulder, thus permitting flexion at both of those joints. Biceps brachii is most effective as an elbow flexor when the forearm is in a supinated position. Biceps brachii is a weak arm flexor, and many texts do not even list arm flexion as an action of the muscle. Because biceps brachii inserts on the radial tuberosity, which is located on the medial, proximal radius, contraction pulls the medial aspect of the radius forward, causing a lateral rotation of the bone, which is supination. Biceps brachii is our strongest supinator.

Notable Muscle Facts

Biceps brachii acts upon three joints. It has no attachment to the humerus.

Implications of Shortened and/or Lengthened/ Weak Muscle

Shortened: Elbows are flexed more than is typical. Limited range of motion of elbow extension, pronation of the forearm, and arm extension is noted.
Lengthened: Limited ability to flex elbow is noted.

Palpation and Massage

Because biceps brachii is superficial in the anterior arm, it is easy to palpate and massage. When a client is supine, the anterior arm is readily accessible. Effleurage and pétrissage are both appropriate strokes for this muscle.

How to Stretch This Muscle

Extend the elbow and arm.

Synergists

Elbow flexors: brachialis and brachioradialis
Arm flexors: coracobrachialis, anterior deltoid, and pectoralis major
Supinator: supinator

Antagonists

Elbow extensors: triceps brachii and anconeus
Arm extensors: latissimus dorsi, teres major, infraspinatus, teres minor, posterior deltoid, pectoralis major, and triceps brachii
Pronators: pronator teres and pronator quadratus

Innervation and Arterial Supply

Innervation: musculocutaneous nerve
Arterial supply: brachial artery and axial artery

BRACHIORADIALIS (bra-ke-o-ra-de-a-lis)

Meaning of Name

Brachii refers to the arm, where this muscle originates, and *radialis* refers to the radius, informing us that this muscle lies in the lateral forearm.

Location

Superficial, lateral forearm

Origin and Insertion

Origin: lateral supracondylar ridge of the humerus
Insertion: styloid process of the radius

Actions

Flexes the elbow when the forearm is in neutral position

Explanation of Actions

Brachioradialis crosses the lateral aspect of the elbow joint; thus, when the forearm is in a neutral position and brachioradialis shortens, elbow flexion results.

Notable Muscle Facts

Brachioradialis has the ability to perform the actions of both pronation and supination. When the forearm is in a pronated position, brachioradialis can supinate the forearm to a neutral position. When the forearm is in a supinated position, brachioradialis can pronate the forearm to a neutral position. A neutral position of the forearm is midway between pronation and supination.

Implications of Shortened and/or Lengthened/ Weak Muscle

Shortened: Elbow is flexed more than is typical.
Lengthened: A deficit in one's ability to flex the elbow when the forearm is in neutral position is noted.

Palpation and Massage

Because brachioradialis is located superficially in the lateral forearm, it can be palpated easily. Providing resistance to elbow flexion in a neutral position and contracting the muscle isometrically makes the outline of the muscle appear. The muscle belly is located in the proximal half of the lateral forearm, and the tendon of insertion runs from the midlateral forearm to the styloid process of the radius. Effleurage, pétrissage, and friction are all appropriate strokes to apply to brachioradialis.

How to Stretch This Muscle

Brachioradialis is a difficult muscle to stretch. If the muscle is quite shortened, one can achieve a stretch by extending the elbow while either supinating or pronating the forearm fully.

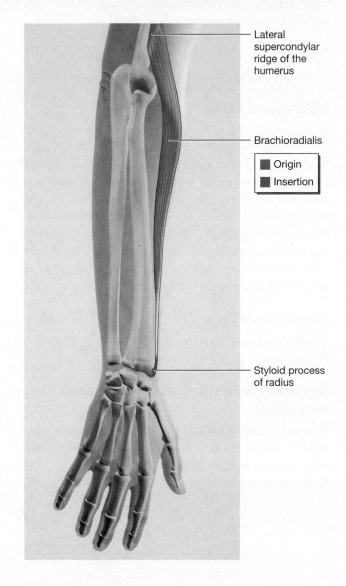

FIGURE 3-35 · Brachioradialis

Synergists

Elbow flexors: biceps brachii and brachialis

Antagonists

Elbow extensors: triceps brachii and anconeus

Innervation and Arterial Supply

Innervation: radial nerve
Arterial supply: brachial artery and radial artery

ANCONEUS (ang-ko-ne-us)

Meaning of Name

Anconeus means "elbow."

Location

Anconeus is located in the posterior elbow.

Origin and Insertion

Origin: lateral epicondyle of the humerus
Insertion: olecranon process of the ulna

Actions

Extends elbow

Explanation of Actions

Anconeus crosses the posterior aspect of the shoulder joint; thus, its shortening causes elbow extension.

Notable Muscle Facts

Some texts suggest that anconeus is an extension of triceps brachii, rather than a separate muscle. Anconeus is a weak elbow extensor, assisting triceps brachii in this task.

Implications of Shortened and/or Lengthened/Weak Muscle

There are no typical postural or functional implications of a shortened or lengthened anconeus muscle.

Palpation and Massage

Anconeus may be palpated in the posterior elbow area between the lateral epicondyle of the humerus and the olecranon process.

How to Stretch This Muscle

Flex the elbow.

Synergists

Triceps brachii

Antagonists

Elbow flexors: brachialis, biceps brachii, and brachioradialis

Innervation and Arterial Supply

Innervation: radial nerve
Arterial supply: deep brachial artery

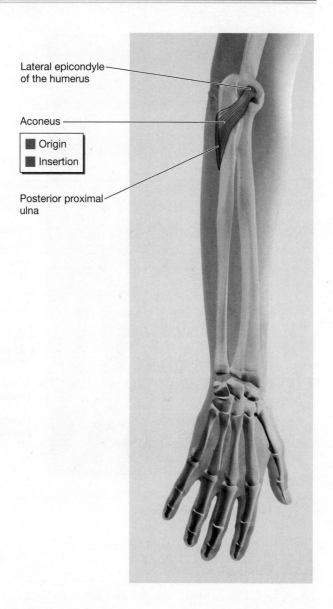

Lateral epicondyle of the humerus

Aconeus

Origin
Insertion

Posterior proximal ulna

FIGURE 3-36 · Anconeus

TRICEPS BRACHII (tri-seps bra-ke-i)

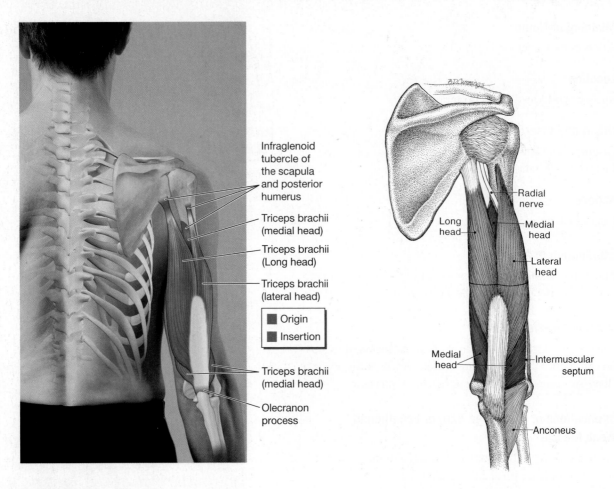

Infraglenoid tubercle of the scapula and posterior humerus

Triceps brachii (medial head)

Triceps brachii (Long head)

Triceps brachii (lateral head)

■ Origin
■ Insertion

Triceps brachii (medial head)

Olecranon process

Radial nerve

Long head

Medial head

Lateral head

Medial head

Intermuscular septum

Anconeus

FIGURE 3-37 · Triceps brachii

Meaning of Name

Triceps means "three heads," and *brachii* refers to the arm.

Location

Triceps brachii is located in the posterior arm and forms the contour of the posterior arm.

Origin and Insertion

Origin: supraglenoid tubercle of the scapula (long head); posterior humerus (medial and lateral heads): the lateral head originates above the spiral groove and the medial head originates below the spiral groove.

Insertion: olecranon process

Actions

Extends elbow and arm

Explanation of Actions

Because triceps brachii crosses the posterior aspect of the elbow joint, it is an elbow extensor. The long head crosses the posterior shoulder joint and thus assists in arm extension.

Notable Muscle Facts

Some sources list the long head of triceps brachii as an arm adductor, as well as an arm extensor. The medial head is the strongest portion of this muscle in regards to elbow extension.

Implications of Shortened and/or Lengthened/ Weak Muscle

Shortened: Shortened triceps brachii may cause the elbow to appear locked and may lead to a limited range of motion of elbow flexion.

Lengthened: Limited elbow extension is noted.

Palpation and Massage

Triceps brachii is easy to palpate and massage in the posterior arm, as it is the only muscle in this location. It is possible to access this muscle when the client is in a supine position by bringing the arm out to the side of the table, or by bringing the arm up over the client's head. Effleurage and petrissage of the muscle belly, and friction of the tendon of insertion are suggestions for massage of this muscle.

How to Stretch This Muscle

Flex the elbow and arm simultaneously.

Synergists

Elbow extensor: anconeus
Arm extensors: latissimus dorsi, teres major, infraspinatus, teres minor, posterior deltoid, and pectoralis major

Antagonists

Elbow flexors: biceps brachii, brachialis, and brachioradialis
Arm flexors: coracobrachialis, anterior deltoid, and pectoralis major

Innervation and Arterial Supply

Innervation: radial nerve
Arterial supply: brachial artery and subscapular artery

REGIONAL ILLUSTRATIONS OF MUSCLES

Figures 3-38 and 3-39 provide regional pictures (anterior and posterior) of the muscles that move the elbow.

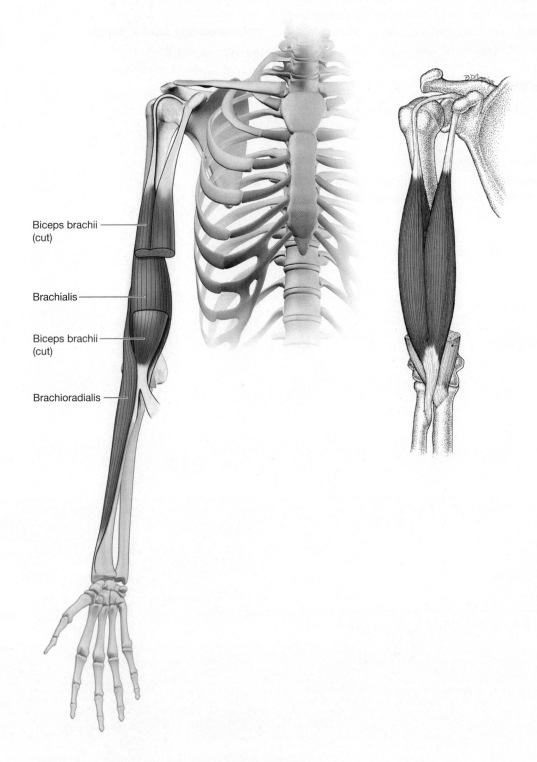

Biceps brachii
(cut)

Brachialis

Biceps brachii
(cut)

Brachioradialis

FIGURE 3-38 · Anterior view of the muscles that move the elbow

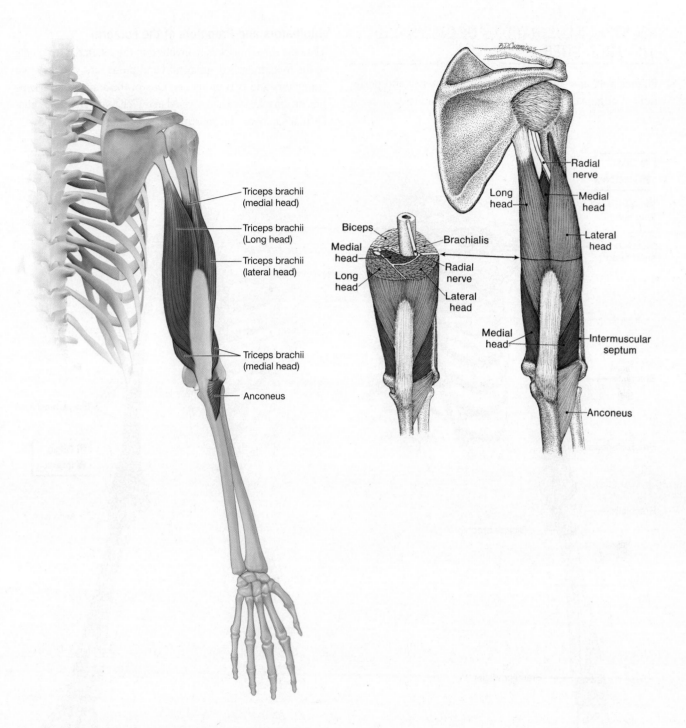

FIGURE 3-39 · Posterior view of the muscles that move the elbow

REGIONAL ILLUSTRATIONS OF ORIGIN AND INSERTION SITES

Figures 3-40 and 3-41 provide pictures (anterior and posterior) of origin and insertion sites of these muscles.

Supinators and Pronators of the Forearm

The next three muscles are involved in the rotation movements of the forearm, called supination and pronation. We have two supinators and two pronators. One of the supinators, biceps brachii, has already been covered in this chapter. The other muscle that supinates the forearm is the first muscle listed below.

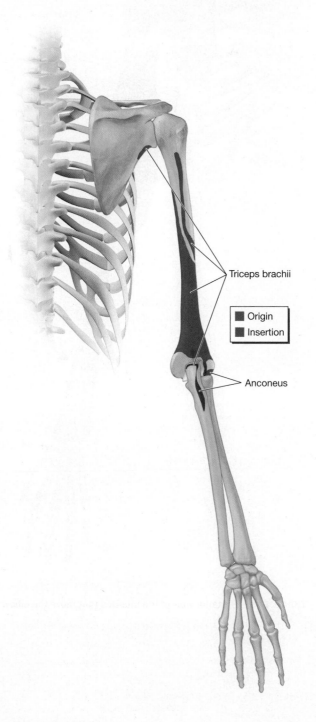

■ Origin
■ Insertion

Biceps brachii
long head

Biceps brachii
short head

Brachialis

Brachioradialis

Brachialis

Biceps brachii

Brachioradialis

Triceps brachii

■ Origin
■ Insertion

Anconeus

FIGURE 3-40 · Anterior view of origin and insertion sites of the elbow

FIGURE 3-41 · Posterior view of origin and insertion sites of the elbow muscles

SUPINATOR (su-pi-na-tor)

Meaning of Name
This muscle's name is based on the fact that it performs the action of supination.

Location
The supinator wraps around the lateral aspect of the proximal forearm from the lateral epicondyle of the humerus and proximal ulna to the radius. It is deep to the wrist extensors and brachioradialis.

Origin and Insertion
Origin: lateral epicondyle of the humerus and proximal ulna
Insertion: proximal third of the anterior, lateral radius

Actions
Supination of the forearm

Explanation of Actions
The supinator pulls the radius laterally toward the lateral epicondyle of the humerus. Lateral turning of the radius is supination.

Notable Muscle Facts
Although biceps brachii is a stronger muscle in regards to the action of supination, the supinator is the muscle that has the primary role of holding the forearm in a neutral position.

Implications of Shortened and/or Lengthened/ Weak Muscle
Shortened: Limited ability to pronate the forearm is noted.
Lengthened: Limited ability to supinate the forearm is noted.

Palpation and Massage
The supinator is deep to the wrist extensors and brachioradialis, so to palpate or massage this muscle it is necessary to press through or between the superficial muscles against the middle third of the lateral radius to find the supinator. Find the lateral epicondyle of the humerus. Trace the muscle as it wraps around the lateral aspect of the proximal forearm to its insertion spot on the anterolateral radius. Friction is the easiest stroke to apply to the supinator.

How to Stretch This Muscle
Pronate the forearm.

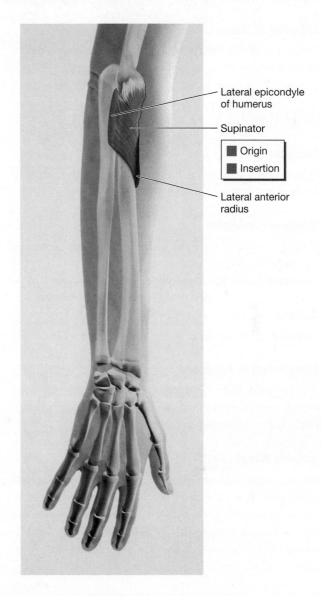

Lateral epicondyle of humerus

Supinator

■ Origin
■ Insertion

Lateral anterior radius

FIGURE 3-42 · Supinator

Synergists
Biceps brachii

Antagonists
Pronator quadratus and pronator teres

Innervation and Arterial Supply
Innervation: radial nerve
Arterial supply: radial artery and interosseus branches of the ulnar artery

PRONATOR TERES (pro-na-tor ter-ez)

Meaning of Name

Pronator indicates that the action of this muscle is pronation of the forearm. *Teres* means "rounded." Although pronator teres does not have an obviously round shape, it is much more rounded and cylindrical than the square-shaped pronator quadrates muscle.

Location

Pronator teres is located in the superficial, proximal, anterior forearm.

Origin and Insertion

Origin: medial epicondyle of the humerus and coronoid process of the ulna
Insertion: lateral mid-shaft of the radius

Actions

Pronation of the forearm

Explanation of Actions

Pronator teres pulls the anterior radius toward the ulna and medial epicondyle of the humerus, causing a medial rotation of the radius, or pronation of the forearm.

Notable Muscle Facts

Pronator teres is the stronger of the two pronator muscles and is engaged whenever a strong pronation movement is needed. The median nerve passes between the two heads of pronator teres and can be compressed by this muscle, leading to pronator teres syndrome. Overuse and/or trauma related to the pronator teres muscle are the most common causes of this condition.

Implications of Shortened and/or Lengthened/ Weak Muscle

Shortened: Limited ability to supinate the forearm is noted.
Lengthened: Limited ability to pronate the forearm is noted.

Palpation and Massage

In the anterior forearm, palpate from the medial epicondyle of the humerus toward the middle of the anterior radius. Effleurage and friction are easy strokes to perform on this muscle.

How to Stretch This Muscle

Supinate the forearm.

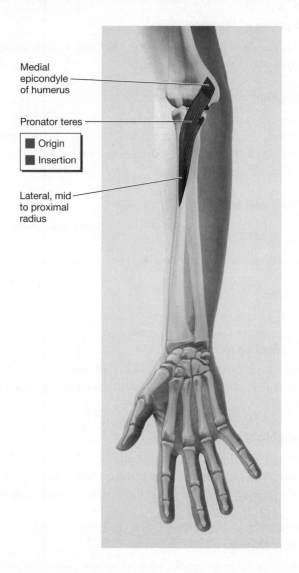

Medial epicondyle of humerus

Pronator teres

■ Origin
■ Insertion

Lateral, mid to proximal radius

FIGURE 3-43 · Pronator teres

Synergists

Pronator quadratus

Antagonists

Supinator and biceps brachii

Innervation and Arterial Supply

Innervation: median nerve
Arterial supply: ulnar and radial arteries

PRONATOR QUADRATUS (pro-na-tor kwa-dra-tus)

Meaning of Name

Pronator indicates that the action of this muscle is pronation of the forearm. *Quadratus* means "four-sided" or "square-shaped."

Location

Pronator quadratus is located deep in the distal, anterior forearm.

Origin and Insertion

Origin: distal fourth of the anterior ulna
Insertion: distal fourth of the anterior radius

Actions

Pronation of the forearm

Explanation of Actions

Pronator quadratus pulls the distal anterior radius toward the distal ulna, resulting in a medial rotation of the radius, which is equivalent to supination.

Notable Muscle Facts

This muscle is the prime pronator, which means that it is engaged whenever we pronate the forearm. The stronger pronator teres is used when additional strength is needed.

Implications of Shortened and/or Lengthened/ Weak Muscle

Shortened: Inability to fully supinate the forearm is present.
Lengthened: Reduction in ability to pronate the forearm is noted, but not as much loss of function as when the pronator teres is weak/lengthened.

Palpation and Massage

Pronator quadratus is deep to all flexor tendons in the distal fourth of the anterior forearm. This area is tender to the touch, so pronator quadratus must be palpated or massaged with care. Gentle friction or direct pressure is perhaps the most appropriate stroke to use for this muscle.

How to Stretch This Muscle

Supinate the forearm.

Synergists

Pronator teres

Antagonists

Supinator and biceps brachii

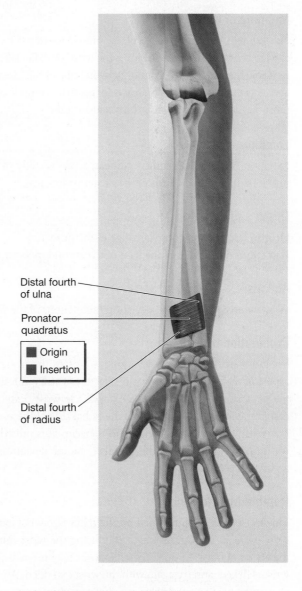

Distal fourth of ulna

Pronator quadratus

■ Origin
■ Insertion

Distal fourth of radius

FIGURE 3-44 · Pronator quadratus

Innervation and Arterial Supply

Innervation: median nerve
Arterial supply: anterior interosseus artery

Wrist Movers

The next group of muscles to be discussed is the wrist movers. These muscles are all located superficially in the forearm: three in the anterior forearm, which flex the wrist, and three in the posterior forearm, which extend the wrist.

EXTENSOR CARPI RADIALIS LONGUS (eks-ten-sor kar-pe ra-de-a-lis long-guss)

Meaning of Name

Extensor tells us that the action of this muscle is extension, and *carpi* tells us that this muscle moves the wrist joint. *Radialis* lets us know that this muscle lies on the radial side of the forearm, and *longus* tells us that this muscle is longer than a muscle of almost the same name, extensor carpi radialis brevis.

Location

Extensor carpi radialis longus is located superficially in the proximal half to two-thirds of the posterior forearm.

Origin and Insertion

Origin: lateral supracondylar ridge of the humerus
Insertion: dorsal side of the base of the second metacarpal

Actions

Wrist extension and radial deviation (abduction) of the wrist

Explanation of Actions

Because extensor carpi radialis longus crosses the posterior aspect of the wrist, it pulls the dorsal side of the hand toward the posterior forearm and thus extends the wrist. Extensor carpi radialis longus also crosses the radial side of the posterior wrist, so that when the second metacarpal is pulled toward the radial side of the forearm, radial deviation or abduction occurs.

Notable Muscle Facts

This muscle, in conjunction with the other two wrist extensors, plays an important role in stabilizing the wrist during the action of finger flexion. Try to flex your fingers when your wrist is flexed, and try again with the wrist extended. Almost every time we flex our fingers, we engage our wrist extensors isometrically to enable the finger flexors to contract with greater ease. Thus, repetitive finger flexion leads to repetitive wrist extension and the potential to irritate the common extensor tendon.

Implications of Shortened and/or Lengthened/ Weak Muscle

Shortened: Limited ability to flex the wrist is noted.
Lengthened: If extensor carpi radialis longus and brevis are lengthened, one would expect to have difficulty with both wrist extension and radial deviation. If extensor carpi ulnaris were lengthened, one might also have difficulty fully adducting the wrist. Inability to fully extend the wrist leads to difficulty accomplishing finger flexion, as the wrist extensors serve as stabilizers for the finger flexors.

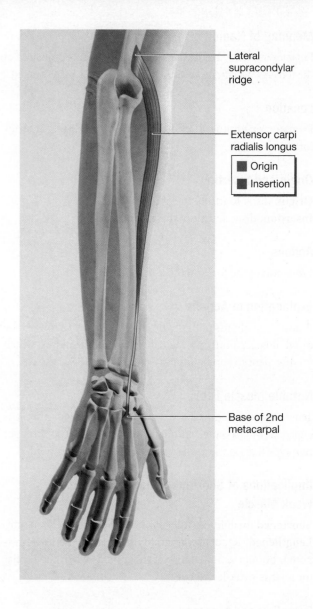

Lateral supracondylar ridge

Extensor carpi radialis longus

■ Origin
■ Insertion

Base of 2nd metacarpal

FIGURE 3-45 · Extensor carpi radialis longus

Palpation and Massage

The wrist extensors are easy to palpate as a unit. Find the lateral epicondyle of the humerus and palpate distally, feeling for the mound of tissue in the proximal posterior forearm. Friction to the wrist extensors' tendons of origin can be an effective way to loosen the muscles, as well as effleurage, digital pétrissage, and friction to the muscle bellies.

How to Stretch This Muscle

Flex the wrist.

Synergists

Wrist extensors: extensor carpi radialis brevis, and extensor carpi ulnaris

Antagonists

Wrist flexors: flexor carpi radialis, flexor carpi ulnaris, and palmaris longus

Innervation and Arterial Supply

Innervation: radial nerve
Arterial supply: branches of the brachial artery

EXTENSOR CARPI RADIALIS BREVIS (eks-ten-sor kar-pe ra-de-a-lis brev-is)

Meaning of Name

Extensor tells us the action of this muscle, and *carpi* tells us that this muscle moves the wrist. *Radialis* lets us know that this muscle lies on the radial side of the forearm, and *brevis* tells us that this muscle is shorter than extensor carpi radialis longus.

Location

Extensor carpi radialis brevis is located superficially in the proximal half to two-thirds of the posterior forearm.

Origin and Insertion

Origin: lateral epicondyle of the humerus via the common extensor tendon
Insertion: dorsal side of the base of the third metacarpal

Actions

Wrist extension and radial deviation (abduction) of the wrist

Explanation of Actions

Because extensor carpi radialis brevis crosses the posterior aspect of the wrist, it pulls the dorsal side of the hand toward the posterior forearm, and thus extends the wrist. Extensor carpi radialis brevis also crosses the radial side of the posterior wrist, so that when the third metacarpal is pulled toward the radial side of the forearm, radial deviation or abduction occurs.

Notable Muscle Facts

Tendonitis in the tendons of origin of extensor carpi radialis brevis and extensor carpi ulnaris can lead to a condition called *tennis elbow* or sometimes called *lateral epicondylitis*. This condition is typically caused by overuse of the wrist extensors, which puts strain on the tendons of origin of these muscles. Tennis elbow that is no longer acute may benefit from the use of friction, which can assist scar tissue fiber realignment.

Implications of Shortened and/or Lengthened/ Weak Muscle

Same as for extensor carpi radialis longus, above.

Palpation and Massage

Same as for extensor carpi radialis longus, above.

How to Stretch This Muscle

Flex the wrist.

Synergists

Wrist extensors: extensor carpi radialis longus, and extensor carpi ulnaris

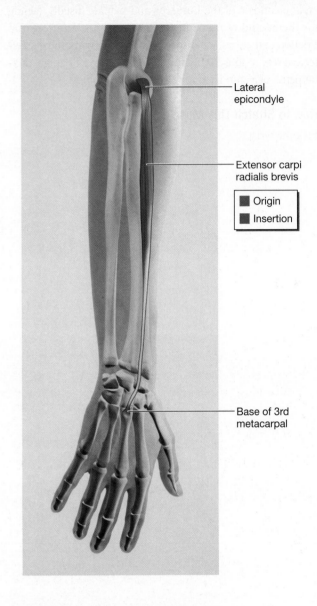

Lateral epicondyle

Extensor carpi radialis brevis

■ Origin
■ Insertion

Base of 3rd metacarpal

FIGURE 3-46 · Extensor carpi radialis brevis

Antagonists

Wrist flexors: flexor carpi radialis, flexor carpi ulnaris, and palmaris longus

Innervation and Arterial Supply

Innervation: radial nerve
Arterial supply: branches of the brachial artery

EXTENSOR CARPI ULNARIS (eks-ten-sor kar-pe ul-na-ris)

Meaning of Name

Extensor tells us the action of this muscle, and *carpi* tells us that this muscle moves the wrist. *Ulnaris* lets us know that this muscle lies on the ulnar side of the forearm.

Location

Extensor carpi ulnaris is located superficially in the posterior forearm.

Origin and Insertion

Origin: lateral epicondyle of the humerus, via the common extensor tendon and posterior ulna
Insertion: dorsal side of the base of the fifth metacarpal

Actions

Wrist extension and ulnar deviation (adduction) of the wrist

Explanation of Actions

Because extensor carpi ulnaris crosses the posterior aspect of the wrist, it pulls the dorsal side of the hand toward the posterior forearm, and thus extends the wrist. Extensor carpi ulnaris also crosses the ulnar side of the posterior wrist, so that when the fifth metacarpal is pulled toward the ulnar side of the forearm, ulnar deviation or adduction occurs.

Notable Muscle Facts

See notable muscle facts for both extensor carpi radialis longus and extensor carpi radialis brevis, above.

Implications of Shortened and/or Lengthened/Weak Muscle

Same as for extensor carpi radialis longus, above.

Palpation and Massage

Same as for extensor carpi radialis longus, above.

How to Stretch This Muscle

Flex the wrist.

Synergists

Extensor carpi radialis longus and extensor carpi radialis brevis

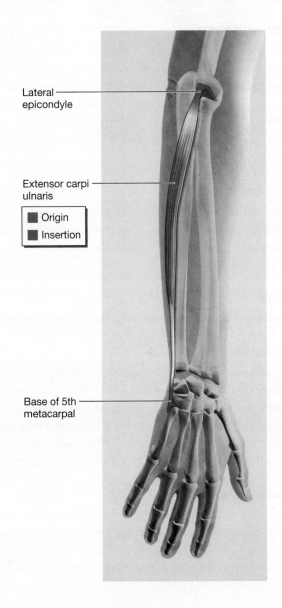

Lateral epicondyle

Extensor carpi ulnaris

- ■ Origin
- ■ Insertion

Base of 5th metacarpal

FIGURE 3-47 · Extensor carpi ulnaris

Antagonists

Wrist flexors: Flexor carpi radialis, flexor carpi ulnaris, and palmaris longus

Innervation and Arterial Supply

Innervation: radial nerve
Arterial supply: branch of the ulnar artery

FLEXOR CARPI RADIALIS (flex-sor kar-pe ra-de-a-lis)

Meaning of Name

Flexor tells us that the action of this muscle is flexion, and *carpi* tells us that this muscle moves the wrist. *Radialis* lets us know that this muscle lies on the radial side of the forearm.

Location

Flexor carpi radialis is located superficially in the anterior forearm.

Origin and Insertion

Origin: medial epicondyle of the humerus
Insertion: palmar side of the base of the second and third metacarpals. *Note:* Some sources list only the second metacarpal as the insertion.

Actions

Wrist flexion and radial deviation (abduction) of the wrist

Explanation of Actions

Because flexor carpi radialis crosses the anterior aspect of the wrist, it pulls the palmar side of the hand toward the anterior forearm, and thus flexes the wrist. Flexor carpi radialis also crosses the radial side of the anterior wrist, so that when the second and third metacarpals are pulled toward the radial side of the forearm, radial deviation or abduction occurs.

Notable Muscle Facts

This muscle is the strongest wrist flexor. The tendon of insertion of flexor carpi radialis passes through the carpal tunnel on its way to the second and third metacarpals. Thus, inflammation of this tendon can irritate the median nerve and cause carpal tunnel syndrome.

Implications of Shortened and/or Lengthened/ Weak Muscle

Shortened: If the wrist flexors are shortened, it is difficult to extend the wrist fully.
Lengthened: If flexor carpi radialis and flexor carpi ulnaris are lengthened, one would expect to have difficulty with both wrist flexion and radial and ulnar deviation.

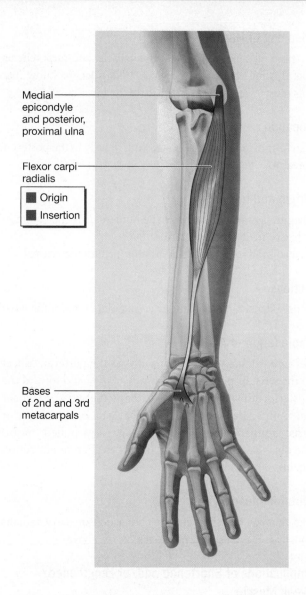

Medial epicondyle and posterior, proximal ulna

Flexor carpi radialis

■ Origin
■ Insertion

Bases of 2nd and 3rd metacarpals

FIGURE 3-48 · Flexor carpi radialis

Palpation and Massage

The wrist flexors are easy to palpate as a unit. Find the medial epicondyle of the humerus and palpate distally, feeling for the mound of tissue on the medial side of the proximal anterior forearm. Friction to the tendons of origin can be an effective way to loosen the muscle, as well as effleurage, digital pétrissage, and friction of the muscle bellies.

How to Stretch This Muscle

Extend the wrist.

Synergists

Wrist flexors: flexor carpi ulnaris and palmaris longus

Antagonists

Wrist extensors: extensor carpi radialis longus, extensor carpi radialis brevis, and extensor carpi ulnaris

Innervation and Arterial Supply

Innervation: median nerve
Arterial supply: branches of the ulnar and radial arteries

FLEXOR CARPI ULNARIS (flex-sor kar-pe ul-na-ris)

Meaning of Name
Flexor tells us that the action of this muscle is flexion, and *carpi* tells us that this muscle moves the wrist. *Ulnaris* lets us know that this muscle lies on the ulnar side of the forearm.

Location
Flexor carpi ulnaris is located superficially in the anterior forearm.

Origin and Insertion
Origin: medial epicondyle of the humerus
Insertion: palmar side of the base of the fifth metacarpal and the pisiform

Actions
Wrist flexion and ulnar deviation (adduction) of the wrist

Explanation of Actions
Because flexor carpi ulnaris crosses the anterior aspect of the wrist, it pulls the palmar side of the hand toward the anterior forearm, and thus flexes the wrist. Flexor carpi ulnaris also crosses the ulnar side of the anterior wrist, so that when the fifth metacarpal and pisiform are pulled toward the ulnar side of the forearm, ulnar deviation or adduction occurs.

Notable Muscle Facts
This muscle is located so medially in the forearm that it is easy to view and palpate from both anterior and posterior perspectives.

Implications of Shortened and/or Lengthened/ Weak Muscle
Same as for flexor carpi radialis, above.

Palpation and Massage
Same as for flexor carpi radialis, above.

How to Stretch This Muscle
Extend the wrist.

Synergists
Wrist flexors: flexor carpi radialis and palmaris longus

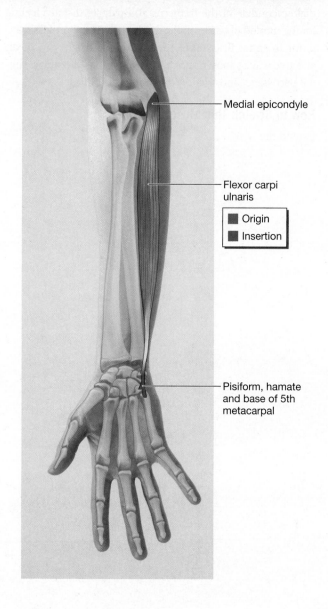

FIGURE 3-49 · Flexor carpi ulnaris

Labels on figure:
- Medial epicondyle
- Flexor carpi ulnaris
- Origin
- Insertion
- Pisiform, hamate and base of 5th metacarpal

Antagonists
Wrist extensors: extensor carpi radialis longus, extensor carpi radialis brevis, and extensor carpi ulnaris

Innervation and Arterial Supply
Innervation: ulnar nerve
Arterial supply: branches of the ulnar artery

PALMARIS LONGUS (pahl-mar-ex long-gus)

Meaning of Name

Palmaris means that the muscle inserts into the palm, and *longus* lets us know that there is another muscle called palmaris brevis, and that palmaris longus is longer than palmaris brevis.

Location

Palmaris longus is located superficially in the anterior forearm.

Origin and Insertion

Origin: medial epicondyle of the humerus
Insertion: palmar aponeurosis

Actions

Wrist flexion

Explanation of Actions

Because palmaris longus crosses the anterior aspect of the wrist, it pulls the palmar side of the hand toward the anterior forearm, and thus flexes the wrist.

Notable Muscle Facts

Palmaris longus is not present in about 15% of the population. The muscle's long tendon of insertion is frequently used in tendon or ligament replacement surgery. Thus, those of us who do have palmaris longus muscles can be considered to have "spare parts," which may be useful in a time of need.

Implications of Shortened and/or Lengthened/ Weak Muscle

Shortened: One may experience difficulty fully extending the wrist.
Lengthened: One would not experience any functional loss, as the muscle is inherently weak.

Palpation and Massage

Same as for flexor carpi radialis, above.

How to Stretch This Muscle

Extend the wrist.

Synergists

Wrist flexors: flexor carpi radialis and flexor carpi ulnaris

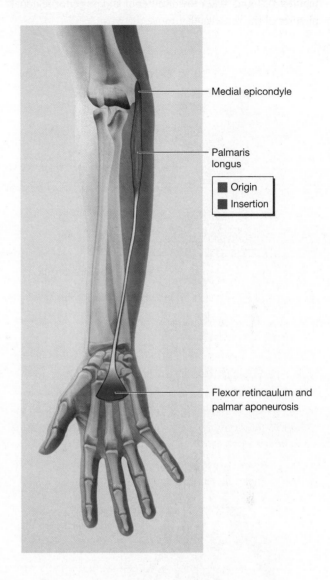

Medial epicondyle

Palmaris longus

Origin
Insertion

Flexor retincaulum and palmar aponeurosis

FIGURE 3-50 · Palmaris longus

Antagonists

Wrist extensors: extensor carpi radialis longus, extensor carpi radialis brevis, and extensor carpi ulnaris

Innervation and Arterial Supply

Innervation: median nerve
Arterial supply: branches of the ulnar artery

REGIONAL ILLUSTRATIONS OF MUSCLES

Figures 3-51 and 3-52 provide anterior and posterior regional pictures of the muscles that move the wrist.

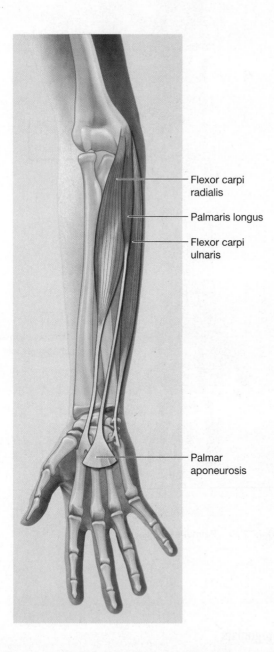

Flexor carpi radialis

Palmaris longus

Flexor carpi ulnaris

Palmar aponeurosis

FIGURE 3-51 · **Anterior view of the muscles that move the wrist**

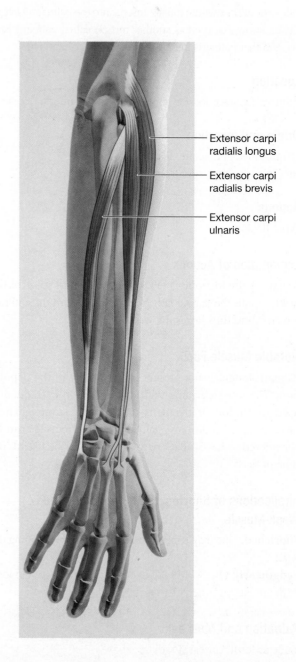

Extensor carpi radialis longus

Extensor carpi radialis brevis

Extensor carpi ulnaris

FIGURE 3-52 · **Posterior view of the muscles that move the wrist**

REGIONAL ILLUSTRATIONS OF ORIGIN AND INSERTION SITES

Figures 3-53 and 3-54 provide anterior and posterior pictures of the origin and insertion sites of these muscles.

Forearm Muscles That Move Fingers and Thumb

The next group of muscles are located in the forearm and move the fingers or digits 1 to 5. Some move only one digit, and some move four digits. The muscles that are located in the posterior forearm tend to extend the fingers or thumb, and the muscles that are located in the anterior forearm flex the fingers or thumb.

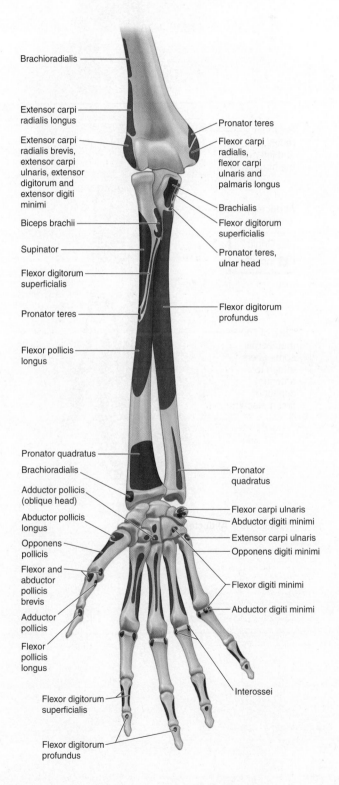

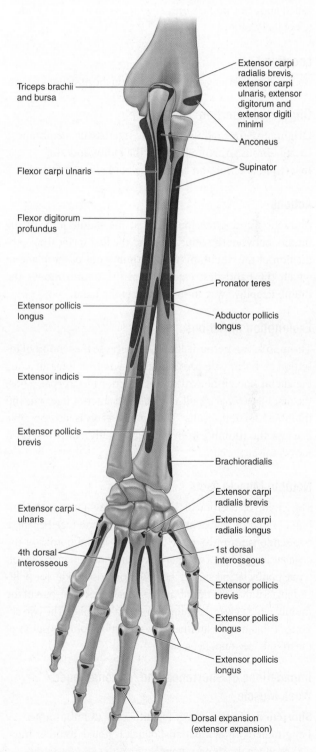

FIGURE 3-54 · Posterior view: origin and insertion sites of muscles that move the wrist

ABDUCTOR POLLICIS LONGUS (ab-duk-tor pol-i-sis long-gus)

Meaning of Name

Abductor tells us that the action of this muscle is abduction. *Pollicis* tells us that this muscle moves the thumb or first digit. *Longus* means "longer" and tells us that there is a muscle called abductor pollicis brevis, which is shorter than abductor pollicis longus.

Location

Abductor pollicis longus is located deep in the posterior forearm.

Origin and Insertion

Origin: posterior radius, ulna, and interosseus membrane, a strong fibrous structure between the radius and ulna
Insertion: anterior and lateral side of the first metacarpal

Actions

Abduction and extension occur at the saddle joint of the thumb, between the trapezium and the first metacarpal. Abduction of the thumb moves the thumb out of the plane in which the hand lies; extension of the thumb moves the thumb laterally away from the side of the hand.

Explanation of Actions

The muscle can perform abduction because the tendon of insertion of this muscle passes from the posterior forearm along the lateral side of the wrist to the anterior metacarpal. Thus, the first metacarpal is pulled toward the anterior forearm, and thumb abduction results. Thumb extension is also possible because the thumb can be pulled laterally when insertion moves toward origin.

Notable Muscle Facts

The tendon of insertion of this muscle lies right next to the tendon of insertion of extensor pollicis brevis, and together these two tendons form the more anterior or lateral border of the *anatomical snuff box*. The snuff box is the indentation in the soft tissue on the lateral side of the posterior wrist. Abductor pollicis longus moves the thumb at the specialized saddle joint of the thumb, which gives the thumb its special mobility. The two actions of this muscle are the opposite actions of opposition of the thumb (see opponens pollicis).

Implications of Shortened and/or Lengthened/Weak Muscle

Shortened: Limited ability to adduct the thumb is noted.
Lengthened: Little functional deficit is noted, as other muscles produce the same actions.

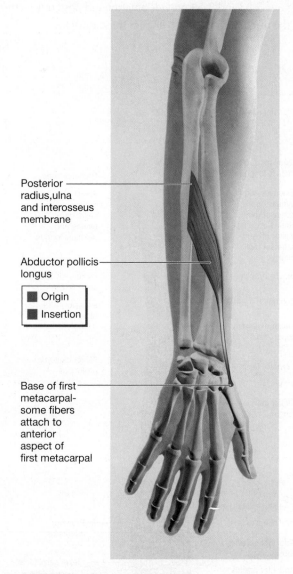

Posterior radius, ulna and interosseus membrane

Abductor pollicis longus

■ Origin
■ Insertion

Base of first metacarpal- some fibers attach to anterior aspect of first metacarpal

FIGURE 3-55 · Abductor pollicis longus

Palpation and Massage

Typically, the four deep posterior forearm muscles that move digits are addressed as a unit during massage. It is difficult to distinguish abductor pollicis longus from the other deep posterior forearm muscles. However, providing deep effleurage or friction to the distal half of the posterior forearm will address abductor pollicis longus.

How to Stretch This Muscle

Adduct and flex the thumb.

Synergists

Thumb abductor: abductor pollicis brevis

Thumb extensors: extensor pollicis brevis and extensor pollicis longus

Antagonists

Thumb adductor: adductor pollicis
Thumb flexors: flexor pollicis longus and flexor pollicis brevis

Innervation and Arterial Supply

Innervation: radial nerve
Arterial supply: posterior interosseus artery

EXTENSOR POLLICIS BREVIS (eks-ten-sor pol-i-sis brev-is)

Meaning of Name

Extensor refers to the action of the muscle, *pollicis* refers to the thumb, and *brevis* tells us that this muscle is the shorter of a pair of thumb extensors.

Location

Deep in the distal, posterior forearm

Origin and Insertion

Origin: distal, posterior radius and interosseus membrane
Insertion: base of the proximal phalanx of the thumb. The tendon of insertion of this muscle, along with the tendon of insertion of abductor pollicis brevis, form the more anterior or lateral border of the anatomical snuff box.

Actions

Extension of the thumb at the CMC and MP joints

Explanation of Actions

The tendon of insertion runs along the lateral edge of the first metacarpal to the proximal phalanx. Thus, the line of pull when this muscle shortens is to pull the thumb out to the lateral side of the hand, or to extend the thumb.

Notable Muscle Facts

The tendon of insertion of extensor pollicis brevis is often enclosed in a common tendon sheath with abductor pollicis longus, and together, the tendons of insertion of these two muscles form the lateral border of the anatomical snuff box.

Implications of Shortened and/or Lengthened/Weak Muscle

Shortened: Limited ability to flex the thumb is noted.
Lengthened: If this muscle is weak/lengthened, there is no significant loss of function.

Palpation and Massage

Typically, the four deep posterior forearm muscles that move digits are addressed as a unit during massage. It is difficult to distinguish extensor pollicis brevis from the other deep posterior forearm muscles. However, providing deep effleurage or friction to the distal half of the posterior forearm will address extensor pollicis brevis.

How to Stretch This Muscle

Flex the thumb.

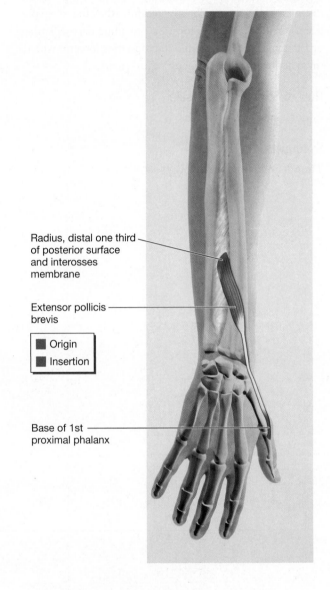

Radius, distal one third of posterior surface and interosses membrane

Extensor pollicis brevis

■ Origin
■ Insertion

Base of 1st proximal phalanx

FIGURE 3-56 · Extensor pollicis brevis

Synergists

Thumb extensor: extensor pollicis longus

Antagonists

Thumb flexors: flexor pollicis longus and flexor pollicis brevis

Innervation and Arterial Supply

Innervation: radial nerve
Arterial supply: posterior interosseus artery

EXTENSOR POLLICIS LONGUS (eks-ten-sor pol-i-sis long-gus)

Meaning of Name

Extensor refers to the action of the muscle, *pollicis* refers to the thumb, and *longus* tells us that this muscle is the longer of a pair of thumb extensors.

Location

Deep in the distal, posterior forearm

Origin and Insertion

Origin: middle third of the posterior ulna and interosseus membrane
Insertion: base of the distal phalanx of the thumb. The tendon of insertion forms the more posterior border of the anatomical snuff box.

Actions

Extension of the thumb at the MP and IP joints

Explanation of Actions

The tendon of insertion runs along the posterior surface of the first metacarpal to the distal phalanx. Thus, when this muscle shortens, it pulls the thumb out to the lateral side of the hand, or extends the thumb.

Notable Muscle Facts

The tendon of insertion of extensor pollicis longus forms the more posterior border of the anatomical snuff box. This muscle is the only thumb extensor to act upon the IP joint of the thumb.

Implications of Shortened and/or Lengthened/ Weak Muscle

Shortened: Limited ability to flex the thumb is noted.
Lengthened: Weakness of thumb extension is noted, particularly at the IP joint of the thumb.

Palpation and Massage

Typically, the four deep posterior forearm muscles that move digits are addressed as a unit during massage. It is difficult to distinguish extensor pollicis longus from the other deep posterior forearm muscles. However, providing deep effleurage or friction to the distal half of the posterior forearm will address extensor pollicis longus.

How to Stretch This Muscle

Flex the thumb.

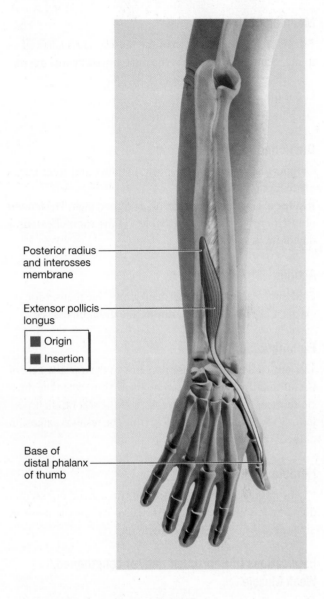

Posterior radius and interosses membrane

Extensor pollicis longus

■ Origin
■ Insertion

Base of distal phalanx of thumb

FIGURE 3-57 · Extensor pollicis longus

Synergists

Thumb extensor: extensor pollicis brevis

Antagonists

Thumb flexors: flexor pollicis longus and flexor pollicis brevis

Innervation and Arterial Supply

Innervation: radial nerve
Arterial supply: posterior interosseus artery

EXTENSOR INDICIS (eks-ten-sor in-di-sis)

Meaning of Name

Extensor refers to the action of the muscle, and *indicis* refers to the second digit, which is the digit moved by this muscle.

Location

Deep in the distal, posterior forearm

Origin and Insertion

Origin: distal third of the posterior ulna and interosseus membrane

Insertion: extensor expansion of the second digit. The tendon of insertion blends with the tendon of insertion of extensor digitorum as well.

Actions

Extension of the second digit at all joints, due to insertion on extensor expansion, which runs to the distal phalanges

Explanation of Actions

This muscle's tendon of insertion crosses the dorsal aspect of the MP and IP joints of the second digit. Thus, when the muscle shortens, it pulls the dorsal side of the second digit posteriorly toward the posterior forearm. The result is extension of the second digit.

Notable Muscle Facts

Extensor indicis gives us greater ability to extend our second digit. Some sources claim that extensor indicis can assist in ulnar deviation of the second digit.

Implications of Shortened and/or Lengthened/ Weak Muscle

Shortened: Limited ability to flex the second digit is noted.
Lengthened: Minor weakness of second digit extension is present. The weakness is minimal due to the presence of extensor digitorum.

Palpation and Massage

Typically, the four deep posterior forearm muscles that move digits are addressed as a unit during massage. It is difficult to distinguish extensor indicis from the other deep posterior forearm muscles. However, providing deep effleurage or friction to the distal half of the posterior forearm will address extensor indicis.

How to Stretch This Muscle

Flex the second digit.

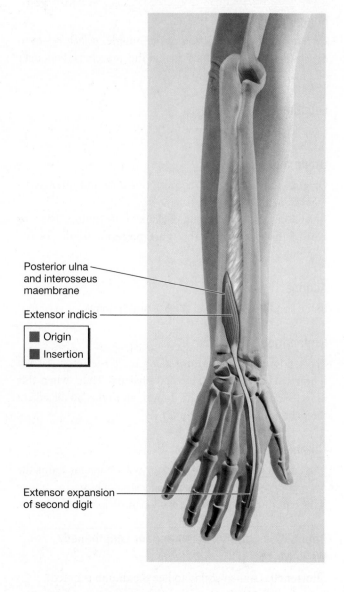

Posterior ulna and interosseus maembrane

Extensor indicis

■ Origin
■ Insertion

Extensor expansion of second digit

FIGURE 3-58 · **Extensor indicis**

Synergists

Extensor: extensor digitorum

Antagonists

Flexors: flexor digitorum profundus and flexor digitorum superficialis

Innervation and Arterial Supply

Innervation: radial nerve
Arterial supply: posterior interosseus artery

EXTENSOR DIGITORUM (eks-ten-sor dij-i-tor-um)

Meaning of Name

Extensor refers to the action of the muscle, and *digitorum* refers to digits 2 through 5 of the hand or foot.

Location

This muscle is located in the superficial, posterior forearm.

Origin and Insertion

Origin: lateral epicondyle of the humerus via the common extensor tendon
Insertion: extensor expansion of digits 2 to 5 of the hand

Actions

Extension of all joints of the four fingers, or digits 2 to 5 of the hand

Explanation of Actions

Because the tendons of insertion cross the posterior side of the CMC, MP, and IP joints of the fingers, the muscle is in position to extend all of these joints.

Notable Muscle Facts

The tendon of origin is part of the common extensor tendon. The tendons of insertion of extensor digitorum use the complex extensor expansion to enable extension of the metacarpal and all IP joints of the fingers. However, the main extension action of this muscle occurs at the MP joints of the four fingers. The lumbrical muscles are primary extensors of the IP joints of the fingers.

Implications of Shortened and/or Lengthened/ Weak Muscle

Shortened: Limited finger flexion is noted.
Lengthened: Limited extension of the MP joints of the fingers is present.

Palpation and Massage

Extensor digitorum has a wide, flat muscle belly, which can be palpated in the superficial, posterior forearm. Effleurage and friction are probably the easiest Swedish strokes to apply to extensor digitorum. Find the lateral epicondyle of the humerus. Friction to the common extensor tendon can be particularly helpful for a client with tightness in this muscle.

How to Stretch This Muscle

Flex the four fingers.

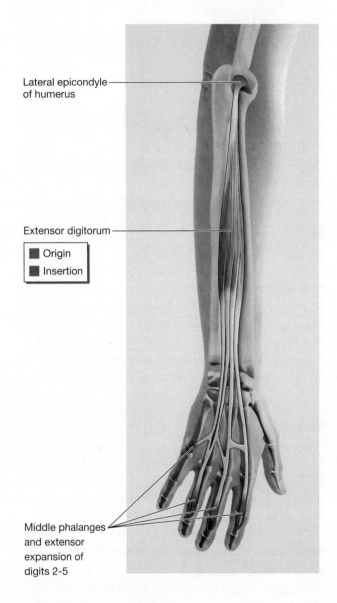

Lateral epicondyle of humerus

Extensor digitorum
■ Origin
■ Insertion

Middle phalanges and extensor expansion of digits 2-5

FIGURE 3-59 · Extensor digitorum

Synergists

Finger extensors: extensor digiti minimi and extensor indicis

Antagonists

Finger flexors: flexor digitorum profundus and flexor digitorum superficialis

Innervation and Arterial Supply

Innervation: radial nerve
Arterial supply: posterior interosseus artery

EXTENSOR DIGITI MINIMI (eks-ten-sor dij-i-ti min-i-mi)

Meaning of Name

Extensor refers to the action of the muscle, and *digiti minimi* means "smallest digit" or the fifth digit.

Location

This muscle is located in the superficial, posterior forearm.

Origin and Insertion

Origin: lateral epicondyle of the humerus, via the common extensor tendon
Insertion: extensor expansion of the fifth digit

Actions

Extension of all joints of the fifth digit

Explanation of Actions

Because this muscle's tendon of insertion crosses the posterior aspect of the fifth digit and pulls the dorsal side of the fifth digit toward the posterior forearm, the muscle performs extension of the fifth digit. The tendon of insertion joins to the extensor mechanism of the fifth digit, thus allowing the muscle to extend all joints of the fifth digit.

Notable Muscle Facts

The tendon of origin is part of the common extensor tendon. The tendon of insertion of extensor digiti minimi is commonly united with the tendon of insertion of extensor digitorum that serves the fifth digit. Thus, some sources claim that extensor digiti minimi is really a part of extensor digitorum.

Implications of Shortened and/or Lengthened/ Weak Muscle

Shortened: Limited flexion of the fifth digit is noted.
Lengthened: If this muscle is lengthened/weak, one would not face any functional limits.

Palpation and Massage

Extensor digiti minimi blends with the medial aspect of extensor digitorum. Effleurage and friction to the superficial posterior forearm will affect extensor digiti minimi. Friction to the common extensor tendon can be helpful as well.

How to Stretch This Muscle

Flex the fifth digit.

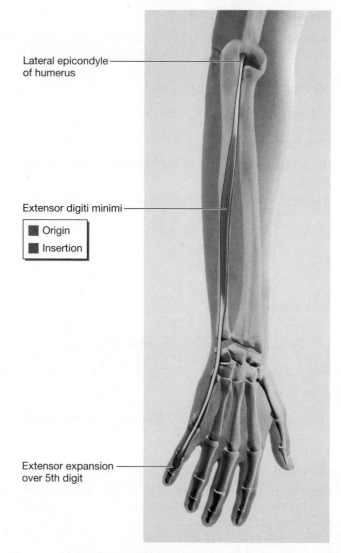

Lateral epicondyle of humerus

Extensor digiti minimi
■ Origin
■ Insertion

Extensor expansion over 5th digit

FIGURE 3-60 · Extensor digiti minimi

Synergists

Extensor digitorum

Antagonists

Flexor digiti minimi, flexor digitorum profundus, and flexor digitorum superficialis

Innervation and Arterial Supply

Innervation: radial nerve
Arterial supply: posterior interosseus artery

FLEXOR POLLICIS LONGUS (flex-sor pol-i-sis long-gus)

Meaning of Name

Flexor refers to the action of flexion, *pollicis* means "thumb," and *longus* means "longer" and lets us know that there is a shorter muscle called flexor pollicis brevis.

Location

Flexor pollicis longus is located deep in the anterior forearm.

Origin and Insertion

Origin: anterior surface of the middle third of the radius and interosseus membrane
Insertion: distal phalanx of the thumb

Actions

Thumb flexion at the MP and IP joints

Explanation of Actions

The tendon of insertion of flexor pollicis longus crosses the anterior aspect of the wrist, passes through the carpal tunnel, crosses the CMC joints, and then runs laterally along the first metacarpal and crosses the MP and IP joints. This muscle thus pulls the thumb medially in the frontal plane, which is flexion.

Notable Muscle Facts

Flexor pollicis longus is the only muscle that is able to flex the IP joint of the thumb. It is an important muscle in the action of grasping. Because the tendon of insertion passes through the carpal tunnel, it can cause carpal tunnel syndrome. This typically occurs when the tendon becomes inflamed and thus irritates the median nerve.

Implications of Shortened and/or Lengthened/Weak Muscle

Shortened: Inability to fully extend the thumb is noted.
Lengthened: Limited ability to flex the IP joint of the thumb is present.

Palpation and Massage

To address the client's anterior forearm, it is probably easiest to have the client in a supine position. When massaging the anterior forearm, it is difficult to distinguish flexor pollicis longus, flexor digitorum profundus, and flexor digitorum superficialis, as all three muscles lie deep to the wrist flexors. However, the distal portions of the muscles are easier to palpate. Flexor pollicis longus is palpable on the lateral side of the distal anterior forearm. Friction is an appropriate stroke for this portion of the muscle. Flexor pollicis longus can also be addressed by performing deep effleurage to the anterior forearm, with the intention of addressing the deeper muscles.

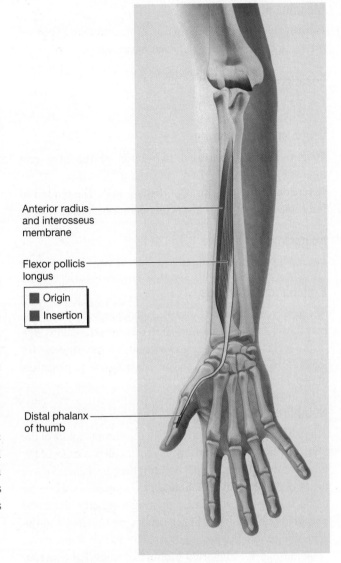

Anterior radius
and interosseus
membrane

Flexor pollicis
longus

■ Origin
■ Insertion

Distal phalanx
of thumb

FIGURE 3-61 · Flexor pollicis longus

How to Stretch This Muscle

Extend the thumb.

Synergists

Flexor pollicis brevis

Antagonists

Extensor pollicis longus and extensor pollicis brevis

Innervation and Arterial Supply

Innervation: median nerve
Arterial supply: radial artery

FLEXOR DIGITORUM PROFUNDUS (flex-sor dij-i-tor-rum pro-fun-dus)

Meaning of Name

Flexor refers to flexion, the action of this muscle. *Digitorum* means "four digits," and *profundus* mean "deep."

Location

Deep anterior forearm

Origin and Insertion

Origin: anterior, proximal two-thirds of the ulna and interosseus membrane
Insertion: distal phalanges of digits 2 to 5. The tendon of insertion splits into four distinct tendons, one for each finger.

Actions

Flexes all phalanges of digits 2 to 5 of the hand

Explanation of Actions

The tendons of insertion cross the anterior aspect of the wrist, pass through the carpal tunnel, and then cross the palmar side of the metacarpophalangeal (MP) and interphalangeal (IP) joints of the hand, allowing the muscle to flex all 12 phalanges of the hand.

Notable Muscle Facts

This is the only muscle that can flex the distal IP joints of the fingers, although it has the capacity to flex all phalanges of the fingers. The tendons of insertion run deep to the tendons of flexor digitorum superficialis and pass through a split in the tendons of insertion of flexor digitorum superficialis at the proximal phalanx. Both finger flexors are important in the action of grasping.

Because flexor digitorum profundus' tendon of insertion passes through the carpal tunnel, it can cause carpal tunnel syndrome. This typically occurs when the tendon becomes inflamed and thus irritates the median nerve.

Implications of Shortened and/or Lengthened/ Weak Muscle

Shortened: Limited ability to extend the fingers is noted.
Lengthened: One would notice a deficit in flexion of the DIP joints of the hand.

Palpation and Massage

To address the client's anterior forearm, it is probably easiest to have the client in a supine position. When massaging the anterior forearm, it is difficult to distinguish flexor pollicis longus, flexor digitorum profundus, and flexor digitorum superficialis, as all three muscles lie deep to the wrist flexors.

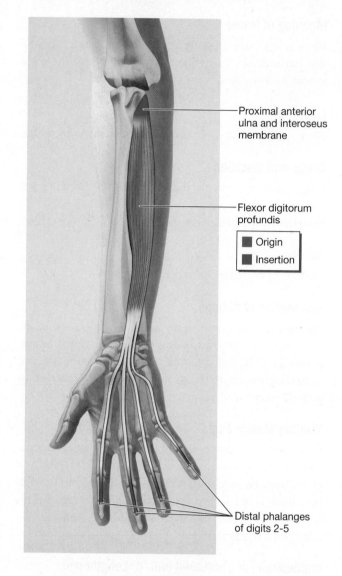

Proximal anterior ulna and interoseus membrane

Flexor digitorum profundis

■ Origin
■ Insertion

Distal phalanges of digits 2-5

FIGURE 3-62 · Flexor digitorum profundus

However, the distal portion of the muscles is easier to palpate. Flexor digitorum profundus is palpable in the medial aspect of the distal anterior forearm. Friction is an appropriate stroke for this portion of the muscle. Flexor digitorum profundus can also be addressed by performing deep effleurage to the anterior forearm, with the intention of addressing the deeper muscles.

How to Stretch This Muscle
Extend fingers and wrist together.

Synergists
Flexor digitorum superficialis

Antagonists
Extensor digitorum

Innervation and Arterial Supply
Innervation: median and ulnar nerves
Arterial supply: ulnar and radial arteries

FLEXOR DIGITORUM SUPERFICIALIS (flex-sor dij-i-tor-rum su-per-fish-e-al-is)

Meaning of Name

Flexor refers to flexion, the action of this muscle. *Digitorum* means "four digits," and *superficialis* means "superficial," as flexor digitorum superficialis is superficial to flexor digitorum profundus.

Location

Midlayer anterior forearm

Origin and Insertion

Origin: medial epicondyle of the humerus, proximal anterior ulna, and anterior radius just distal to the radial tuberosity
Insertion: both sides of the proximal phalanges of digits 2 to 5.

Actions

Flexion of the MP and PIP joints of digits 2 to 5

Explanation of Actions

The tendons of insertion of flexor digitorum superficialis cross the anterior aspect of the wrist, pass through the carpal tunnel, and then cross the palmar side of the MP and proximal interphalangeal (PIP) joints. Because the muscle pulls the palmar surface of the proximal phalanges toward the anterior forearm, the resulting action is flexion of the MP and PIP joints.

Notable Muscle Facts

The very distal aspect of the tendons of insertion of flexor digitorum superficialis split to create a small tunnel, through which pass the tendons of insertion of the deeper flexor digitorum profundus. Flexor digitorum superficialis is the stronger finger flexor at the PIP joints, and is an important muscle in grasping.

Because flexor digitorum superficialis' tendon of insertion passes through the carpal tunnel, it can cause carpal tunnel syndrome. This typically occurs when the tendon becomes inflamed and thus irritates the median nerve.

Implications of Shortened and/or Lengthened/ Weak Muscle

Shortened: Inability to fully extend the fingers is noted.
Lengthened: One could expect to have reduced ability to flex the PIP joints of the hand.

Palpation and Massage

To address the anterior forearm, it is probably easiest to have the client in a supine position. When massaging the

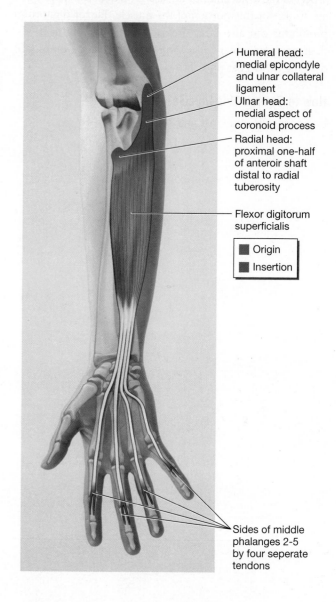

Humeral head: medial epicondyle and ulnar collateral ligament
Ulnar head: medial aspect of coronoid process
Radial head: proximal one-half of anteroir shaft distal to radial tuberosity
Flexor digitorum superficialis

■ Origin
■ Insertion

Sides of middle phalanges 2-5 by four seperate tendons

FIGURE 3-63 · Flexor digitorum superficialis

anterior forearm, it is difficult to distinguish flexor pollicis longus, flexor digitorum profundus, and flexor digitorum superficialis, as all three muscles lie deep to the wrist flexors. Flexor digitorum superficialis can perhaps best be addressed by performing deep effleurage and/or friction to the anterior forearm, with the intention of addressing the mid-layer muscle.

How to Stretch This Muscle
Extend fingers and wrist together.

Synergists
Flexor digitorum profundus

Antagonists
Extensor digitorum

Innervation and Arterial Supply
Innervation: median nerve
Arterial supply: ulnar and radial arteries

REGIONAL ILLUSTRATIONS OF MUSCLES

Figures 3-64 and 3-65 provide anterior and posterior regional pictures of the muscles that are located in the forearm and move the fingers, thumb, or rotate the forearm.

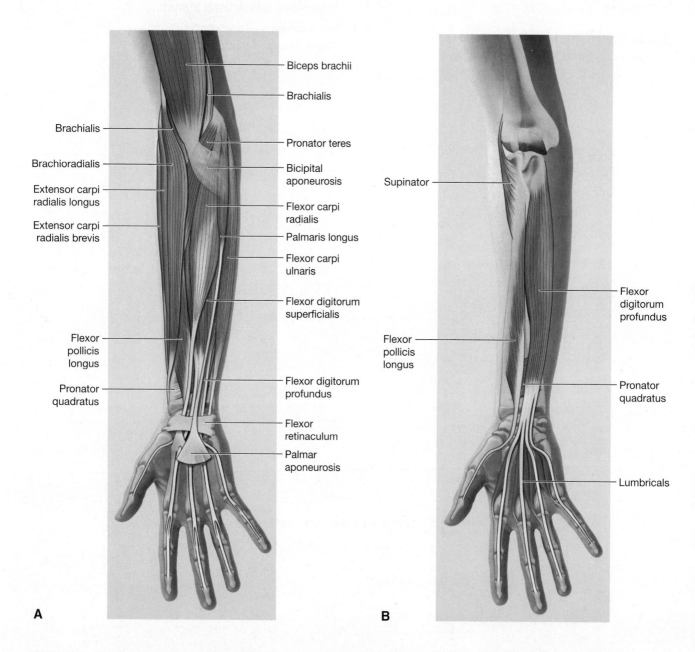

A

B

FIGURE 3-64 · Muscles that are located in the anterior forearm and move the fingers or thumb, or supinate or pronate the forearm

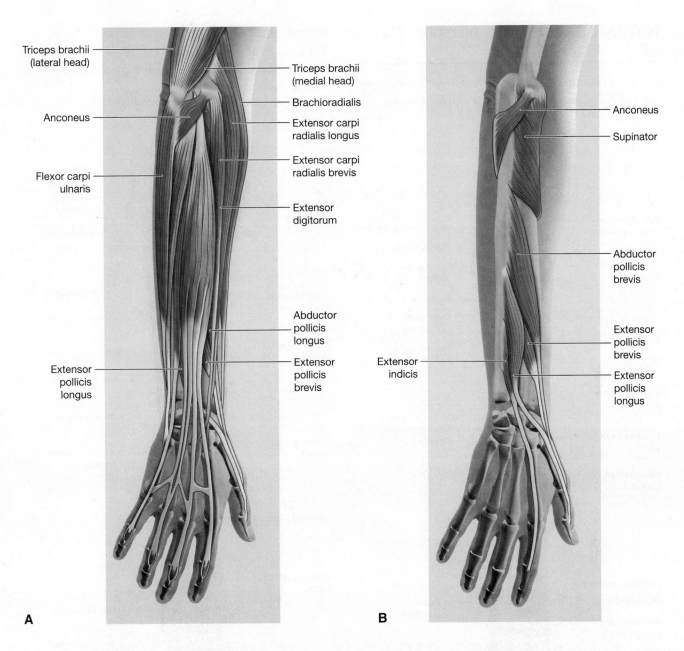

Triceps brachii
(lateral head)

Anconeus

Flexor carpi
ulnaris

Extensor
pollicis
longus

Triceps brachii
(medial head)

Brachioradialis

Extensor carpi
radialis longus

Extensor carpi
radialis brevis

Extensor
digitorum

Abductor
pollicis
longus

Extensor
pollicis
brevis

Anconeus

Supinator

Abductor
pollicis
brevis

Extensor
pollicis
brevis

Extensor
pollicis
longus

Extensor
indicis

A

B

FIGURE 3-65 · Muscles that are located in the posterior forearm and move the fingers or thumb, or supinate the forearm

REGIONAL ILLUSTRATIONS OF ORIGIN AND INSERTION SITES

Figures 3-66 and 3-67 provide anterior and posterior pictures of the origin and insertion sites of these muscles.

Intrinsic Hand Muscles

The next group of muscles are located entirely within the hand and are thus called the intrinsic hand muscles. These muscles move the fingers and thumb.

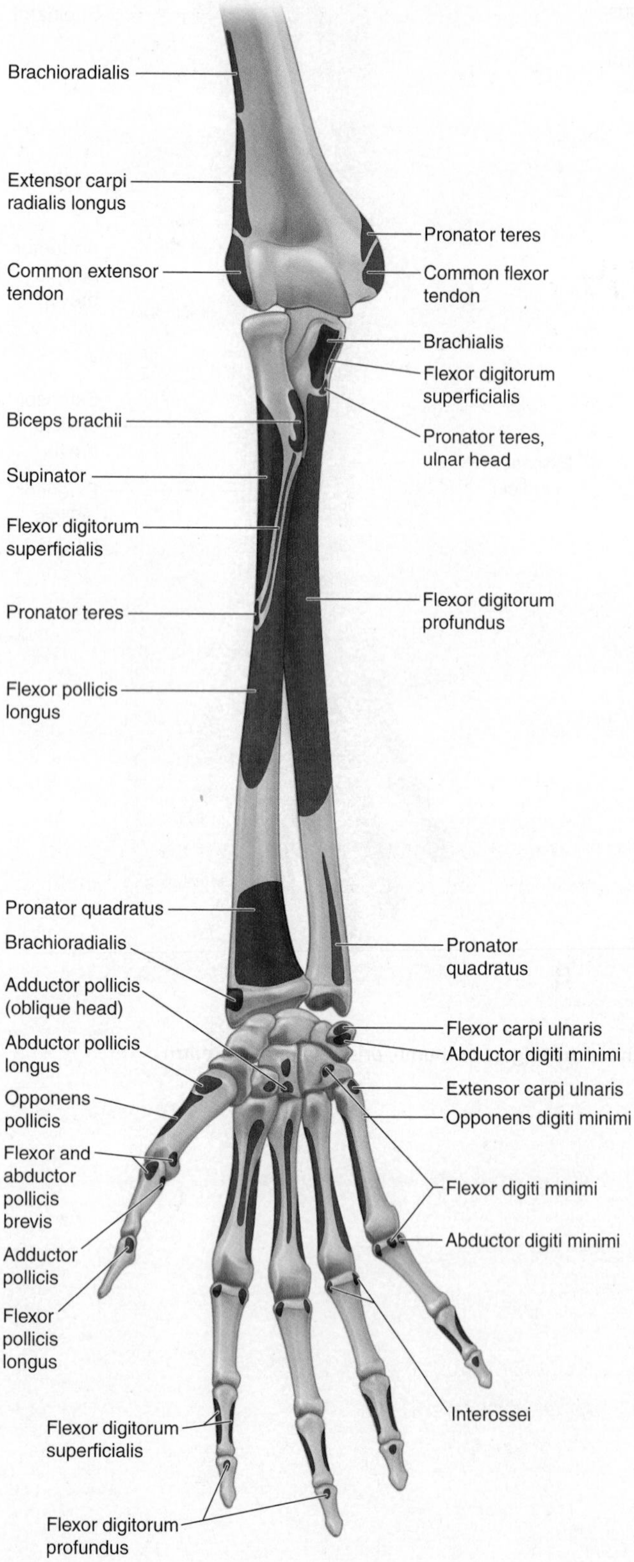

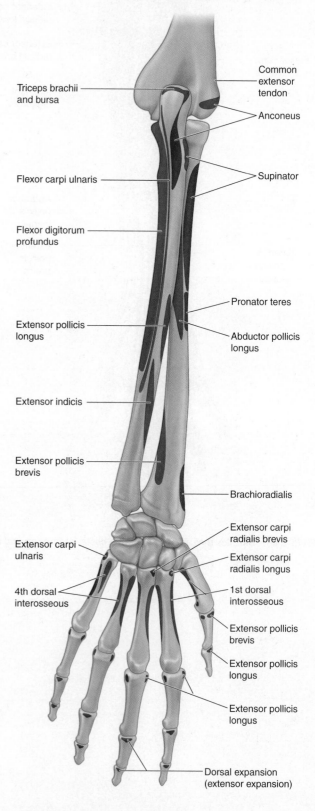

FIGURE 3-66 · Origin and insertion sites of the muscles located in the anterior forearm that move the fingers or thumb

FIGURE 3-67 · Origin and insertion sites of the muscles located in the posterior forearm that move fingers or thumb

DORSAL INTEROSSEI (dor-sal in-ter-ahse)

Meaning of Name

Dorsal refers to the back side of the hand, where this muscle is located. *Interossei* means "between bones," and this muscle is located between the metatarsals. The dorsal interossei are a group of four interosseus muscles, each of which moves a single digit in one direction.

Location

Between the metatarsals on the dorsal side of the hand

Origin and Insertion

Origin: adjacent sides of the metacarpals between which this muscle lies

Insertion: base of the proximal phalanx of a certain digit and the extensor mechanism that supports that digit

Actions

The collective action of the dorsal interossei is usually said to be finger abduction, which is the movement of the digits away from the midline of the hand or third digit. In reality, each interosseus muscle moves a single digit either medially or laterally. One muscle moves the fourth digit medially (ulnar deviation), one muscle moves the second digit laterally (radial deviation), one muscle moves the third digit medially (ulnar deviation), and one muscle moves the third digit laterally (radial deviation).

Explanation of Actions

Each interosseus muscle is located on one particular side (either the radial side or the ulnar side) of the phalanx it moves and inserts into the same side of the base of a proximal phalanx. The interossei located on the radial side of a digit pull the proximal phalanx toward the radius, thus producing radial deviation. The interossei located on the ulnar side of a digit pull the proximal phalanx toward the ulna, thus producing ulnar deviation.

Notable Muscle Facts

DAB is a useful acronym to remember that Dorsal interossei ABduct the fingers.

Implications of Shortened and/or Lengthened/ Weak Muscle

Shortened: Limited ability to adduct the fingers is noted.
Lengthened: Limited ability to abduct the fingers is noted.

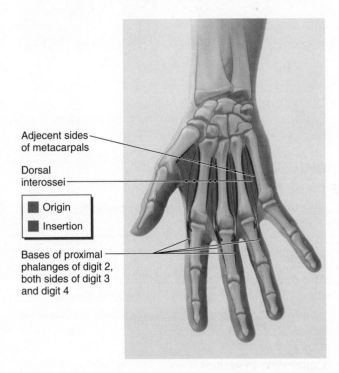

Adjacent sides of metacarpals

Dorsal interossei

■ Origin
■ Insertion

Bases of proximal phalanges of digit 2, both sides of digit 3 and digit 4

FIGURE 3-68 · Dorsal interossei

Palpation and Massage

Palpating and frictioning deep between the metacarpals on the dorsal side of the hand will find and address dorsal interossei.

How to Stretch This Muscle

Adduct the fingers.

Synergists

According to some sources, the lumbricals can assist the action of dorsal interossei by allowing radial deviation of digits 2 and 3. Dorsal interossei has no other synergist.

Antagonists

Palmar interossei

Innervation and Arterial Supply

Innervation: ulnar nerve
Arterial supply: radial and ulnar arteries

PALMAR INTEROSSEI (pahl-mar in-ter-ahse)

Meaning of Name

Palmar refers to the palmar or anterior side of the hand, and *interossei* means "between bones."

Location

Palmar interossei are located on the palmar side of the hand, deep between the metacarpals.

Origin and Insertion

Origin: metacarpals 2, 3, and 5
Insertion: palmar sides of the proximal phalanges of digits 2, 3, and 5

Actions

As a group, palmar interossei adduct the fingers. Individually, each palmar interosseus moves either the second, third, or fifth digit toward the third digit, which is the midline of the hand.

Explanation of Actions

The palmar interosseus that originates on the second metacarpal attaches to the ulnar or medial side of the second metacarpal. This interosseus muscle inserts on the ulnar or medial side of the proximal phalanx of the second digit. When the muscle shortens, it pulls the proximal phalanx of the second digit medially. The palmar interosseus muscle that originates on the fourth metacarpal attaches to the radial or lateral side of the metacarpal and inserts on the lateral side of the proximal phalanx of the fourth digit. Thus, when it shortens, it pulls the proximal phalanx of the fourth digit laterally. The palmar interosseus muscle that originates on the fifth metacarpal attaches to the radial or lateral side of the metacarpal. It inserts on the lateral side of the proximal phalanx of the fifth digit and thus pulls the fifth digit laterally when it shortens. The combined movements of the three interossei muscles are to bring digits 2, 4, and 5 closer to digit 3, which is the same as adducting the fingers.

Notable Muscle Facts

PAD is a useful acronym to remember that Palmar interossei ADduct the fingers.

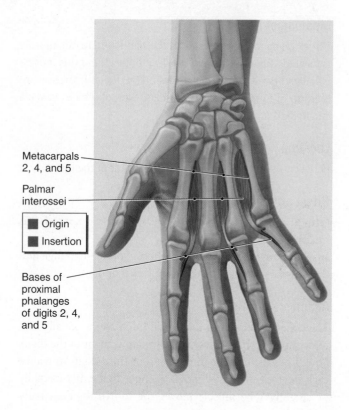

Metacarpals 2, 4, and 5

Palmar interossei

■ Origin
■ Insertion

Bases of proximal phalanges of digits 2, 4, and 5

FIGURE 3-69 · Palmar interossei

Implications of Shortened and/or Lengthened/Weak Muscle

Lengthened: If palmar interossei were lengthened or weak, one would experience difficulty in adducting the fingers.

Palpation and Massage

Palpating and providing friction to the palmar side of the hand, deep between the metacarpals, allows us to access and massage palmar interossei.

How to Stretch This Muscle

Abduct the fingers.

Synergists

According to some sources, the lumbricals can assist the action of palmar interossei by allowing radial deviation of digit 4. Palmar interossei has no other synergists.

Antagonists

Dorsal interossei

Innervation and Arterial Supply

Innervation: ulnar nerve
Arterial supply: radial and ulnar arteries

LUMBRICALS (lum-bri-kals)

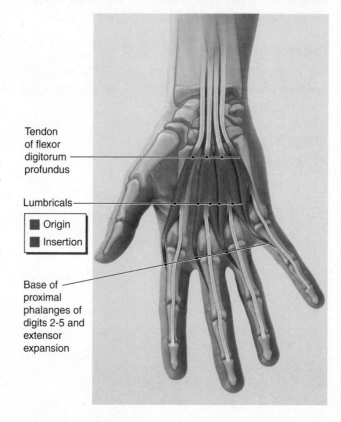

Tendon of flexor digitorum profundus

Lumbricals

■ Origin
■ Insertion

Base of proximal phalanges of digits 2-5 and extensor expansion

FIGURE 3-70 · **Lumbricals**

Meaning of Name
Earthworms

Location
In the palm of the hand

Origin and Insertion
Origin: tendon of origin of flexor digitorum profundus
Insertion: anterior aspect of the proximal phalanges of digits 2 to 5 and extensor expansion, which covers the posterior aspect of the fingers

Actions
Flexion of the MP joints of digits 2 to 5 and extension of the PIP and DIP joints of digits 2 to 5

Explanation of Actions
Lumbricals flex the MP joints because the tendons of origin cross the anterior aspect of these joints. Lumbricals extend the DIP and PIP joints of digits 2 to 5, because they pull on the extensor expansion, which pulls the dorsal sides of the fingers toward the dorsal side of the hand.

Notable Muscle Facts
Lumbricals are unique in that the muscle originates and inserts into connective tissue. Lumbricals are located in both the hands and the feet.

Implications of Shortened and/or Lengthened/Weak Muscle
There are no common or obvious implications of shortened or lengthened lumbrical muscles.

Palpation and Massage
Lumbricals can be palpated and massaged by providing friction to the palm of the hand between the thenar eminence and hypothenar eminence, deep to the palmar fascia.

How to Stretch This Muscle
Extend the MP joints and flex the IP joints.

Synergists
Extensor digitorum serves as a synergist at the IP joints, and flexor digitorum profundus serves as a synergist at the MP joints.

Antagonists
Flexor digitorum profundus and flexor digitorum superficialis serve as antagonists to lumbricals at the IP joints. Extensor digitorum is an antagonist at the metacarpophalangeal (MP) joints.

Innervation and Arterial Supply
Innervation: median and ulnar nerves
Arterial supply: radial and ulnar arteries

ADDUCTOR POLLICIS (a-duk-tor pol-i-sis)

Meaning of Name

Adductor refers to the action of adduction, and *pollicis* means "thumb."

Location

Adductor pollicis is located in the webbing between the first and second digits.

Origin and Insertion

Origin: bases of the second and third metacarpals, the capitate, and trapezoid (oblique head); shaft of the third metacarpal (transverse head)
Insertion (both heads): proximal phalanx of the thumb

Actions

Adduction of the thumb at the CMC joint

Explanation of Actions

This muscle pulls the proximal phalanx toward the center of the palm, causing thumb adduction.

Notable Muscle Facts

Adductor pollicis is the largest of the intrinsic hand muscles.

Implications of Shortening and/or Lengthening/ Weak Muscle

Shortened: Limited abduction of the thumb is noted.
Lengthened: Limited adduction of the thumb is noted.

Palpation and Massage

Adductor pollicis may be addressed by applying pressure into the webbing of the hand between the first and second metacarpals. Pressure in this location can ease headache pain, jaw pain, and sinus pressure.

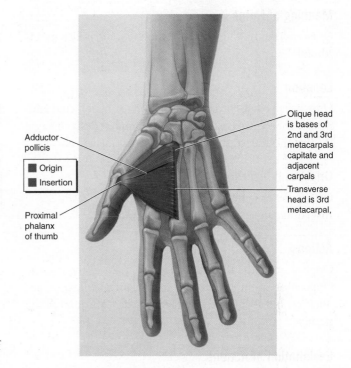

Adductor pollicis

■ Origin
■ Insertion

Oblique head is bases of 2nd and 3rd metacarpals capitate and adjacent carpals

Transverse head is 3rd metacarpal,

Proximal phalanx of thumb

FIGURE 3-71 · Adductor pollicis

How to Stretch This Muscle

Abduct the thumb.

Synergists

Adductor pollicis is the only thumb adductor.

Antagonists

Abductor pollicis brevis and abductor pollicis longus

Innervation and Arterial Supply

Innervation: ulnar nerve
Arterial supply: radial artery

OPPONENS POLLICIS (o-po-nenz pol-i-sis)

Meaning of Name

Opponens refers to the action of opposition, and *pollicis* means "thumb."

Location

Opponens pollicis is located deepest in the hypothenar eminence. The thenar eminence is the mound of flesh covering the first metacarpal and medial to the first metacarpal.

Origin and Insertion

Origin: flexor retinaculum and trapezium
Insertion: lateral aspect of the first metacarpal

Actions

Opposition of the thumb at the CMC joint of the thumb. Opposition of the thumb is a combination of flexion, abduction, and slight medial rotation at the CMC joint of the thumb.

Explanation of Actions

This muscle pulls the lateral aspect of the first metacarpal toward the trapezium and flexor retinaculum, causing opposition of the thumb.

Notable Muscle Facts

This muscle allows us to perform the action of opposition, which is the basis of our opposable thumb.

Implications of Shortened and/or Lengthened/ Weak Muscle

Shortened: Limited extension and adduction of the thumb is noted.
Lengthened: Difficulty performing opposition of the thumb may be present.

Palpation and Massage

Opponens pollicis may be addressed by applying pressure to the thenar eminence and focusing on the tissue deep to flexor pollicis brevis and abductor pollicis brevis.

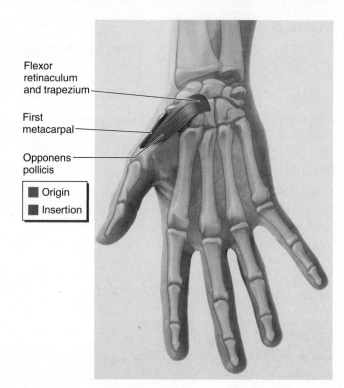

Flexor retinaculum and trapezium

First metacarpal

Opponens pollicis

■ Origin
■ Insertion

FIGURE 3-72 · Opponens pollicis

How to Stretch This Muscle

Adduct and extend the thumb.

Synergists

Abductor pollicis longus, abductor pollicis brevis, flexor pollicis brevis, and flexor pollicis longus

Antagonists

Extensor pollicis longus, extensor pollicis brevis, and adductor pollicis

Innervation and Arterial Supply

Innervation: medial and ulnar nerves
Arterial supply: radial artery

FLEXOR POLLICIS BREVIS (flek-sor pol-i-sis brev-is)

Meaning of Name
Flexor refers to the action of flexion, *pollicis* means "thumb," and *brevis* means "shorter."

Location
Flexor pollicis brevis is located in the medial, superficial aspect of the thenar eminence.

Origin and Insertion
Origin: trapezium and flexor retinaculum
Insertion: base of the proximal phalanx of the thumb

Actions
Flexion of the thumb at the MP joint

Explanation of Actions
By pulling the proximal phalanx of the thumb toward the flexor retinaculum and trapezium, the thumb moves toward and across the palm, thus accomplishing flexion.

Notable Muscle Facts
Flexor pollicis brevis and abductor pollicis brevis lie side by side, making up the superficial portion of the mound that is the thenar eminence.

Implications of Shortening and/or Lengthening/ Weak Muscle
Shortened: Limited ability to extending the thumb is noted.
Lengthened: Limited ability to flex the thumb is noted.

Palpation and Massage
Palpating and applying pressure to the medial, superficial aspect of the thenar eminence will address flexor pollicis brevis.

How to Stretch This Muscle
Extending the thumb at the MP joint.

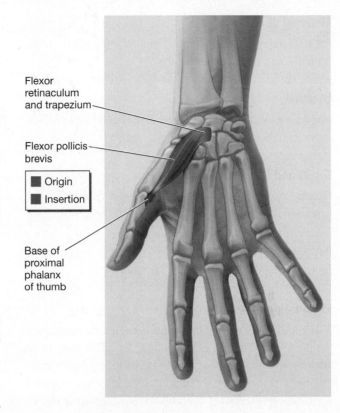

Flexor retinaculum and trapezium

Flexor pollicis brevis

■ Origin
■ Insertion

Base of proximal phalanx of thumb

FIGURE 3-73 · Flexor pollicis brevis

Synergists
Flexor pollicis longus

Antagonists
Extensor pollicis longus and extensor pollicis brevis

Innervation and Arterial Supply
Innervation: medial and ulnar nerves
Arterial supply: radial artery

ABDUCTOR POLLICIS BREVIS (ab-duk-tor pol-i-sis)

Meaning of Name

Abductor refers to the action of abduction, *pollicis* means "thumb," and *brevis* means "shorter."

Location

Abductor pollicis brevis is located in the lateral aspect of the superficial thenar eminence.

Origin and Insertion

Origin: scaphoid, trapezium, and the flexor retinaculum
Insertion: base of the proximal phalanx of the thumb

Actions

Abduction of the thumb at the CMC joint

Explanation of Actions

This muscle pulls the proximal phalanx of the thumb toward the flexor retinaculum, causing abduction. This movement takes the thumb out of the plane of the hand and moves it anteriorly. The more lateral position of the muscle, compared with flexor pollicis brevis, accounts for the difference in the actions of these two muscles.

Notable Muscle Facts

Abductor pollicis brevis and flexor pollicis brevis lie side by side, making up the superficial portion of the mound that is the thenar eminence.

Implications of Shortened and/or Lengthened/Weak Muscle

Shortened: Limited adduction of the thumb is noted.
Lengthened: Limited ability to abduct the thumb is noted.

Palpation and Massage

Palpating and applying pressure to the lateral aspect of the superficial thenar eminence allows us to find and address abductor pollicis brevis.

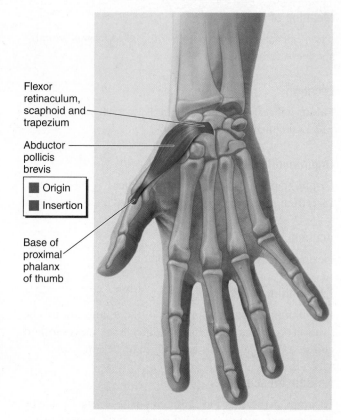

Flexor retinaculum, scaphoid and trapezium

Abductor pollicis brevis

■ Origin
■ Insertion

Base of proximal phalanx of thumb

FIGURE 3-74 · Abductor pollicis brevis

How to Stretch This Muscle

Adduct the thumb.

Synergists

Abductor pollicis longus

Antagonists

Adductor pollicis

Innervation and Arterial Supply

Innervation: median nerve
Arterial supply: radial artery

OPPONENS DIGITI MINIMI (o-po-nenz dij-i-ti min-i-mi)

Meaning of Name

Opponens refers to the action of opposition. *Digiti* means "digit," and *minimi* means "smallest." Thus, this muscle performs opposition of the smallest or fifth digit.

Location

This muscle is the deepest in the hypothenar eminence, which is the mound of tissue that covers the area superficial to the fifth metacarpal.

Origin and Insertion

Origin: flexor retinaculum and hook of the hamate
Insertion: medial border of the fifth metacarpal

Actions

Opposition of the fifth digit at the CMC joint, including flexion, adduction, and very slight lateral rotation of the CMC joint

Explanation of Actions

This muscle pulls the lateral border of the fifth metacarpal toward the flexor retinaculum, and thus the fifth digit is pulled anteriorly and laterally, resulting in opposition of the fifth digit.

Notable Muscle Facts

Only two muscles in the body are said to perform the action of opposition, opponens pollicis and opponens digiti minimi. Thus, only two joints are said to permit opposition. The CMC joint of the fifth digit allows a slight bit of lateral rotation, as well as flexion and adduction (radial deviation). When these movements are combined with opposition of the thumb, the palmar surface over the distal phalanx of the fifth digit meets the palmar surface of the first digit.

Implications of Shortening and/or Lengthening/ Weak Muscle

Shortened: Limited extension and/or abduction of the fifth digit is noted.
Lengthened: Difficulty performing the action of opposition of the fifth digit is present.

Palpation and Massage

Providing pressure into the hypothenar eminence, intending to affect the muscle deep to flexor digiti minimi and abductor digiti minimi, will affect opponens digit minimi.

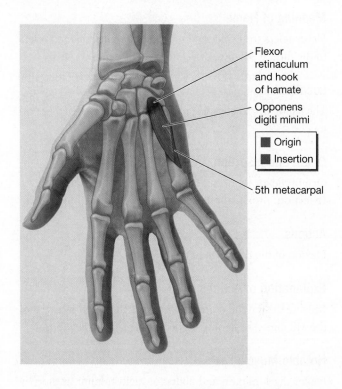

Flexor retinaculum and hook of hamate
Opponens digiti minimi
■ Origin
■ Insertion
5th metacarpal

FIGURE 3-75 · Opponens digiti minimi

How to Stretch This Muscle

Abduct and extend the fifth digit.

Synergists

Flexor digiti minimi and palmar interossei

Antagonists

Extensor digiti minimi and abductor digiti minimi

Innervation and Arterial Supply

Innervation: ulnar nerve
Arterial supply: ulnar artery

FLEXOR DIGITI MINIMI (flek-sor dij-i-ti min-i-mi)

Meaning of Name

Flexor refers to the action of flexion, and *digiti minimi* refers to the fifth or smallest digit.

Location

The lateral or radial aspect of the superficial hypothenar eminence

Origin and Insertion

Origin: flexor retinaculum and hook of the hamate
Insertion: proximal phalanx of the fifth digit

Actions

Flexion of the fifth digit at the MP joint

Explanation of Actions

Because the tendon of insertion crosses the anterior aspect of the MP joint, shortening of the muscle permits flexion.

Notable Muscle Facts

Flexor digiti minimi and abductor digiti minimi lie side by side, making up the superficial portion of the mound that is the hypothenar eminence.

Implications of Shortening and/or Lengthening/ Weak Muscle

Shortened: Limited ability to extend the fifth digit is noted.
Lengthened: No particular postural or functional limits is noticed.

Palpation and Massage

Palpating and applying pressure to the lateral aspect of the hypothenar eminence will address flexor digiti minimi.

How to Stretch This Muscle

Extend the fifth digit.

Synergists

Flexor digitorum profundus and flexor digitorum superficialis

Antagonists

Extensor digiti minimi

Innervation and Arterial Supply

Innervation: ulnar nerve
Arterial supply: ulnar artery

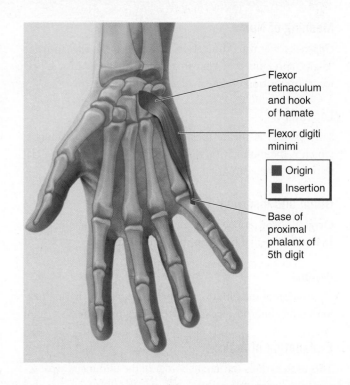

Flexor retinaculum and hook of hamate

Flexor digiti minimi

■ Origin
■ Insertion

Base of proximal phalanx of 5th digit

FIGURE 3-76 · Flexor digiti minimi

ABDUCTOR DIGITI MINIMI (ab-duk-tor dij-i-ti min-i-mi)

Meaning of Name

Abductor refers to the action of abduction, and *digiti minimi* refers to the fifth or smallest digit.

Location

Abductor digiti minimi is located in the medial aspect of the hypothenar eminence.

Origin and Insertion

Origin: pisiform
Insertion: medial aspect of the base of the proximal phalanx of the fifth digit

Actions

Abduction of the fifth digit

Explanation of Actions

This muscle pulls the medial side of the proximal phalanx of the fifth digit toward the pisiform, causing the fifth digit to be pulled medially, resulting in abduction. This muscle works in conjunction with dorsal interossei to allow abduction of all of the fingers of the hand.

Notable Muscle Facts

Abductor digiti minimi and flexor digiti minimi lie side by side, making up the superficial portion of the mound that is the hypothenar eminence.

Implications of Shortening and/or Lengthening/ Weak Muscle

Shortened: Difficulty adducting the fifth digit is present.
Lengthened: Difficulty abducting the fifth digit fully is present.

Palpation and Massage

Palpating and applying pressure to the medial aspect of the hypothenar eminence allow us to find and address this muscle.

How to Stretch This Muscle

Adduct the fifth digit.

Synergists

No synergists

Antagonists

One of the palmar interosseus muscles

Innervation and Arterial Supply

Innervation: ulnar nerve
Arterial supply: ulnar artery

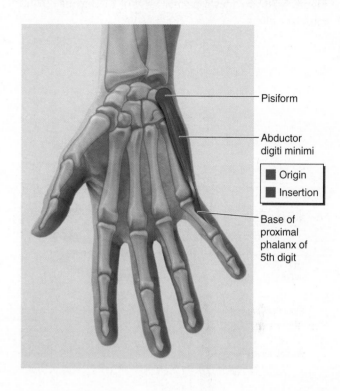

Pisiform

Abductor digiti minimi

■ Origin
■ Insertion

Base of proximal phalanx of 5th digit

FIGURE 3-77 · Abductor digiti minimi

REGIONAL ILLUSTRATIONS OF MUSCLES

Figure 3-78 provides a palmar view of the intrinsic hand muscles.

ILLUSTRATIONS OF NERVE SUPPLY AND ARTERIAL SUPPLY TO UPPER LIMB

Figure 3-79 shows the nerves and arterial supply of the upper limb.

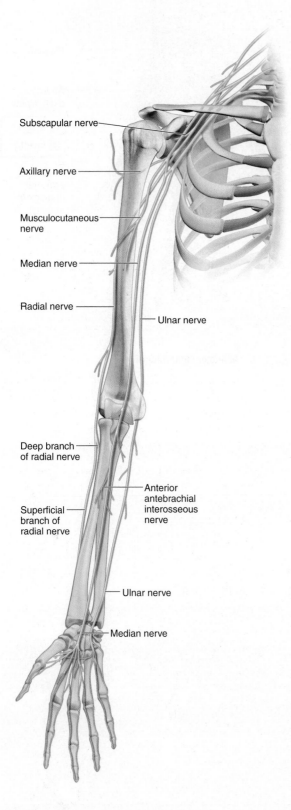

FIGURE 3-78 · **Nerve supply to upper limb**

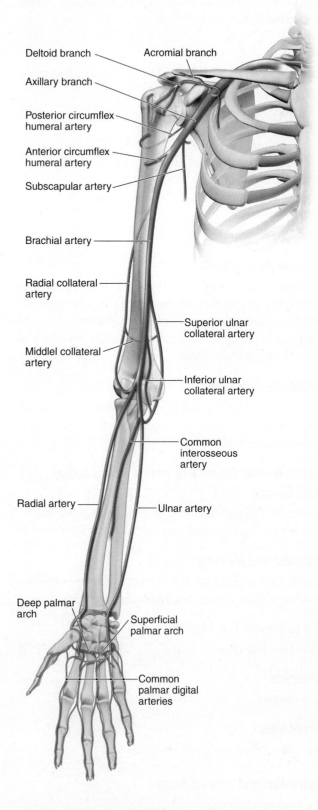

FIGURE 3-79 · **Arterial supply to upper limb**

This chapter provides you with a multitude of information about the bones and joints of the upper extremity and the muscles that move the arm, scapula, elbow, wrist, fingers, and thumb. Much of the information presented is straightforward and factual in nature and can be memorized. However, the application of this knowledge to massage therapy requires a thorough understanding of the muscles' movements and careful thinking about their ability to produce postural and functional imbalances in the body.

■ WORKBOOK

Muscle Drawing Exercises

CORACOBRACHIALIS

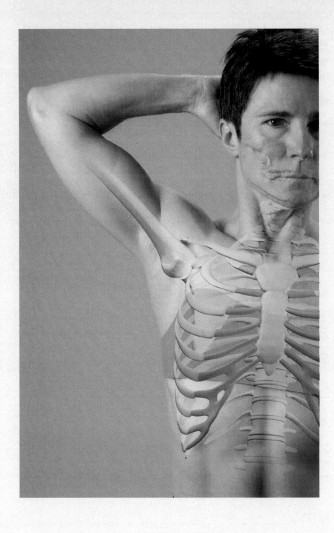

ORIGIN: _____

INSERTION: _____

ACTION(S): _____

NERVE: _____

ARTERIAL SUPPLY: _____

LOCATION AND/OR HOW TO PALPATE:

_____
_____
_____
_____

WHEN MUSCLE IS SHORTENED:

_____
_____
_____

WHEN MUSCLE IS LENGTHENED:

_____
_____
_____

HOW TO STRETCH THIS MUSCLE:

_____
_____

SYNERGIST(S):

_____
_____

ANTAGONIST(S):

_____
_____
_____

NOTES: _____

_____
_____
_____

PECTORALIS MAJOR

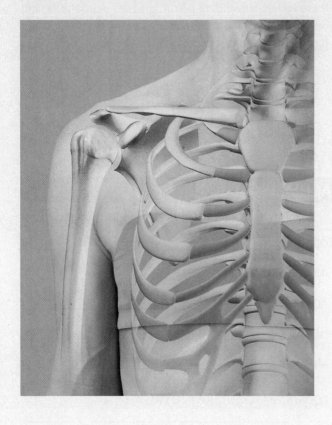

ORIGIN: _____

INSERTION: _____

ACTION(S): _____

NERVE: _____

ARTERIAL SUPPLY: _____

LOCATION AND/OR HOW TO PALPATE:
_____
_____
_____
_____
_____

WHEN MUSCLE IS SHORTENED:
_____
_____
_____
_____

WHEN MUSCLE IS LENGTHENED:
_____
_____
_____
_____

HOW TO STRETCH THIS MUSCLE:
_____
_____

SYNERGIST(S):
_____
_____

ANTAGONIST(S):
_____
_____
_____

NOTES: _____
_____
_____
_____
_____
_____
_____

DELTOID (Anterior)

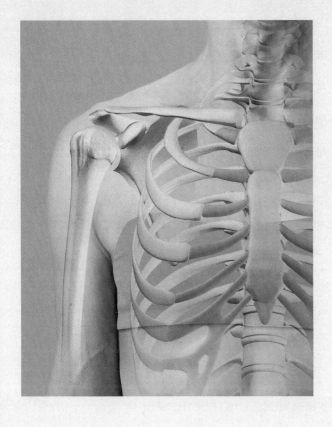

ORIGIN: _____

INSERTION: _____

ACTION(S): _____

NERVE: _____

ARTERIAL SUPPLY: _____

LOCATION AND/OR HOW TO PALPATE:
_____
_____
_____
_____
_____

WHEN MUSCLE IS SHORTENED:
_____
_____
_____
_____

WHEN MUSCLE IS LENGTHENED:
_____
_____
_____
_____

HOW TO STRETCH THIS MUSCLE:
_____
_____

SYNERGIST(S):
_____
_____

ANTAGONIST(S):
_____
_____
_____
_____

NOTES: _____
_____
_____
_____
_____
_____

DELTOID (Middle)

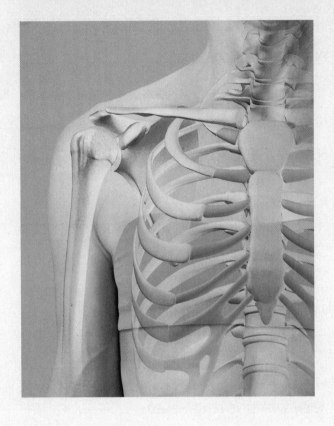

ORIGIN: _____

INSERTION: _____

ACTION(S): _____

NERVE: _____

ARTERIAL SUPPLY: _____

LOCATION AND/OR HOW TO PALPATE:

_____
_____
_____
_____
_____

WHEN MUSCLE IS SHORTENED:

_____
_____
_____
_____

WHEN MUSCLE IS LENGTHENED:

_____
_____
_____
_____

HOW TO STRETCH THIS MUSCLE:

_____
_____

SYNERGIST(S):

_____
_____

ANTAGONIST(S):

_____
_____
_____
_____

NOTES: _____

_____
_____
_____
_____
_____

DELTOID (Posterior)

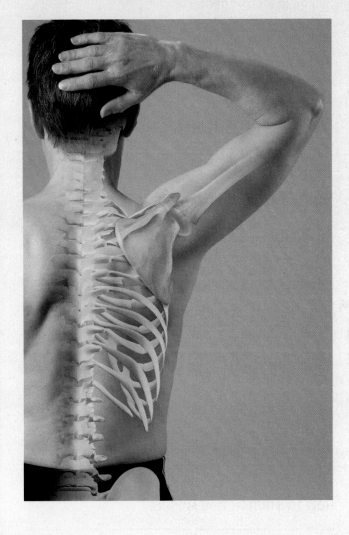

ORIGIN: _____

INSERTION: _____

ACTION(S): _____

NERVE: _____

ARTERIAL SUPPLY: _____

LOCATION AND/OR HOW TO PALPATE:
_____
_____
_____
_____
_____

WHEN MUSCLE IS SHORTENED:
_____
_____
_____
_____

WHEN MUSCLE IS LENGTHENED:
_____
_____
_____
_____

HOW TO STRETCH THIS MUSCLE:
_____
_____

SYNERGIST(S):
_____
_____

ANTAGONIST(S):
_____
_____
_____

NOTES: _____
_____
_____
_____
_____
_____

SUPRASPINATUS

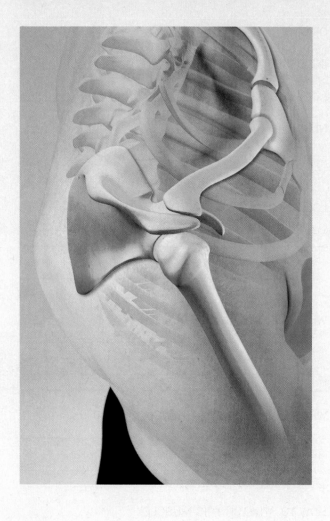

ORIGIN: _____

INSERTION: _____

ACTION(S): _____

NERVE: _____

ARTERIAL SUPPLY: _____

LOCATION AND/OR HOW TO PALPATE:
_____
_____
_____
_____
_____

WHEN MUSCLE IS SHORTENED:
_____
_____
_____
_____

WHEN MUSCLE IS LENGTHENED:
_____
_____
_____
_____

HOW TO STRETCH THIS MUSCLE:
_____
_____

SYNERGIST(S):
_____
_____

ANTAGONIST(S):
_____
_____
_____

NOTES: _____
_____
_____
_____
_____
_____

INFRASPINATUS

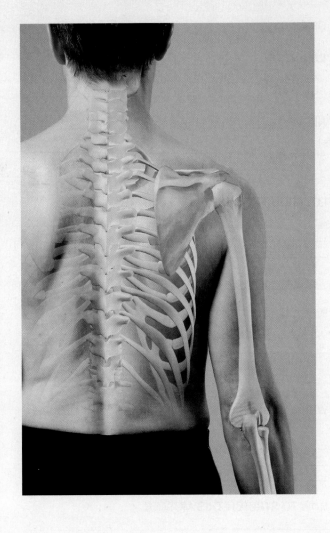

ORIGIN: _____

INSERTION: _____

ACTION(S): _____

NERVE: _____

ARTERIAL SUPPLY: _____

LOCATION AND/OR HOW TO PALPATE:
_____
_____
_____
_____
_____

WHEN MUSCLE IS SHORTENED:
_____
_____
_____
_____

WHEN MUSCLE IS LENGTHENED:
_____
_____
_____
_____

HOW TO STRETCH THIS MUSCLE:
_____
_____

SYNERGIST(S):
_____
_____

ANTAGONIST(S):
_____
_____
_____

NOTES: _____
_____
_____
_____
_____
_____

TERES MINOR

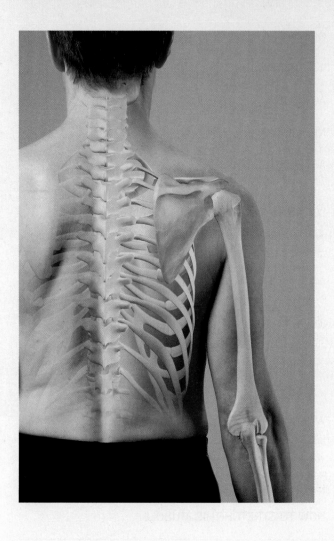

ORIGIN: _____

INSERTION: _____

ACTION(S): _____

NERVE: _____

ARTERIAL SUPPLY: _____

LOCATION AND/OR HOW TO PALPATE:

_____
_____
_____
_____
_____

WHEN MUSCLE IS SHORTENED:

_____
_____
_____
_____

WHEN MUSCLE IS LENGTHENED:

_____
_____
_____
_____

HOW TO STRETCH THIS MUSCLE:

_____
_____

SYNERGIST(S):

_____
_____

ANTAGONIST(S):

_____
_____
_____

NOTES: _____
_____
_____
_____
_____
_____

SUBSCAPULARIS

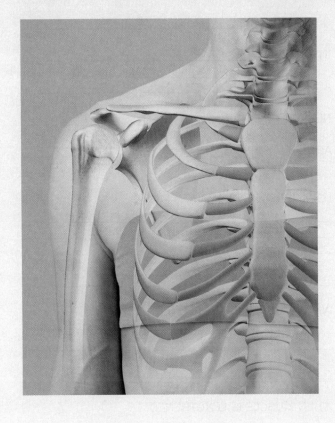

ORIGIN: _____

INSERTION: _____

ACTION(S): _____

NERVE: _____

ARTERIAL SUPPLY: _____

LOCATION AND/OR HOW TO PALPATE:

_____
_____
_____
_____
_____

WHEN MUSCLE IS SHORTENED:

_____
_____
_____
_____

WHEN MUSCLE IS LENGTHENED:

_____
_____
_____
_____

HOW TO STRETCH THIS MUSCLE:

_____
_____

SYNERGIST(S):

_____
_____

ANTAGONIST(S):

_____
_____
_____

NOTES: _____
_____
_____
_____
_____
_____

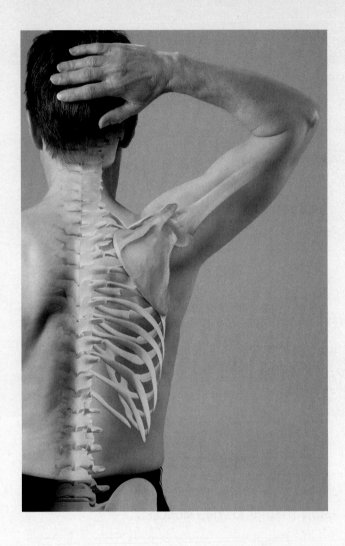

ORIGIN: _____

INSERTION: _____

ACTION(S): _____

NERVE: _____

ARTERIAL SUPPLY: _____

LOCATION AND/OR HOW TO PALPATE:
_____
_____
_____
_____
_____

WHEN MUSCLE IS SHORTENED:
_____
_____
_____
_____

WHEN MUSCLE IS LENGTHENED:
_____
_____
_____
_____

HOW TO STRETCH THIS MUSCLE:
_____
_____

SYNERGIST(S):
_____
_____

ANTAGONIST(S):
_____
_____
_____
_____

NOTES: _____
_____
_____
_____
_____
_____
_____

TERES MAJOR

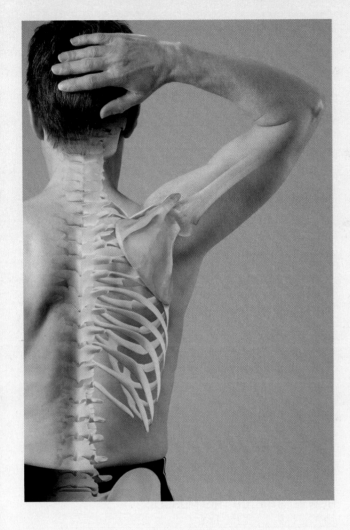

ORIGIN: _____

INSERTION: _____

ACTION(S): _____

NERVE: _____

ARTERIAL SUPPLY: _____

LOCATION AND/OR HOW TO PALPATE:
_____
_____
_____
_____
_____

WHEN MUSCLE IS SHORTENED:
_____
_____
_____
_____

WHEN MUSCLE IS LENGTHENED:
_____
_____
_____
_____

HOW TO STRETCH THIS MUSCLE:
_____
_____

SYNERGIST(S):
_____
_____

ANTAGONIST(S):
_____
_____
_____

NOTES: _____
_____
_____
_____
_____
_____

SERRATUS ANTERIOR

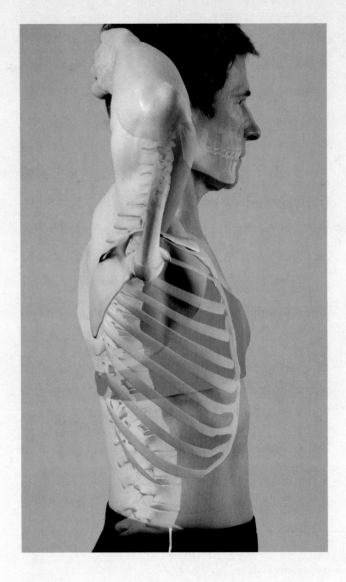

ORIGIN: _____

INSERTION: _____

ACTION(S): _____

NERVE: _____

ARTERIAL SUPPLY: _____

LOCATION AND/OR HOW TO PALPATE:
_____
_____
_____
_____
_____

WHEN MUSCLE IS SHORTENED:
_____
_____
_____
_____

WHEN MUSCLE IS LENGTHENED:
_____
_____
_____
_____

HOW TO STRETCH THIS MUSCLE:
_____
_____

SYNERGIST(S):
_____
_____

ANTAGONIST(S):
_____
_____
_____
_____

NOTES: _____
_____
_____
_____
_____
_____

PECTORALIS MINOR

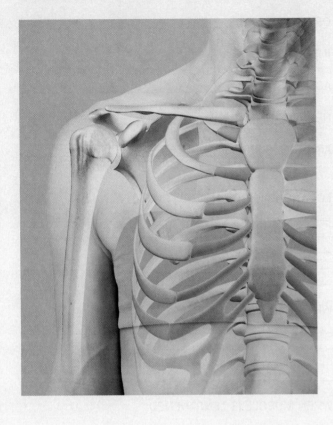

ORIGIN: _____

INSERTION: _____

ACTION(S): _____

NERVE: _____

ARTERIAL SUPPLY: _____

LOCATION AND/OR HOW TO PALPATE:

_____
_____
_____
_____
_____

WHEN MUSCLE IS SHORTENED:

_____
_____
_____
_____

WHEN MUSCLE IS LENGTHENED:

_____
_____
_____
_____

HOW TO STRETCH THIS MUSCLE:

_____
_____

SYNERGIST(S):

_____
_____

ANTAGONIST(S):

_____
_____
_____

NOTES: _____
_____
_____
_____
_____
_____

LEVATOR SCAPULA

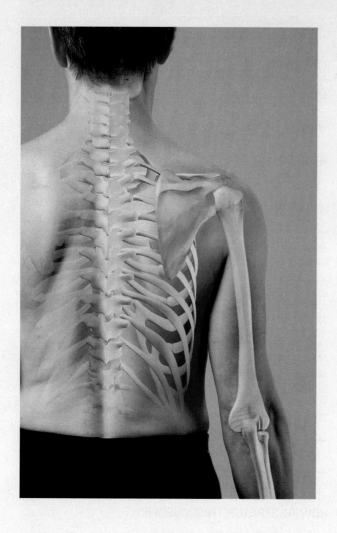

ORIGIN: _____

INSERTION: _____

ACTION(S): _____

NERVE: _____

ARTERIAL SUPPLY: _____

LOCATION AND/OR HOW TO PALPATE:

_____
_____
_____
_____
_____

WHEN MUSCLE IS SHORTENED:

_____
_____
_____
_____

WHEN MUSCLE IS LENGTHENED:

_____
_____
_____
_____

HOW TO STRETCH THIS MUSCLE:

_____
_____

SYNERGIST(S):

_____
_____

ANTAGONIST(S):

_____
_____
_____
_____

NOTES: _____
_____
_____
_____
_____
_____

RHOMBOIDS MAJOR AND MINOR

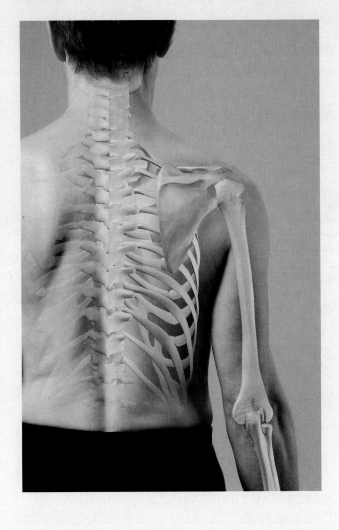

ORIGIN: _____

INSERTION: _____

ACTION(S): _____

NERVE: _____

ARTERIAL SUPPLY: _____

LOCATION AND/OR HOW TO PALPATE:
_____
_____
_____
_____
_____

WHEN MUSCLE IS SHORTENED:
_____
_____
_____
_____

WHEN MUSCLE IS LENGTHENED:
_____
_____
_____
_____

HOW TO STRETCH THIS MUSCLE:
_____
_____

SYNERGIST(S):
_____
_____

ANTAGONIST(S):
_____
_____
_____
_____

NOTES: _____
_____
_____
_____
_____
_____

TRAPEZIUS

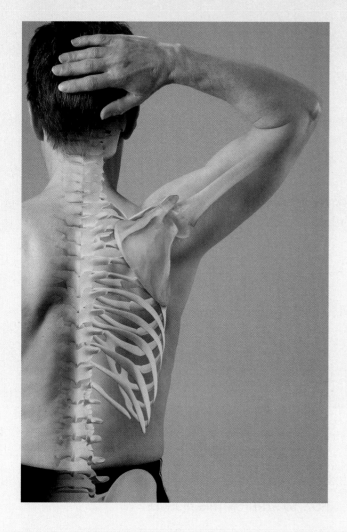

ORIGIN: _____

INSERTION: _____

ACTION(S): _____

NERVE: _____

ARTERIAL SUPPLY: _____

LOCATION AND/OR HOW TO PALPATE:
_____
_____
_____
_____
_____

WHEN MUSCLE IS SHORTENED:
_____
_____
_____
_____

WHEN MUSCLE IS LENGTHENED:
_____
_____
_____
_____

HOW TO STRETCH THIS MUSCLE:
_____
_____

SYNERGIST(S):
_____
_____

ANTAGONIST(S):
_____
_____
_____

NOTES: _____
_____
_____
_____
_____
_____

BRACHIALIS

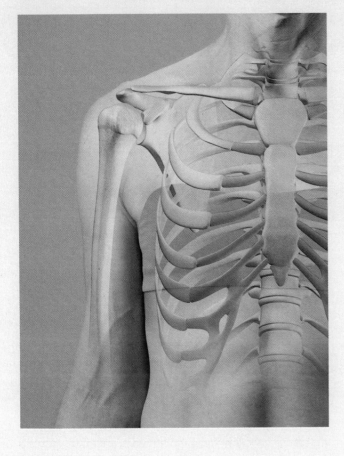

ORIGIN: _____

INSERTION: _____

ACTION(S): _____

NERVE: _____

ARTERIAL SUPPLY: _____

LOCATION AND/OR HOW TO PALPATE:
_____
_____
_____
_____
_____

WHEN MUSCLE IS SHORTENED:
_____
_____
_____
_____

WHEN MUSCLE IS LENGTHENED:
_____
_____
_____
_____

HOW TO STRETCH THIS MUSCLE:
_____
_____

SYNERGIST(S):
_____
_____

ANTAGONIST(S):
_____
_____
_____

NOTES: _____
_____
_____
_____
_____
_____

BICEPS BRACHII

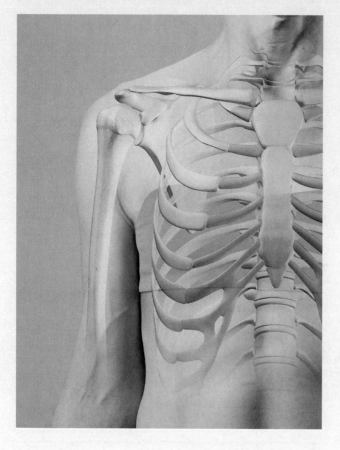

ORIGIN: _____

INSERTION: _____

ACTION(S): _____

NERVE: _____

ARTERIAL SUPPLY: _____

LOCATION AND/OR HOW TO PALPATE:
_____
_____
_____
_____
_____

WHEN MUSCLE IS SHORTENED:
_____
_____
_____
_____

WHEN MUSCLE IS LENGTHENED:
_____
_____
_____
_____

HOW TO STRETCH THIS MUSCLE:
_____
_____

SYNERGIST(S):
_____
_____

ANTAGONIST(S):
_____
_____
_____

NOTES: _____
_____
_____
_____
_____
_____
_____

BRACHIORADIALIS

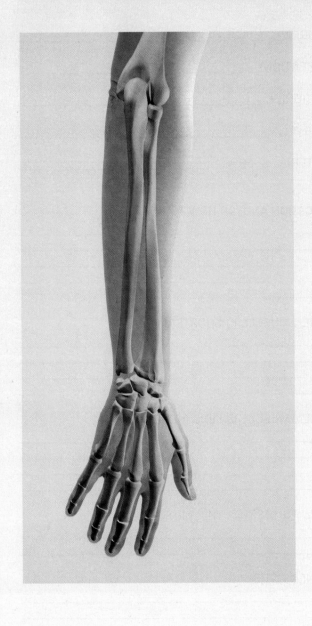

ORIGIN: _____

INSERTION: _____

ACTION(S): _____

NERVE: _____

ARTERIAL SUPPLY: _____

LOCATION AND/OR HOW TO PALPATE:
_____
_____
_____
_____
_____

WHEN MUSCLE IS SHORTENED:
_____
_____
_____
_____

WHEN MUSCLE IS LENGTHENED:
_____
_____
_____
_____

HOW TO STRETCH THIS MUSCLE:
_____
_____

SYNERGIST(S):
_____
_____

ANTAGONIST(S):
_____
_____
_____

NOTES: _____
_____
_____
_____
_____
_____

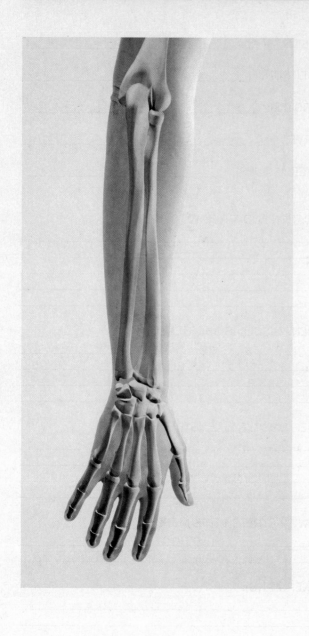

ORIGIN: _____

INSERTION: _____

ACTION(S): _____

NERVE: _____

ARTERIAL SUPPLY: _____

LOCATION AND/OR HOW TO PALPATE:
_____
_____
_____
_____
_____

WHEN MUSCLE IS SHORTENED:
_____
_____
_____
_____

WHEN MUSCLE IS LENGTHENED:
_____
_____
_____
_____

HOW TO STRETCH THIS MUSCLE:
_____
_____

SYNERGIST(S):
_____
_____

ANTAGONIST(S):
_____
_____
_____

NOTES: _____
_____
_____
_____
_____
_____
_____

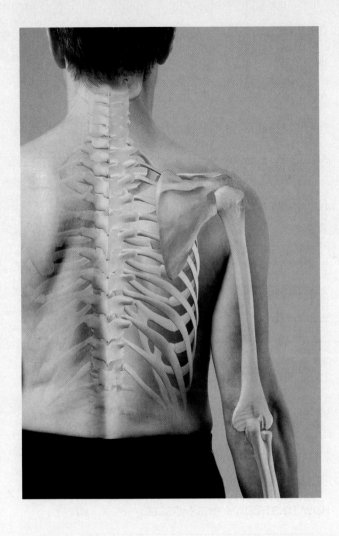

ORIGIN: _____

INSERTION: _____

ACTION(S): _____

NERVE: _____

ARTERIAL SUPPLY: _____

LOCATION AND/OR HOW TO PALPATE:
_____
_____
_____
_____
_____

WHEN MUSCLE IS SHORTENED:
_____
_____
_____
_____

WHEN MUSCLE IS LENGTHENED:
_____
_____
_____
_____

HOW TO STRETCH THIS MUSCLE:
_____
_____

SYNERGIST(S):
_____
_____

ANTAGONIST(S):
_____
_____
_____
_____

NOTES: _____
_____
_____
_____
_____
_____

SUPINATOR

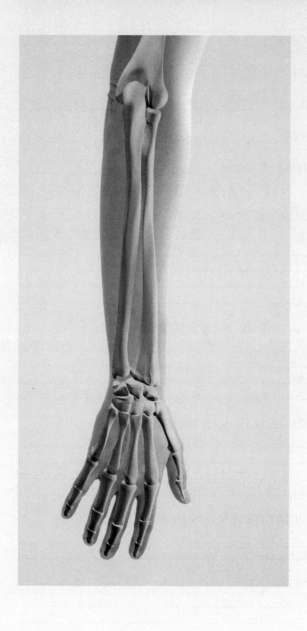

ORIGIN: _____

INSERTION: _____

ACTION(S): _____

NERVE: _____

ARTERIAL SUPPLY: _____

LOCATION AND/OR HOW TO PALPATE:
_____
_____
_____
_____
_____

WHEN MUSCLE IS SHORTENED:
_____
_____
_____

WHEN MUSCLE IS LENGTHENED:
_____
_____
_____
_____

HOW TO STRETCH THIS MUSCLE:
_____
_____

SYNERGIST(S):
_____
_____

ANTAGONIST(S):
_____
_____
_____
_____

NOTES: _____
_____
_____
_____
_____
_____

PRONATOR TERES

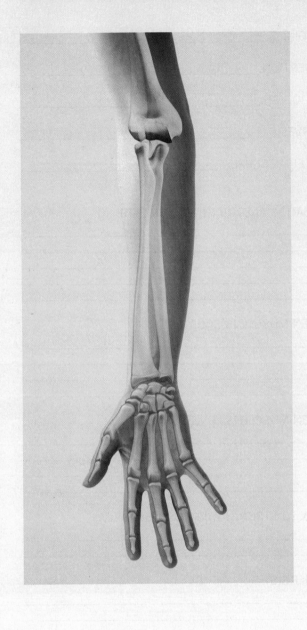

ORIGIN: _____

INSERTION: _____

ACTION(S): _____

NERVE: _____

ARTERIAL SUPPLY: _____

LOCATION AND/OR HOW TO PALPATE:
_____
_____
_____
_____
_____

WHEN MUSCLE IS SHORTENED:
_____
_____
_____
_____

WHEN MUSCLE IS LENGTHENED:
_____
_____
_____
_____

HOW TO STRETCH THIS MUSCLE:
_____
_____

SYNERGIST(S):
_____
_____

ANTAGONIST(S):
_____
_____
_____
_____

NOTES: _____
_____
_____
_____
_____
_____

PRONATOR QUADRATUS

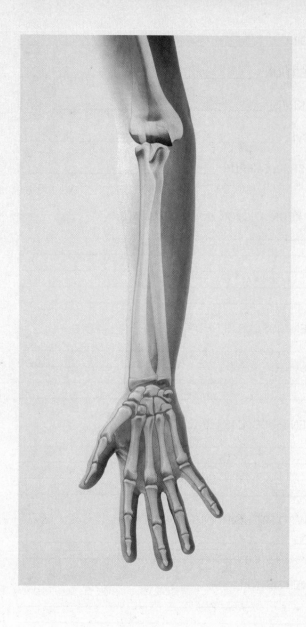

ORIGIN: _____

INSERTION: _____

ACTION(S): _____

NERVE: _____

ARTERIAL SUPPLY: _____

LOCATION AND/OR HOW TO PALPATE:
_____
_____
_____
_____
_____

WHEN MUSCLE IS SHORTENED:
_____
_____
_____
_____

WHEN MUSCLE IS LENGTHENED:
_____
_____
_____
_____

HOW TO STRETCH THIS MUSCLE:
_____
_____

SYNERGIST(S):
_____
_____

ANTAGONIST(S):
_____
_____
_____
_____

NOTES: _____
_____
_____
_____
_____
_____

EXTENSOR CARPI RADIALIS LONGUS

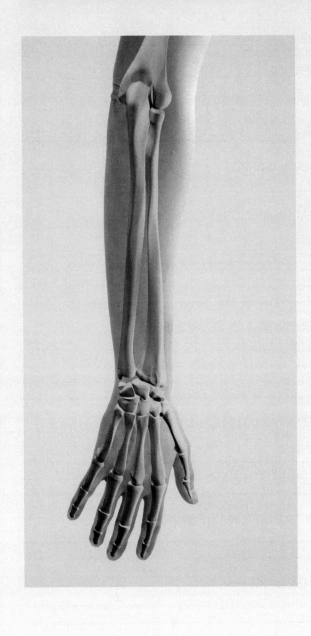

ORIGIN: _____

INSERTION: _____

ACTION(S): _____

NERVE: _____

ARTERIAL SUPPLY: _____

LOCATION AND/OR HOW TO PALPATE:
_____
_____
_____
_____
_____

WHEN MUSCLE IS SHORTENED:
_____
_____
_____
_____

WHEN MUSCLE IS LENGTHENED:
_____
_____
_____
_____

HOW TO STRETCH THIS MUSCLE:
_____
_____

SYNERGIST(S):
_____
_____

ANTAGONIST(S):
_____
_____
_____
_____

NOTES: _____
_____
_____
_____
_____
_____
_____

EXTENSOR CARPI RADIALIS BREVIS

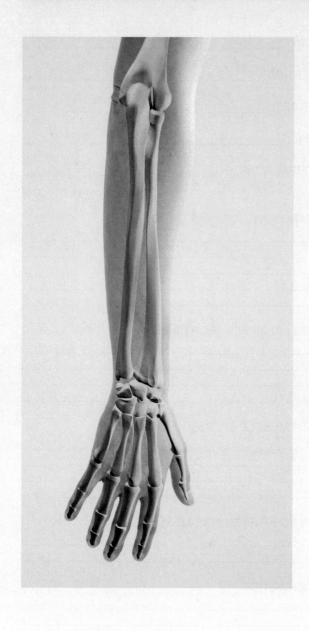

ORIGIN: _____

INSERTION: _____

ACTION(S): _____

NERVE: _____

ARTERIAL SUPPLY: _____

LOCATION AND/OR HOW TO PALPATE:

_____
_____
_____
_____

WHEN MUSCLE IS SHORTENED:

_____
_____
_____
_____

WHEN MUSCLE IS LENGTHENED:

_____
_____
_____
_____

HOW TO STRETCH THIS MUSCLE:

_____
_____

SYNERGIST(S):

_____

ANTAGONIST(S):

_____
_____
_____
_____

NOTES: _____
_____
_____
_____
_____
_____
_____

EXTENSOR CARPI ULNARIS

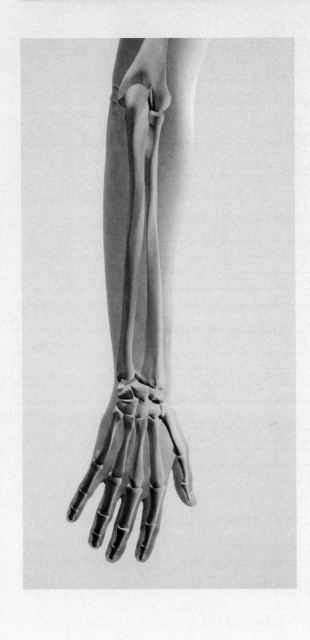

ORIGIN: _____

INSERTION: _____

ACTION(S): _____

NERVE: _____

ARTERIAL SUPPLY: _____

LOCATION AND/OR HOW TO PALPATE:
_____
_____
_____
_____
_____

WHEN MUSCLE IS SHORTENED:
_____
_____
_____
_____

WHEN MUSCLE IS LENGTHENED:
_____
_____
_____
_____

HOW TO STRETCH THIS MUSCLE:
_____
_____

SYNERGIST(S):
_____
_____

ANTAGONIST(S):
_____
_____
_____
_____

NOTES: _____
_____
_____
_____
_____
_____

FLEXOR CARPI RADIALIS

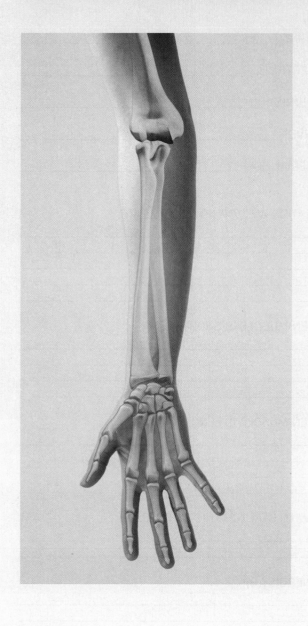

ORIGIN: _____

INSERTION: _____

ACTION(S): _____

NERVE: _____

ARTERIAL SUPPLY: _____

LOCATION AND/OR HOW TO PALPATE:
_____
_____
_____
_____
_____

WHEN MUSCLE IS SHORTENED:
_____
_____
_____
_____

WHEN MUSCLE IS LENGTHENED:
_____
_____
_____
_____

HOW TO STRETCH THIS MUSCLE:
_____
_____

SYNERGIST(S):
_____
_____

ANTAGONIST(S):
_____
_____
_____
_____

NOTES: _____
_____
_____
_____
_____
_____
_____

FLEXOR CARPI ULNARIS

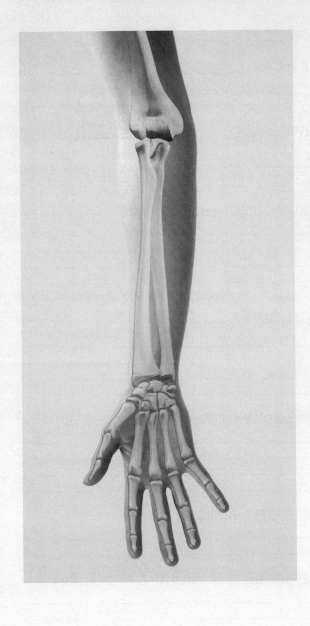

ORIGIN: _____

INSERTION: _____

ACTION(S): _____

NERVE: _____

ARTERIAL SUPPLY: _____

LOCATION AND/OR HOW TO PALPATE:

_____
_____
_____
_____
_____

WHEN MUSCLE IS SHORTENED:

_____
_____
_____
_____

WHEN MUSCLE IS LENGTHENED:

_____
_____
_____
_____

HOW TO STRETCH THIS MUSCLE:

_____
_____

SYNERGIST(S):

_____

ANTAGONIST(S):

_____
_____
_____
_____

NOTES: _____

_____
_____
_____
_____
_____

PALMARIS LONGUS

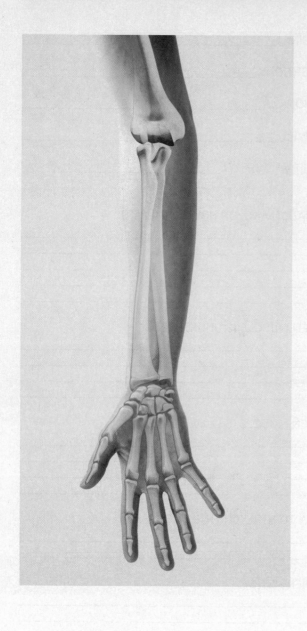

ORIGIN: _____

INSERTION: _____

ACTION(S): _____

NERVE: _____

ARTERIAL SUPPLY: _____

LOCATION AND/OR HOW TO PALPATE:
_____
_____
_____
_____

WHEN MUSCLE IS SHORTENED:
_____
_____
_____
_____

WHEN MUSCLE IS LENGTHENED:
_____
_____
_____
_____

HOW TO STRETCH THIS MUSCLE:
_____
_____

SYNERGIST(S):
_____
_____

ANTAGONIST(S):
_____
_____
_____
_____

NOTES: _____
_____
_____
_____
_____
_____
_____
_____

ABDUCTOR POLLICIS LONGUS

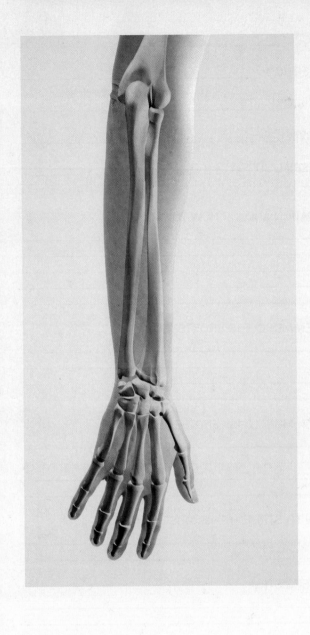

ORIGIN: _____

INSERTION: _____

ACTION(S): _____

NERVE: _____

ARTERIAL SUPPLY: _____

LOCATION AND/OR HOW TO PALPATE:
_____
_____
_____
_____
_____

WHEN MUSCLE IS SHORTENED:
_____
_____
_____
_____

WHEN MUSCLE IS LENGTHENED:
_____
_____
_____
_____

HOW TO STRETCH THIS MUSCLE:
_____
_____

SYNERGIST(S):
_____
_____

ANTAGONIST(S):
_____
_____
_____
_____

NOTES: _____
_____
_____
_____
_____
_____

EXTENSOR POLLICIS BREVIS

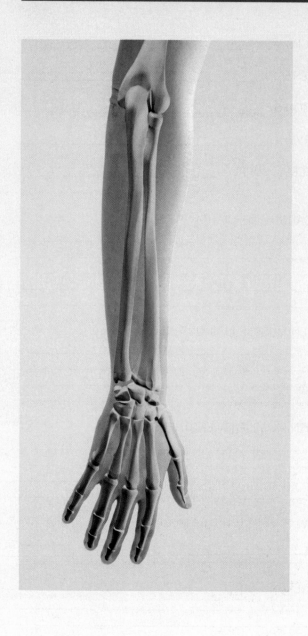

ORIGIN: _____

INSERTION: _____

ACTION(S): _____

NERVE: _____

ARTERIAL SUPPLY: _____

LOCATION AND/OR HOW TO PALPATE:
_____
_____
_____
_____
_____

WHEN MUSCLE IS SHORTENED:
_____
_____
_____
_____

WHEN MUSCLE IS LENGTHENED:
_____
_____
_____
_____

HOW TO STRETCH THIS MUSCLE:
_____
_____

SYNERGIST(S):
_____
_____

ANTAGONIST(S):
_____
_____
_____
_____

NOTES: _____
_____
_____
_____
_____
_____
_____
_____

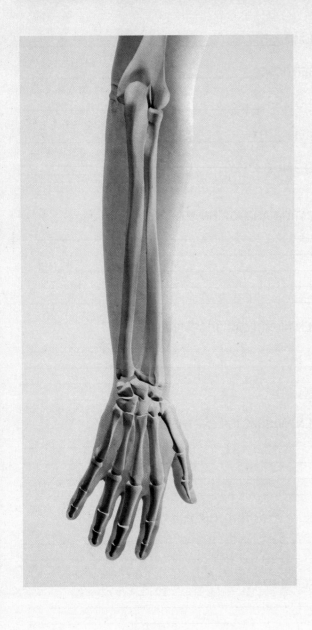

ORIGIN: _____

INSERTION: _____

ACTION(S): _____

NERVE: _____

ARTERIAL SUPPLY: _____

LOCATION AND/OR HOW TO PALPATE:
_____
_____
_____
_____
_____

WHEN MUSCLE IS SHORTENED:
_____
_____
_____
_____

WHEN MUSCLE IS LENGTHENED:
_____
_____
_____
_____

HOW TO STRETCH THIS MUSCLE:
_____
_____

SYNERGIST(S):
_____
_____

ANTAGONIST(S):
_____
_____
_____
_____

NOTES: _____
_____
_____
_____
_____
_____
_____

EXTENSOR INDICIS

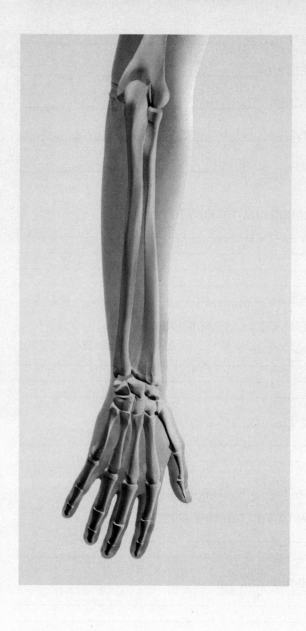

ORIGIN: _____

INSERTION: _____

ACTION(S): _____

NERVE: _____

ARTERIAL SUPPLY: _____

LOCATION AND/OR HOW TO PALPATE:
_____
_____
_____
_____
_____

WHEN MUSCLE IS SHORTENED:
_____
_____
_____
_____

WHEN MUSCLE IS LENGTHENED:
_____
_____
_____
_____

HOW TO STRETCH THIS MUSCLE:
_____
_____

SYNERGIST(S):
_____
_____

ANTAGONIST(S):
_____
_____
_____
_____

NOTES: _____
_____
_____
_____
_____
_____

EXTENSOR DIGITORUM

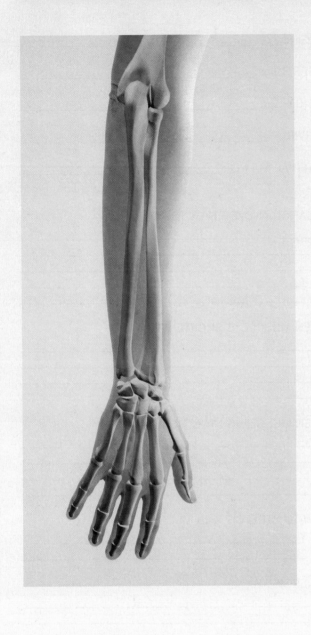

ORIGIN: _____

INSERTION: _____

ACTION(S): _____

NERVE: _____

ARTERIAL SUPPLY: _____

LOCATION AND/OR HOW TO PALPATE:
_____
_____
_____
_____
_____

WHEN MUSCLE IS SHORTENED:
_____
_____
_____
_____

WHEN MUSCLE IS LENGTHENED:
_____
_____
_____
_____

HOW TO STRETCH THIS MUSCLE:
_____
_____

SYNERGIST(S):
_____
_____

ANTAGONIST(S):
_____
_____
_____

NOTES: _____
_____
_____
_____
_____
_____

EXTENSOR DIGITI MINIMI

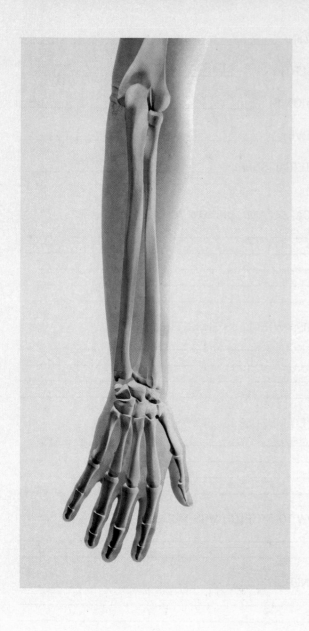

ORIGIN: _____

INSERTION: _____

ACTION(S): _____

NERVE: _____

ARTERIAL SUPPLY: _____

LOCATION AND/OR HOW TO PALPATE:
_____
_____
_____
_____
_____

WHEN MUSCLE IS SHORTENED:
_____
_____
_____
_____

WHEN MUSCLE IS LENGTHENED:
_____
_____
_____
_____

HOW TO STRETCH THIS MUSCLE:
_____
_____

SYNERGIST(S):
_____
_____

ANTAGONIST(S):
_____
_____
_____

NOTES: _____
_____
_____
_____
_____
_____

FLEXOR POLLICIS LONGUS

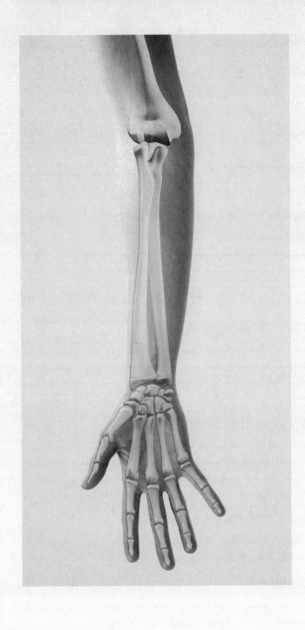

ORIGIN: _____

INSERTION: _____

ACTION(S): _____

NERVE: _____

ARTERIAL SUPPLY: _____

LOCATION AND/OR HOW TO PALPATE:
_____
_____
_____
_____
_____

WHEN MUSCLE IS SHORTENED:
_____
_____
_____
_____

WHEN MUSCLE IS LENGTHENED:
_____
_____
_____
_____

HOW TO STRETCH THIS MUSCLE:
_____
_____

SYNERGIST(S):
_____
_____

ANTAGONIST(S):
_____
_____
_____
_____

NOTES: _____
_____
_____
_____
_____
_____

FLEXOR DIGITORUM PROFUNDUS

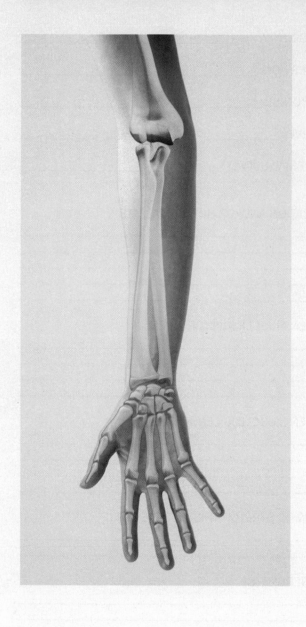

ORIGIN: _____

INSERTION: _____

ACTION(S): _____

NERVE: _____

ARTERIAL SUPPLY: _____

LOCATION AND/OR HOW TO PALPATE:
_____
_____
_____
_____
_____

WHEN MUSCLE IS SHORTENED:
_____
_____
_____
_____

WHEN MUSCLE IS LENGTHENED:
_____
_____
_____
_____

HOW TO STRETCH THIS MUSCLE:
_____
_____

SYNERGIST(S):
_____
_____

ANTAGONIST(S):
_____
_____
_____

NOTES: _____
_____
_____
_____
_____
_____

FLEXOR DIGITORUM SUPERFICIALIS

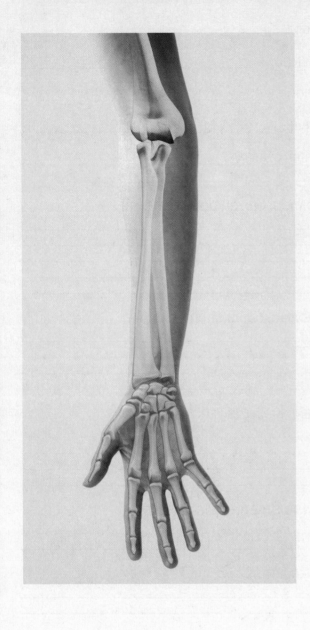

ORIGIN: _____

INSERTION: _____

ACTION(S): _____

NERVE: _____

ARTERIAL SUPPLY: _____

LOCATION AND/OR HOW TO PALPATE:
_____
_____
_____
_____
_____

WHEN MUSCLE IS SHORTENED:
_____
_____
_____
_____

WHEN MUSCLE IS LENGTHENED:
_____
_____
_____
_____

HOW TO STRETCH THIS MUSCLE:
_____
_____

SYNERGIST(S):
_____
_____

ANTAGONIST(S):
_____
_____
_____
_____

NOTES: _____
_____
_____
_____
_____
_____
_____

DORSAL INTEROSSEI

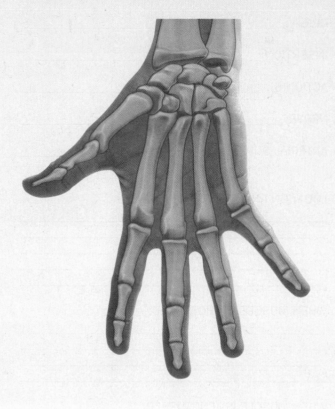

ORIGIN: _____

INSERTION: _____

ACTION(S): _____

NERVE: _____

ARTERIAL SUPPLY: _____

LOCATION AND/OR HOW TO PALPATE:
_____
_____
_____
_____
_____

WHEN MUSCLE IS SHORTENED:
_____
_____
_____
_____

WHEN MUSCLE IS LENGTHENED:
_____
_____
_____
_____

HOW TO STRETCH THIS MUSCLE:
_____
_____
_____

SYNERGIST(S):
_____
_____

ANTAGONIST(S):
_____
_____
_____
_____

NOTES: _____
_____
_____
_____
_____
_____

PALMAR INTEROSSEI

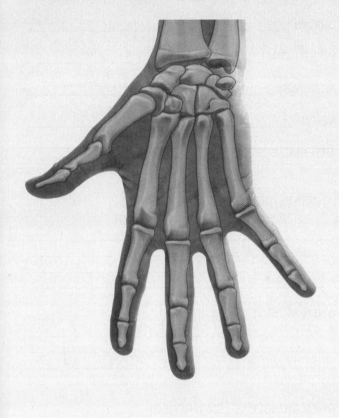

ORIGIN: _____

INSERTION: _____

ACTION(S): _____

NERVE: _____

ARTERIAL SUPPLY: _____

LOCATION AND/OR HOW TO PALPATE:
_____
_____
_____
_____
_____

WHEN MUSCLE IS SHORTENED:
_____
_____
_____
_____

WHEN MUSCLE IS LENGTHENED:
_____
_____
_____
_____

HOW TO STRETCH THIS MUSCLE:
_____
_____

SYNERGIST(S):
_____
_____

ANTAGONIST(S):
_____
_____
_____

NOTES: _____
_____
_____
_____
_____

LUMBRICALS

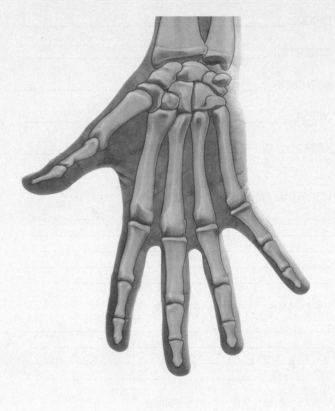

ORIGIN: _____

INSERTION: _____

ACTION(S): _____

NERVE: _____

ARTERIAL SUPPLY: _____

LOCATION AND/OR HOW TO PALPATE:

_____
_____
_____
_____
_____

WHEN MUSCLE IS SHORTENED:

_____
_____
_____
_____

WHEN MUSCLE IS LENGTHENED:

_____
_____
_____
_____

HOW TO STRETCH THIS MUSCLE:

_____
_____

SYNERGIST(S):

_____
_____

ANTAGONIST(S):

_____
_____
_____
_____

NOTES: _____
_____
_____
_____
_____
_____

ADDUCTOR POLLICIS

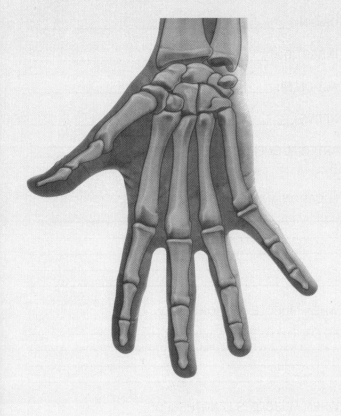

ORIGIN: _____

INSERTION: _____

ACTION(S): _____

NERVE: _____

ARTERIAL SUPPLY: _____

LOCATION AND/OR HOW TO PALPATE:
_____
_____
_____
_____
_____

WHEN MUSCLE IS SHORTENED:
_____
_____
_____
_____

WHEN MUSCLE IS LENGTHENED:
_____
_____
_____
_____

HOW TO STRETCH THIS MUSCLE:
_____
_____

SYNERGIST(S):
_____
_____

ANTAGONIST(S):
_____
_____
_____
_____

NOTES: _____
_____
_____
_____
_____
_____
_____

OPPONENS POLLICIS

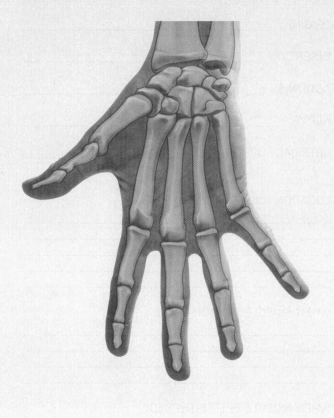

ORIGIN: _____

INSERTION: _____

ACTION(S): _____

NERVE: _____

ARTERIAL SUPPLY: _____

LOCATION AND/OR HOW TO PALPATE:

_____
_____
_____
_____
_____

WHEN MUSCLE IS SHORTENED:

_____
_____
_____
_____

WHEN MUSCLE IS LENGTHENED:

_____
_____
_____
_____

HOW TO STRETCH THIS MUSCLE:

_____
_____

SYNERGIST(S):

_____
_____

ANTAGONIST(S):

_____
_____
_____
_____

NOTES: _____

_____
_____
_____
_____
_____

FLEXOR POLLICIS BREVIS

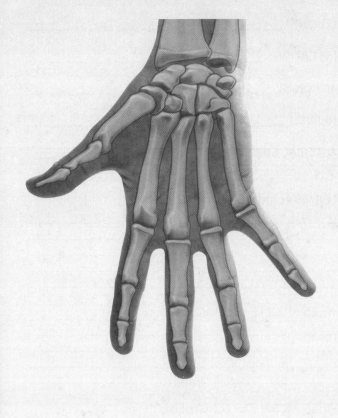

ORIGIN: _____

INSERTION: _____

ACTION(S): _____

NERVE: _____

ARTERIAL SUPPLY: _____

LOCATION AND/OR HOW TO PALPATE:

_____
_____
_____
_____
_____

WHEN MUSCLE IS SHORTENED:

_____
_____
_____
_____

WHEN MUSCLE IS LENGTHENED:

_____
_____
_____
_____

HOW TO STRETCH THIS MUSCLE:

_____
_____

SYNERGIST(S):

_____
_____

ANTAGONIST(S):

_____
_____
_____
_____

NOTES: _____

_____
_____
_____
_____
_____

ABDUCTOR POLLICIS BREVIS

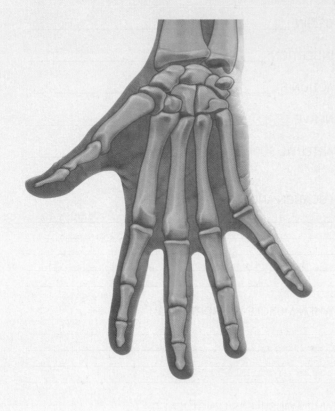

ORIGIN: _____

INSERTION: _____

ACTION(S): _____

NERVE: _____

ARTERIAL SUPPLY: _____

LOCATION AND/OR HOW TO PALPATE:
_____
_____
_____
_____
_____

WHEN MUSCLE IS SHORTENED:
_____
_____
_____
_____

WHEN MUSCLE IS LENGTHENED:
_____
_____
_____
_____

HOW TO STRETCH THIS MUSCLE:
_____
_____

SYNERGIST(S):
_____
_____

ANTAGONIST(S):
_____
_____
_____
_____

NOTES: _____
_____
_____
_____
_____
_____

OPPONENS DIGITI MINIMI

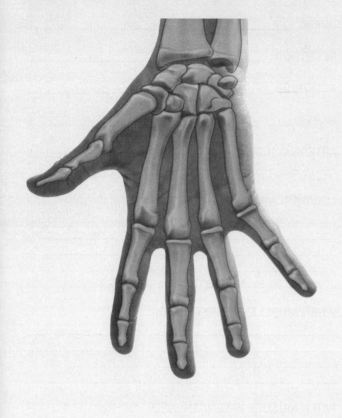

ORIGIN: _____

INSERTION: _____

ACTION(S): _____

NERVE: _____

ARTERIAL SUPPLY: _____

LOCATION AND/OR HOW TO PALPATE:
_____
_____
_____
_____
_____

WHEN MUSCLE IS SHORTENED:
_____
_____
_____
_____

WHEN MUSCLE IS LENGTHENED:
_____
_____
_____
_____

HOW TO STRETCH THIS MUSCLE:
_____
_____

SYNERGIST(S):
_____
_____

ANTAGONIST(S):
_____
_____
_____
_____

NOTES: _____
_____
_____
_____
_____
_____
_____

FLEXOR DIGITI MINIMI

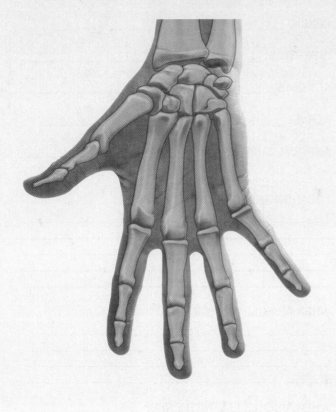

ORIGIN: _____

INSERTION: _____

ACTION(S): _____

NERVE: _____

ARTERIAL SUPPLY: _____

LOCATION AND/OR HOW TO PALPATE:
_____
_____
_____
_____
_____

WHEN MUSCLE IS SHORTENED:
_____
_____
_____
_____

WHEN MUSCLE IS LENGTHENED:
_____
_____
_____
_____

HOW TO STRETCH THIS MUSCLE:
_____
_____

SYNERGIST(S):
_____
_____

ANTAGONIST(S):
_____
_____
_____
_____

NOTES: _____
_____
_____
_____
_____
_____

ABDUCTOR DIGITI MINIMI

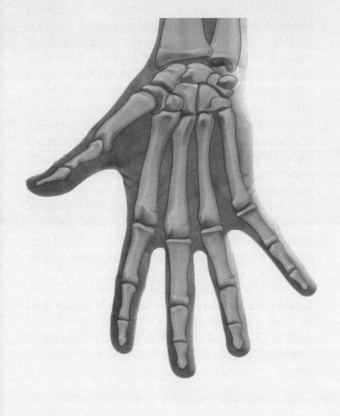

ORIGIN: _____

INSERTION: _____

ACTION(S): _____

NERVE: _____

ARTERIAL SUPPLY: _____

LOCATION AND/OR HOW TO PALPATE:
_____
_____
_____
_____
_____

WHEN MUSCLE IS SHORTENED:
_____
_____
_____
_____

WHEN MUSCLE IS LENGTHENED:
_____
_____
_____
_____

HOW TO STRETCH THIS MUSCLE:
_____
_____

SYNERGIST(S):
_____
_____

ANTAGONIST(S):
_____
_____
_____

NOTES: _____
_____
_____
_____
_____
_____

Palpation Exercises

Palpation of the muscles is important to reinforce their locations and to prepare for the application of muscle knowledge to massage therapy settings.

Palpation Exercise #1

This palpation exercise will require you to locate the bones and bony landmarks related to the following arm-moving muscles: coracobrachialis, pectoralis major, and deltoid. After locating the bony landmarks, you will palpate the muscles, as well.

Bones/Bony Landmarks

1. **Sternum:** Palpate the jugular notch at the superior end of the sternum, and palpate the xiphoid process gently, at the inferior end of the sternum. Where is the gladiolus? Palpate the lateral borders of the sternum, which are joined by the costal cartilage of the ribs. Can you feel the strips of costal cartilage and the spaces between them?

2. **Scapula:** Palpate the whole outline of the scapula, noting the vertebral (medial) and axillary (lateral) borders and the inferior angle. The superior angle is more difficult to palpate, but if you find the spine of the scapula, trace it to its medial edge (this is called the root of the spine of the scapula) and move superiorly about an inch and a half. You will be at the site of the superior angle. Why is the superior angle more difficult to palpate than the inferior angle? Find the acromion by tracing the spine of the scapula laterally until you reach the flattened area of the acromion, or trace the clavicle laterally until you reach the bump at its lateral end, then slip off the clavicle onto the acromion. Finally, find the coracoid process on the anterior scapula. Trace the clavicle laterally until you feel it curve inward; then move inferiorly about an inch and look for the coracoid process. Note the location of the glenoid fossa, where the scapula accepts the head of the humerus.

3. **Clavicle:** Palpate the entire clavicle, noting its shape and noting its medial, lateral, superior, and inferior aspects. Find the AC joint, where the clavicle joins the acromion. (Trace the clavicle laterally. You will likely reach a bump. Slide off this high point onto the flat acromion.) Find the sternoclavicular joint by tracing the clavicle medially until you reach the jugular notch. Move laterally and anteriorly, feeling for the sternoclavicular joint.

4. **Ribs:** Most people have 12 pairs of ribs. Can you trace them from their anterior aspect to their posterior aspect, where they join the thoracic vertebrae? Can you feel the spaces between the ribs?

5. **Bicipital groove of the humerus:** The bicipital groove lies lateral to the coracoid process by less than an inch on most people. The proximal end of the groove is easiest to palpate. Can you feel a tendon lying in the groove? Which tendon would that be?

6. **Deltoid tuberosity, on the anterolateral aspect of the humerus:** It does not feel like a prominent projection. You can find it by asking your partner to abduct his or her arm while you provide resistance and tracing the triangularly shaped deltoid to its inferior point. Is it sensitive?

Muscles

1. **Coracobrachialis:** Have the arm laterally rotated and abducted. Palpate the medial arm carefully, as the median nerve is located there. The origin of coracobrachialis is the coracoid process of the scapula, which is deep to pectoralis major. It is possible to palpate into the axillary region, deep to pectoralis major, reaching toward the coracoid process of the scapula. Do you understand the difference between palpating pectoralis minor and coracobrachialis when pressing into the axillary region?

2. **Pectoralis major:** Palpate the inferior border of the medial clavicle, pressing into the lateral border of the sternum and feeling for the junction of the sternum and the costal cartilages of the upper six ribs. Press between these costal cartilages, applying the pressure toward the sternum. Trace the fibers laterally toward the bicipital groove. The insertion of pectoralis major is the lateral lip of the bicipital groove.

3. **Deltoids:** Find the origin of anterior deltoid, the lateral clavicle. Trace the fibers of anterior deltoid to the deltoid tuberosity. Find the origin of the middle deltoid, the acromion. Trace the fibers of middle deltoid to the deltoid tuberosity. Finally, find the origin of posterior deltoid, the spine of scapula. Trace the fibers of posterior deltoid to the deltoid tuberosity. How sensitive is the deltoid tuberosity to your partner? The deltoid muscle is superficial and forms what is called the *shoulder cap*.

Palpation Exercise #2

This palpation requires you to locate a few new bone markings, review some bone markings already palpated on the humerus and scapula, and palpate the rotator cuff muscles.

Bones/Bony Landmarks

1. Once again, find the bicipital groove. Look for a groove in the anterior, proximal, medial humerus.

2. Find the greater and lesser tubercles of the humerus. The two tubercles are found on either side of the bicipital groove. The greater tubercle is lateral to the bicipital groove and includes both the anterior and posterior aspects of the lateral proximal humerus. However, the lateral aspect of the greater tubercle is covered by the deltoid muscle and is thus difficult to palpate. The lesser tubercle is located on the medial side of the bicipital groove. It is the only anterior projection on the proximal humerus. Do you know that the bicipital groove is also called the *intertubercular groove*? Do you understand why? The greater and lesser tubercles are the insertion spots for the four rotator cuff muscles.

3. Please palpate the spine of the scapula. We will use the spine of the scapula as a landmark when we are looking for supraspinatus and infraspinatus.

4. Palpate the entire outline of the scapula once again. Note the vertebral border. It is easier to find the vertebral border of the scapula if your partner can put his or her hand behind the back. Find the axillary border of the scapula as well.

Muscles

1. **Supraspinatus:** Find the spine of the scapula and press into the muscle just superior to the spine of the scapula. You will be pressing into the supraspinous fossa.

2. **Infraspinatus:** Find the spine of the scapula and press into the muscle just inferior to the spine of the scapula. Press up right into the inferior border of the spine of the scapula and see if you find any trigger points. Then massage the whole muscle, which fills the infraspinous fossa.

3. **Teres minor:** Find the axillary border of the scapula and find the muscle that is along this border. The superior aspect of teres minor is deep to posterior deltoid.

4. **Subscapularis:** Have your client supine. Feel for the axillary border of the scapula. Press your thumbs between the ribs and the scapula, and then press down onto the anterior aspect of the scapula. You can only access the lateral aspect of this muscle.

Palpation Exercise #3

This palpation requires you to locate and palpate bones and bone markings related to latissimus dorsi and teres major.

Bones/Bony Landmarks

1. The spine is a stack of vertebrae. Each vertebra has a posterior projection called a *spinous process* and two lateral projections called *transverse processes*. The vertebral column is divided into a cervical region (with seven vertebrae), a thoracic region (12 vertebrae), a lumbar region (five vertebrae), a sacrum (five fused vertebrae), and a coccyx (generally four fused vertebrae). Palpate as many spinous processes as you can. Can you find the spinous process of C7? It is quite prominent in most people in the inferior neck. Once you find the spinous process of C7, count down the spinous processes until you find T7. From T7 count all the way down to L5. Palpate the sacrum. Covering the sacrum is a fascial structure called the *thoracolumbar aponeurosis or thoracolumbar fascia*.

2. Palpate the posterior iliac crest, which is the superior border of the posterior ilium (one of the fused hip bones that we will discuss in more detail later in the course).

3. Feel for the lower two to three ribs, posteriorly.

4. Find the inferior angle of the scapula.

5. Remember the location of the bicipital groove on the proximal, medial humerus.

Muscles

1. **Latissimus dorsi:** Have partner prone, with arm out to side. To find the borders of latissimus dorsi, first find the sacrum and posterior iliac crest and lumbar and thoracic vertebrae (spinous processes T7 through L5). Latissimus dorsi spreads laterally from its origin toward the axilla, and ultimately to the bicipital groove. Next, find the inferior angle of scapula and recall that, in many people, latissimus dorsi attaches here.

2. **Teres major:** The inferior angle of the scapula is also the origin of teres major. Place a thumb on the axillary border of scapula and the fingers beneath the mass of muscle in the

axilla region. Squeeze gently. This is latissimus dorsi and teres major. Ask the client to medially rotate the arm against your resistance and see if you feel muscle fibers contract.

Palpation Exercise #4

These bones and bone markings are related to the following scapula-moving muscles: serratus anterior, pectoralis minor, levator scapula, rhomboids, and trapezius.

Bones/Bony Landmarks

1. Palpate the lateral trunk to feel as many ribs as you can. Remember that serratus anterior originates on lateral ribs 1 to 8.

2. Palpate the vertebral border of the scapula. Remember that serratus anterior inserts on the anterior aspect of this bone marking and that rhomboids insert on the posterior aspect of this bone marking.

3. Palpate the coracoid process again, and palpate ribs 3, 4, and 5 near the costal cartilage.

4. Palpate the spine of the scapula and find the most medial aspect of the spine of the scapula. Remember that this bony landmark is called the root of the scapula. Find the superior angle of the scapula by palpating an inch to two directly superior to the root of the spine of the scapula.

5. Palpate as many transverse processes of the vertebrae as you can. Find the transverse processes of C1 to C4.

6. Palpate the spinous processes of C7 to T5, recalling that this is the origin of the rhomboids.

7. Palpate the external occipital protuberance, a projection in the posterior occiput (our most inferior, posterior skull bone). The ligamentum nuchae is a ligament joining the external occipital protuberance with all seven cervical spinous processes. Can you palpate it?

Muscles

1. **Pectoralis minor:** Pectoralis minor is located deep to pectoralis major, running from ribs 3, 4, and 5 to the coracoid process. Pectoralis minor connects to ribs 3, 4, and 5 quite near the costal cartilage of these ribs. Much of rib 1 is directly behind (deep to) the clavicle. Pectoralis minor can be palpated directly through pectoralis major, when pectoralis major is relaxed. The lateral aspect of pectoralis minor can be accessed by pressing medially into the axilla, just deep to pectoralis major.

2. **Serratus anterior:** Palpate the lateral chest wall, just lateral to pectoralis major's lateral border. Can you feel the ribs? Palpate between them and against them to access serratus anterior.

3. **Levator scapula:** Find the root of the spine of scapula. Move your finger up about an inch or an inch and a half. Here is the superior angle of the scapula, the insertion of levator scapula. At this point, levator scapula is deep to trapezius. Trace the muscle upward to its origin on the transverse processes of C1 to C4. The superior portion of levator scapula (near the origin on the transverse processes) is deep to splenius capitis and superficial to scalenes. Be gentle.

4. **Rhomboids:** Locate the medial (vertebral) border of scapula and spinous processes of C7 to T5. Palpate through the trapezius muscles to find the rhomboids. Can you feel the direction of the fibers?

5. **Trapezius:** With partner prone, find the occipital protuberance, ligamentum nuchae, and spinous processes of C7 to T12. This is the origin of the entire trapezius muscle. It is helpful to think of the trapezius in three sections: upper, middle, and lower. Each of these sections has a different insertion and different actions. Upper trapezius runs from the occiput and ligamentum nuchae to the lateral clavicle and acromion. Middle trapezius runs from the spinous processes of T1 to T5 to the spine of the scapula. Lower trapezius runs from the spinous processes of T6 to T12 to the root of the spine of the scapula. Trace each section of the trapezius. It is a broad, yet relatively thin, superficial back muscle.

Palpation Exercise #5

Muscles

1. **Biceps brachii:** Palpate the mound of muscle in the anterior arm. Biceps brachii is the superficial muscle in this mound. Flex your elbow, and you can feel the tendon of insertion as it crosses the anterior elbow joint quite superficially on its way to the radial tuberosity. There is a second tendon just medial to the tendon of insertion of biceps brachii. That is the tendon of brachialis. You can also palpate the coracoid process of the scapula to access one of the origins of biceps brachii.

2. **Brachialis:** This muscle lies deep to biceps brachii in the distal half of the anterior arm. The muscle belly of brachialis is more distal than that of biceps brachii, so as you palpate the distal end of the mound of muscle in the anterior arm, you will be accessing brachialis. Find the tendon of insertion just medial and a bit deeper than the tendon of biceps brachii.

3. **Brachioradialis:** Place your left forearm in a neutral position (halfway between supination and pronation). Place your right hand around the radial aspect of your left wrist to provide resistance. Isometrically contract your left brachioradialis, and it will likely be visible along the lateral aspect of your forearm.

4. **Anconeus:** Palpate between the lateral epicondyle of the humerus and the olecranon process to find anconeus.

5. **Triceps brachii:** Palpate the entire posterior arm, and you will feel the belly of triceps brachii. The tendon of origin of the long head of triceps brachii passes between teres major and teres minor on its way to the infraglenoid tubercle of the scapula. The tendon of insertion can be palpated just proximal to the olecranon process.

Palpation Exercise #6

Muscles

1. **Supinator:** Palpate from the lateral epicondyle of the humerus and the proximal, posterior ulna. Trace around the lateral aspect of the proximal forearm to the proximal to mid anterior radius. You have traced the supinator. This muscle is deep to brachialis and the wrist extensors.

2. **Pronator teres:** Find the medial epicondyle of the humerus. From this bone marking, trace distally and laterally to the midshaft of the anterior radius. Pronator teres is superficial and typically has some thickness to it.

3. **Pronator quadratus:** Carefully palpate the distal fourth of the anterior forearm to find pronator quadratus. The muscle is flat and deep to all the flexor tendons in the anterior wrist area.

Palpation Exercise #7

Muscles

1. **Extensor carpi radialis longus:** Find the lateral supracondylar ridge of the humerus, and trace along the superficial, lateral aspect of the posterior forearm. Can you feel where the muscle belly ends and tendon begins? The tendon of insertion travels to the base of the second metacarpal.

2. **Extensor carpi radialis brevis and extensor carpi ulnaris:** Trace distally from the lateral epicondyle of the humerus down the superficial, posterior forearm. The muscle bellies cover the proximal half of the posterior forearm. Contracting the wrist extensors isometrically makes it easier to feel the muscle fibers as they tighten.

3. **Flexor carpi radialis, flexor carpi ulnaris, and palmaris longus:** Palpate the medial epicondyle of the humerus and trace distally down the superficial, anterior forearm. These three muscles are difficult to distinguish from each other but can easily be palpated as a group. The tendons of insertion of the three wrist flexors are palpable and distinguishable as they cross the wrist joint. The tendon of insertion of flexor carpi radialis is quite central and decidedly superficial at the anterior wrist. The tendon of insertion of flexor carpi ulnaris can be palpated just proximal to the pisiform. Not everyone has a palmaris longus, but those who do can find the tendon of insertion when flexing the wrist. It lies quite superficial and between the tendons of insertion of flexor carpi radialis and flexor carpi ulnaris.

Palpation Exercise #8

Muscles

1. **Abductor pollicis longus, extensor pollicis brevis, extensor pollicis longus, and extensor indicis:** Palpate the distal half to two-thirds of the posterior forearm, recalling that these four muscles lie deep in the posterior arm.

2. **Extensor digitorum:** This muscle originates on the lateral epicondyle of the humerus and runs along the superficial, posterior forearm, to the extensor expansion on the dorsal side of the fingers. It is located superficially in the posterior forearm, between extensor carpi radialis brevis and extensor carpi ulnaris. Extensor digiti minimi is difficult to distinguish from extensor digitorum, as it is also located in the superficial posterior forearm, and is just medial to extensor digitorum.

3. **Flexor pollicis longus and flexor digitorum profundus:** These two muscles are located deep in the anterior forearm. Flexor digitorum superficialis and the wrist flexors are superficial to flexor pollicis longus and flexor digitorum profundus, making it difficult to find these deeper muscles.

4. **Flexor digitorum superficialis:** This is a midlayer anterior forearm, covered by the wrist flexors. Several of the tendons of flexor digitorum superficialis are palpable at the anterior wrist, if one flexes the fingers to make a fist.

Palpation Exercise #9

Muscles

1. **Dorsal interossei:** Palpate between the metacarpals on the dorsal side of the hand to find dorsal interossei.

2. **Palmar interossei and lumbricals:** Palpate the central area of the palm, between the thenar eminence and the hypothenar eminence. The lumbricals are superficial to palmar interossei, which lie deep between the metacarpals.

3. **Adductor pollicis:** Palpate the webbing between the first and second digits, and you will be accessing adductor pollicis.

4. **Thenar eminence muscles—opponens pollicis, flexor pollicis brevis, abductor pollicis brevis:** The thenar eminence is the mound of flesh proximal to the MP joint of the thumb. Of the three muscles that make up the thenar eminence, opponens pollicis is the deepest. Flexor pollicis brevis and abductor pollicis brevis lie side by side, covering opponens pollicis. The flexor is medial and the abductor is lateral.

5. **Hypothenar eminence muscles—opponens digiti minimi, flexor digiti minimi, abductor digiti minimi:** The hypothenar eminence is just proximal to the MP joint of the fifth digit. Of the three muscles that make up the hypothenar eminence, opponens digiti minimi is the deepest. Flexor digiti minimi and abductor digiti minimi lie side by side, covering opponens digiti minimi. The flexor is lateral, and the abductor is medial.

Clay Work Exercises

These exercises help reinforce the names and locations of muscles. They require the use of small plastic skeletons and clay. In each exercise below, create each of the listed muscles out of clay, one at a time, and attach it to the plastic skeleton where appropriate. Also, list the origin, insertion, and action of each muscle in the spaces provided. Share your understanding of the muscles with your partner as you build them.

Clay Work Exercise #1

Muscle	Origin	Insertion	Location	Action
1. Coracobrachialis				
2. Pectoralis Major				
3. Anterior Deltoid				
4. Middle Deltoid				
5. Posterior Deltoid				

Clay Work Exercise #2

Muscle	Origin	Insertion	Location	Action
1. Supraspinatus				
2. Infraspinatus				
3. Teres Minor				
4. Subscapularis				

Clay Work Exercise #3

Muscle	Origin	Insertion	Location	Action
1. Latissimus Dorsi				
2. Teres Major				

Clay Work Exercise #4

Muscle	Origin	Insertion	Location	Action
1. Serratus Anterior				
2. Pectoralis Minor				
3. Levator Scapula				
4. Rhomboids				
5. Trapezius				

Clay Work Exercise #5

Muscle	Origin	Insertion	Location	Action
1. Brachialis				
2. Biceps Brachii				
3. Brachioradialis				
4. Anconeus				
5. Triceps Brachii				

Clay Work Exercise #6

Muscle	Origin	Insertion	Location	Action
1. Supinator				
2. Pronator Teres				
3. Pronator Quadratus				

Clay Work Exercise #7

Muscle	Origin	Insertion	Location	Action
1. Extensor Carpi Radialis Longus				
2. Extensor Carpi Radialis Brevis				
3. Extensor Carpi Ulnaris				
4. Flexor Carpi Radialis				
5. Flexor Carpi Ulnaris				
6. Palmaris Longus				

Clay Work Exercise #8

Muscle	Origin	Insertion	Location	Action
1. Abductor Pollicis Longus				
2. Extensor Pollicis Brevis				
3. Extensor Pollicis Longus				
4. Extensor Indicis				
5. Extensor Digitorum				
6. Extensor Digiti Minimi				
7. Flexor Pollicis Longus				
8. Flexor Digitorum Profundus				
9. Flexor Digitorum Superficialis				

Case Study Exercises

These exercises require you to apply the information you have learned about muscles that move the arm and scapula to potential cases involving massage clients. The case studies provided in this workbook include both postural and functional issues typically faced by massage therapy clients. When observing and interviewing a massage therapy client in preparation for creating a treatment plan, it is important to observe any postural imbalances and to inquire about any movement limitations the client may be experiencing. You must then determine the likely shortened and lengthened muscles that could be causing the postural or functional issues presented.

To look for postural imbalances due to shortening or lengthening, we need to understand what constitutes a balanced posture. Clients with a balanced posture stand erect with arms at their sides, not in front of the body or behind the body. The arms are slightly away from their body. The radial side of one's hands should face forward. The left and right acromion processes are level. The shoulders are back, so that the acromion processes are in line with the ear lobes. To address range-of-motion limitations, we must remember that shortened muscles lead to the inability to perform the opposite action. For example, shortened arm flexors lead to an inability to extend the arm fully.

Case Study #1

A client comes to your office for a massage therapy session. As you observe her posture, you notice that her right shoulder is raised (right acromion is higher than the left) and the backs (dorsal side) of both hands face forward. Your task is to determine which muscles are out of balance to cause these postural issues.

The client is performing two actions. Which action is indicated by a raised shoulder/acromion on the right side?

_____ of the _____ on the right side.

Which muscles perform the action your client is performing?

_____

These muscles are likely to be shortened and should be massaged to assist in bettering the client's posture.

Which action is indicated by the fact that the back of both hands face forward?

Bilateral _____ of the _____.

Which muscles perform the action your client is performing?

_____

These muscles are likely to be shortened and should be massaged to assist in bettering the client's posture.

Where would you focus your massage to address these shortened muscles?

_____

Case Study #2

A client comes to see you and tells you that he is having difficulty raising his arm fully in front of him.

What action is the client having trouble performing?

_____ of the _____.

What muscle would be shortened and limit the ability of the client to perform the above action?

_____

Remember that limits on performing an action are often caused by shortening of antagonists. The shortened muscles should be massaged to assist the client's range of motion.

Where would you focus your massage to address these shortened muscles?

_____

_____

Case Study #3

Your client has difficulty bringing her arm from a position in which it is abducted to 90 degrees, further out to the side of her body. She cannot raise her arm to a position where her arm is resting against the side of her head.

What action is the client having trouble performing?

_____ of the _____.

What muscle would be shortened and limit the ability of the client to perform the above action?

_____

Remember that limits on performing an action are often caused by shortening of antagonists. The shortened muscles should be massaged to assist the client's range of motion.

Where would you focus your massage to address these shortened muscles?

_____

_____

Case Study #4

As you observe your client's posture, you notice that her shoulders are more anterior than her ear lobes, and her shoulders appear rounded. In addition, you notice that her scapulae seem far away from the spine.

Which action is the client performing?

_____ of the _____.

Which muscles perform this action?

_____

These muscles are likely to be shortened and should be massaged to assist in bettering the client's posture.

Where would you focus your massage to address these shortened muscles?

_____

_____

Case Study #5

As you observe your client's posture, you notice that his elbows appear bent. As you ask your client about his daily activities you learn that he is a bodybuilder who lifts substantial weight as part of his workout.

Which action is the client performing through his posture?

_____ of the _____.

Which muscles perform this action?

_____

These muscles are likely to be shortened and should be massaged to assist in bettering the client's posture.

Where would you focus your massage to address these shortened muscles?

_____

_____

Case Study #6

As you interview your client, she informs you that she cannot fully extend her wrists. She is a massage therapist and uses the muscles in her hands and forearms on a daily basis.

When a client is unable to fully extend her wrist due to shortened muscles, which muscles are likely to be shortened?

_____

_____

Where would you focus your massage to address these shortened muscles?

_____

_____

Review Exercises

These review exercises help you to recall what you have learned in
this chapter and reinforce your learning.

Review Charts to Study

Origin, Insertion, Location, and Action Chart of the Muscles That Move the Arm				
Name of Muscle	Origin	Insertion	Basic Location	Action(s)
Coracobrachialis	Coracoid process of the scapula	Medial humerus	Medial arm (blends with short head of biceps brachii)	Adduction and flexion of the arm
Pectoralis Major	Medial clavicle, sternum, and costal cartilage of ribs 1–6	Bicipital groove of the humerus	Superficial chest	Medial rotation, flexion, extension from a flexed position, adduction, and horizontal adduction of the arm
Deltoid: Anterior	Lateral third of clavicle	Deltoid tuberosity	Anterior shoulder cap	Flexion, medial rotation, and horizontal adduction of the arm
Middle	Acromion	Deltoid tuberosity	Lateral shoulder	Abduction of the arm
Posterior	Spine of the scapula	Deltoid tuberosity	Posterior shoulder cap	Extension, lateral rotation, and horizontal abduction of the arm
Supraspinatus	Supraspinous fossa	Greater tubercle of the humerus	Superior to the spine of the scapula	Initiation of arm abduction
Infraspinatus	Infraspinous fossa	Greater tubercle of the humerus	Inferior to the spine of the scapula	Lateral rotation and extension of the arm
Teres Minor	Axillary border of the scapula	Greater tubercle of the humerus	Along axillary border of the scapula	Lateral rotation and extension of the arm
Subscapularis	Subscapular fossa	Lesser tubercle of the humerus	Anterior scapula	Medial rotation of the arm
Latissimus Dorsi	Thoracolumbar aponeurosis, sacrum, posterior iliac crest, spinous processes of T7–L5, inferior 2–3 ribs, inferior angle of scapula	Bicipital groove of the humerus	Superficial low to mid back and posterior axilla	Extension, medial rotation, and adduction of the arm
Teres Major	Inferior angle of the scapula	Bicipital groove of the humerus	Posterior axilla	Extension, medial rotation, and adduction of the arm

Origin, Insertion, Location, and Action Chart of the Muscles That Move the Scapula

Name of Muscle	Origin	Insertion	Basic Location	Action(s)
Serratus Anterior	Lateral ribs 1–8	Anterior, vertebral border of the scapula	Lateral ribs	Protraction and upward rotation of the scapula
Pectoralis Minor	Ribs 3, 4, 5 close to costal cartilage	Coracoid process of the scapula	Deep anterolateral chest	Protraction, depression, and downward rotation of the scapula
Levator Scapula	Transverse processes of C1–C4	Superior angle of the scapula	Lateral neck	Elevation and downward rotation of the scapula
Rhomboids	Spinous processes of C7–T5	Vertebral border of the scapula	Between the scapula and the spine, mid-layer	Retraction and downward rotation of the scapula
Trapezius: Upper fibers	External occipital protuberance and ligamentum nuchae	Lateral clavicle and acromion	Superficial, posterolateral neck and between neck and acromion	Elevation and upward rotation of the scapula
Middle fibers	Spinous processes of C7–T6	Spine of the scapula	Superficial middle back	Retraction of the scapula
Lower fibers	Spinous Processes of T7–T12	Root of the spine of the scapula	Superficial middle back	Depression and upward rotation of the scapula

Origin, Insertion, Location, and Action Chart of the Muscles That Move the Elbow

Name of Muscle	Origin	Insertion	Basic Location	Action(s)
Brachialis	Distal half of anterior arm	Proximal anterior ulna including coronoid process and ulnar tuberosity	Deep anterior arm	Flexion of the elbow (strongest)
Biceps Brachii	Coracoid process and supraglenoid tubercle of the scapula	Radial tuberosity	Superficial anterior arm	Flexion of the elbow, supination of the forearm, and flexion of the arm
Brachioradialis	Lateral supracondylar ridge of the humerus	Styloid process of the radius	Superficial, lateral forearm	Flexion of the elbow (when the forearm is in neutral position)
Anconeus	Lateral epicondyle of the humerus	Olecranon process and proximal posterior ulna	Posterior elbow	Extension of the elbow
Triceps Brachii	Infraglenoid tubercle of the scapula and posterior humerus	Olecranon process	Posterior arm	Extension of the elbow

Origin, Insertion, Location, and Action Chart of the Muscles That Rotate the Forearm

Name of Muscle	Origin	Insertion	Basic Location	Action(s)
Supinator	Lateral epicondyle of the humerus, supinator crest of the ulna, and ligaments of the elbow	Proximal, anterior radius	Wraps around the lateral aspect of the proximal forearm	Supination of the forearm
Biceps Brachii	Coracoid process and supraglenoid tubercle of the scapula	Radial tuberosity	Superficial anterior arm	Supination of the forearm, flexion of the elbow, and flexion of the arm
Pronator Quadratus	Distal ¼ of the anterior ulna	Distal ¼ of the anterior radius	Deep, distal, anterior forearm	Pronation of the forearm
Pronator Teres	Medial epicondyle of the humerus and coronoid process of the ulna	Mid lateral shaft of the radius	Superficial, proximal, anterior forearm	Pronation of the forearm

Origin, Insertion, Location, and Action Chart of the Muscles That Move the Wrist

Name of Muscle	Origin	Insertion	Location	Action(s)
Extensor Carpi Radialis Longus	Lateral supracondylar ridge of the humerus	Base of the second metacarpal	Superficial, posterior forearm	Extension and radial deviation of the wrist
Extensor Carpi Radialis Brevis	Lateral epicondyle of the humerus	Base of the third metacarpal	Superficial, posterior forearm	Extension and radial deviation of the wrist
Extensor Carpi Ulnaris	Lateral epicondyle of the humerus	Base of the fifth metacarpal	Superficial, posterior forearm	Extension and ulnar deviation of the wrist
Flexor Carpi Radialis	Medial epicondyle of the humerus	Bases of the second and third metacarpals	Superficial, anterior forearm	Flexion and radial deviation of the wrist
Palmaris Longus	Medial epicondyle of the humerus	Palmar aponeurosis	Superficial, anterior forearm	Flexion of the wrist
Flexor Carpi Ulnaris	Medial epicondyle of the humerus and proximal ulna	Pisiform, hamate, and base of the fifth metacarpal	Superficial, anterior forearm, although most proximal aspect is posterior	Flexion and ulnar deviation of the wrist

Origin, Insertion, Location, and Action Chart of the Forearm Muscles That Move the Fingers and Thumb

Name of Muscle	Origin	Insertion	Location	Action(s)
Abductor Pollicis Longus	Posterior radius, ulna, and interosseus membrane	Base of the first metacarpal	Deep posterior forearm	Abduction of the thumb at the CMC joint
Extensor Pollicis Brevis	Posterior radius and interosseus membrane	Base of the proximal phalanx of the thumb	Deep posterior forearm	Extension of the thumb at the MP joint
Extensor Pollicis Longus	Posterior ulna and interosseus membrane	Base of the distal phalanx of the thumb	Deep posterior forearm	Extension of the thumb at the IP joint
Extensor Indicis	Posterior ulna and interosseus membrane	Extensor expansion of the second digit	Deep posterior forearm	Extension of the second digit
Extensor Digitorum	Lateral epicondyle of the humerus	Base of middle phalanges and extensor expansion of digits 2–5	Superficial posterior forearm	Extension of digits 2–5
Extensor Digiti Minimi	Posterior radius, ulna, and interosseus membrane	Base of the first metacarpal	Superficial posterior forearm	Extension of the fifth digit
Flexor Pollicis Longus	Anterior radius and interosseus membrane	Distal phalanx of the thumb	Deep anterior forearm	Flexion of the thumb at the IP joint
Flexor Digitorum Profundus	Anterior ulna and interosseus membrane	Distal phalanges of digits 2–5	Deep anterior forearm	Flexion of digits 2–5 at MP, PIP, and DIP joints
Flexor Digitorum Superficialis	Medial epicondyle of the humerus, coronoid process of the ulna, and anterior radius	Middle phalanges of digits 2–5	Midlayer anterior forearm	Flexion of digits 2–5 at MP and PIP joints

CMC, carpometacarpal; MP, metacarpophalangeal; IP, interphalangeal; PIP, proximal interphalangeal; DIP, distal interphalangeal

Origin, Insertion, Location, and Action Chart of the Intrinsic Hand Muscles

Name of Muscle	Origin	Insertion	Location	Action(s)
Dorsal Interossei	Adjacent sides of metacarpals	Proximal phalanges of digits 2, 3, and 4	Dorsal side of hand, between the metacarpals	Abduction of digits 2, 3, and 4 at the MP joints
Palmar Interossei	Shafts of second, fourth, and fifth metacarpals	Proximal phalanges of digits 2, 4, and 5	Deep, palmar side of the hand, between the metacarpals	Adduction of digits 2, 4, and 5 at the MP joints
Lumbricals	Tendon of insertion of flexor digitorum profundus	Bases of the proximal phalanges of digits 2–5 and extensor expansion	Palmar side of the hand	Flexion of the MP joints and extension of the PIP and DIP joints
Adductor Pollicis	Transverse head: shaft of the third metacarpal. Oblique head: bases of the second and third metacarpals, capitate and adjacent carpals	Base of the proximal phalanx of the thumb	Webbing between the first and second digits	Adduction of the thumb at the CMC joint
Opponens Pollicis	Flexor retinaculum and trapezium	Lateral shaft of the first metacarpal	Thenar eminence (deepest)	Opposition of the thumb: combination of abduction and flexion at the CMC joint
Flexor Pollicis Brevis	Flexor retinaculum and trapezium	Base of the proximal phalanx of the thumb	Thenar eminence	Flexion of the thumb at the MP joint
Abductor Pollicis Brevis	Flexor retinaculum, trapezium, and scaphoid	Base of the proximal phalanx of the thumb	Thenar eminence	Abduction of the thumb at the MP joint
Opponens Digiti Minimi	Hook of hamate and flexor retinaculum	Medial border of the fifth metacarpal	Hypothenar eminence (deepest)	Opposition of the fifth digit: combination of flexion and adduction
Flexor Digiti Minimi	Hook of hamate and flexor retinaculum	Base of the proximal phalanx of the fifth digit	Hypothenar eminence	Flexion of the fifth digit
Abductor Digiti Minimi	Pisiform	Base of the proximal phalanx of the fifth digit	Hypothenar eminence	Abduction of the fifth digit

Review List of Arm and Scapula Movers to Fill In

Please list muscles that move the arm or scapula.

ARM MOVERS	SCAPULA MOVERS
1.	1.
2.	2.
3. Anterior	3.
Middle	
Posterior	
4.	4.
5.	5. Upper fibers of
	Middle fibers of
	Lower fibers of
6.	
7.	
8.	
9.	
10. Biceps brachii (additional arm flexor)	
11. Triceps brachii (additional arm extensor)	

Review Chart to Fill In

LATISSIMUS DORSI AND TERES MAJOR	LEVATOR SCAPULA AND UPPER TRAPEZIUS	RHOMBOIDS AND MIDDLE TRAPEZIUS	SERRATUS ANTERIOR AND PECTORALIS MINOR	LATTISIMUS DORSI AND TERES MAJOR
List some uses of these muscles in daily life.				
If these muscles are SHORTENED, what posture might you notice?				
What would be the effect of LENGTH-ENED or dysfunctional muscles?				
How would you massage these muscles?				

Action Charts of Arm and Scapula Movers

Please fill in the muscles that perform the arm or scapula movements indicated:

ARM EXTENORS	ARM FLEXORS
1.	1.
2.	2.
3.	3.
4.	4.
5.	
6.	
7.	

ARM MEDIAL ROTATORS	ARM LATERAL ROTATORS
1.	1.
2.	2.
3.	3.
4.	
5.	

ARM ADDUCTORS	ARM ABDUCTORS
1.	1.
2.	2.
3.	
4.	

ARM HORIZONTAL ADDUCTORS	ARM HORIZONTAL ABDUCTORS
1.	1.
2.	

SCAPULA ELEVATORS	SCAPULA DEPRESSORS
1.	1.
2.	2.

SCAPULA PROTRACTORS	SCAPULA RETRACTORS
1.	1.
2.	2.

SCAPULA UPWARD ROTATORS	SCAPULA DOWNWARD ROTATORS
1.	1.
2.	2.
3.	3.

Action Charts of Elbow, Forearm, and Wrist Movers

Please fill in the muscles that perform the elbow, forearm, or wrist movements indicated:

ELBOW FLEXORS	ELBOW EXTENSORS
1.	1.
2.	2.
3.	

FOREARM SUPINATORS	FOREARM PRONATORS
1.	1.
2.	2.

WRIST EXTENSORS	WRIST FLEXORS
1.	1.
2.	2.
3.	3.

Review of Muscles Located in the Hand and Forearm That Move the Fingers and Thumb

Fill in the appropriate muscle in the space provided.
Deep posterior forearm muscles:

1. _____ deep posterior forearm muscle that abducts the thumb

2. _____ shorter deep posterior forearm muscle that extends the thumb

3. _____ longer deep posterior forearm muscle that extends the thumb

4. _____ deep posterior forearm muscle that extends the second digit

Superficial posterior forearm muscles:

5. _____ superficial posterior forearm muscle that extends four fingers (digits 2–5); the origin is the lateral epicondyle of the humerus, and the tendon of origin is part of the common extensor tendon.

6. _____ superficial, posterior forearm muscle that extends the fifth digit; the origin is the lateral epicondyle of the humerus, and the tendon of origin is part of the common extensor tendon.

Deep anterior forearm muscles:

7. _____ deep anterior forearm muscle that flexes the thumb

8. _____ deep anterior forearm muscle that flexes 12 phalanges Midlayer, anterior forearm muscle:

9. _____ midlayer anterior forearm muscle that flexes four fingers

Review of Ten Intrinsic Hand Muscles

Fill in the appropriate muscle in the space provided:

Three muscles that move the fingers: (Muscles that move the fingers must insert on the phalanges.)

1. _____ DAB, dorsal side, deep between metacarpals, spreads or abducts the fingers

2. _____ PAD, palmar side, deep between metacarpals, adducts the fingers

3. _____ located on the palmar side of the hand, flexes MP joints, and extends the PIPs and DIPs; this muscle is located in both hands and feet.

Four muscles that move the thumb: (All thumb movers insert on the thumb!)

1. _____ deep to the lumbricals, webbing between the first and second digits (thumb), adducts the thumb

2. _____ part of the thenar eminence, performs opposition of the thumb

3. _____ part of the thenar eminence, performs flexion of the thumb

4. _____ part of the thenar eminence, performs abduction of the thumb

Three muscles that move the little finger (have digiti minimi in name, insert on the fifth digit):

1. _____ hypothenar eminence, performs opposition of the fifth digit

2. _____ hypothenar eminence, performs flexion of the fifth digit

3. _____ hypothenar eminence, performs abduction of the fifth digit

4

Head, Neck, Trunk, Abdomen, and Low Back

■ CHAPTER OUTLINE

OVERVIEW OF THE REGION

It is probably hard to argue that any area of the body is more significant than the head. The head contains the brain, that amazing, unique center of thought, communication, and control. The head contains eyes, ears, nose, mouth, and tongue, and is therefore the focal area of the majority of the senses. We see, hear, smell, and taste by using structures within the head. We express much of who we are by using structures within the head that permit facial expressions and speech. The head also contains the openings of the respiratory and digestive tracts. Yes, the head is infinitely important to us.

So, what do we need to know to plan an appropriate massage of the head and face? Understanding the bone structure and musculature of the head and face is as essential for this body area as it is for all body areas. But, in addition, it is important to be aware of the power of these areas of the body and consider the significance they hold for our clients.

The region that contains our neck, trunk, abdomen, and low back contains the core of the body. It is solid and foundational, and houses the spine as well as many key organs responsible for essential physiological functions of the body. We often speak of the spine as our *back bone*, both literally and figuratively. The spine forms the central axis around which the body moves. The organs of the core are crucial for life. The heart pumps warm, nutrient-filled blood; the lungs fill with air and exchange gases; and the digestive organs absorb nutrients. Despite the fact that these processes go on endlessly, often without our awareness, they are essential to our health. When we do focus on these areas, we may note that our sense of energy and strength often reside in this core, and emanate from this area. It is surely an area that deserves much respect and care.

BONES AND BONE MARKINGS OF THE REGION

We will begin this chapter with an overview of the skull bones. Do you remember the difference between the axial skeleton and appendicular skeleton? The axial skeleton consists of the skull, sternum, ribs, hyoid bone, and vertebral column. The appendicular skeleton consists of bones of the upper and lower extremities, the shoulder girdle, and the pelvic girdle. The skull is the skeletal portion of the head. It surrounds and protects the brain. The skull contains openings into the digestive and respiratory tracts. The human skull comprises eight cranial bones (four single and two paired) and 14 facial bones. The cranial bones surround and protect our brain. The facial bones comprise much of the anterior and lateral face and provide muscle attachment sites for many muscles of facial movement and expression. All bones of the skull are joined together by sutures, except for the mandible, which is attached to the temporal bone at a freely movable joint.

Skull

We will look at the eight cranial bones first. The frontal bone is the main bone of the forehead. It is a large, flat, smooth, curved bone. It forms the roof of the orbits (eye sockets) and has a supraorbital foramen through which passes vessels and nerves (supraorbital nerve and artery). This foramen is palpable near the medial eyebrows, when pressing upward, and is a good point to press for frontal sinus congestion. The frontal bone houses paranasal sinuses. The frontal bone articulates with the parietal bones at the coronal suture, and with the nasal bones, zygomatic bones, lacrimal bones, ethmoid bone, and sphenoid bone.

Figure 4-1 shows an anterior view of the skull bones with frontal bone, maxilla, zygomatic, nasal, sphenoid, and mandible labeled and shown in different colors. The zygomatic arch is also shown.

The two parietal bones meet in the middle of the top of the skull at the sagittal suture. They create most of the superior and lateral walls of the cranium. They articulate with the occiput at the lambdoidal suture (named for its similarity to the shape of the Greek letter *lambda*). The parietal bones also articulate with the temporal bone at the squamous suture and the sphenoid bone.

Figure 4-2 shows a lateral view of the skull bones and markings, including parietal bone, temporal bone, mastoid process, external auditory meatus, styloid process of temporal bone, occiput, mandible, sphenoid, zygomatic, frontal, and nasal bones labeled and shown in different colors.

We have two temporal bones, which are located inferior to the parietal bones and form a sizable part of the sides of the skull. The temporal bones have many important bone markings. The styloid process is a thin, tooth-like projection that serves as a muscle attachment site for some muscles that move the neck and tongue. The zygomatic process is a thin bridge of bone that joins to the zygomatic bones of the cheek. When combined with the temporal process of the zygomatic bone, these two processes form the zygomatic arch, which is the widest part of the face and is a common fracture site. The mastoid process is a projection on the temporal bone located posterior and inferior to the opening of the external auditory meatus. The *external auditory meatus* is a formal name for the ear canal. The jugular foramen is an opening between the temporal bone and the occiput. It allows passage of the internal jugular vein, which drains the brain, and passage of cranial nerves IX, X, and XI. The mandibular fossa is on the zygomatic process and attaches to the mandible at the temporal mandibular joint (see Fig. 4-1).

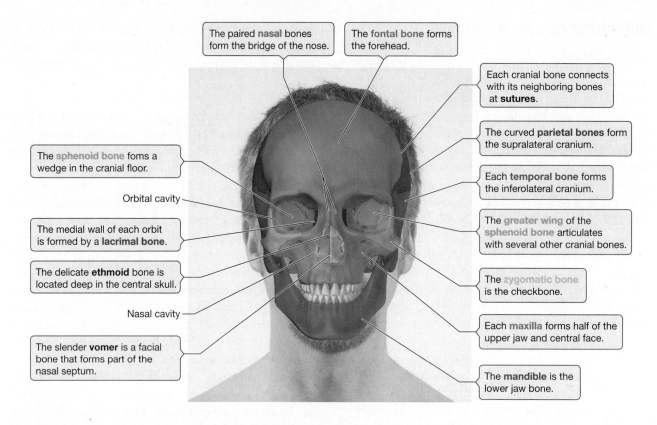

The paired **nasal** bones form the bridge of the nose.

The **fontal bone** forms the forehead.

Each cranial bone connects with its neighboring bones at **sutures**.

The curved **parietal bones** form the supralateral cranium.

Each **temporal bone** forms the inferolateral cranium.

The **sphenoid bone** foms a wedge in the cranial floor.

The **greater wing** of the **sphenoid bone** articulates with several other cranial bones.

Orbital cavity

The medial wall of each orbit is formed by a **lacrimal bone**.

The **zygomatic bone** is the checkbone.

The delicate **ethmoid** bone is located deep in the central skull.

Nasal cavity

Each **maxilla** forms half of the upper jaw and central face.

The slender **vomer** is a facial bone that forms part of the nasal septum.

The **mandible** is the lower jaw bone.

FIGURE 4-1 · **Anterior view of the skull bones.** Frontal bone, maxilla, zygomatic, nasal, sphenoid, and mandible are labeled.

Parietal bone

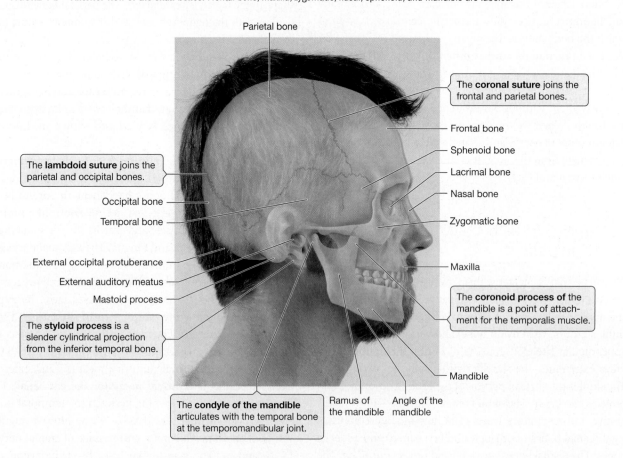

The **coronal suture** joins the frontal and parietal bones.

Frontal bone

Sphenoid bone

Lacrimal bone

Nasal bone

The **lambdoid suture** joins the parietal and occipital bones.

Zygomatic bone

Occipital bone

Temporal bone

External occipital protuberance

External auditory meatus

Mastoid process

Maxilla

The **coronoid process of** the mandible is a point of attachment for the temporalis muscle.

The **styloid process** is a slender cylindrical projection from the inferior temporal bone.

Mandible

The **condyle of the mandible** articulates with the temporal bone at the temporomandibular joint.

Ramus of the mandible

Angle of the mandible

FIGURE 4-2 · **Lateral view of the skull bones.** Parietal bone, temporal bone, mastoid process, external auditory meatus, styloid process of temporal bone, occipital bone, mandible, sphenoid, zygomatic, frontal, and nasal bones are labeled.

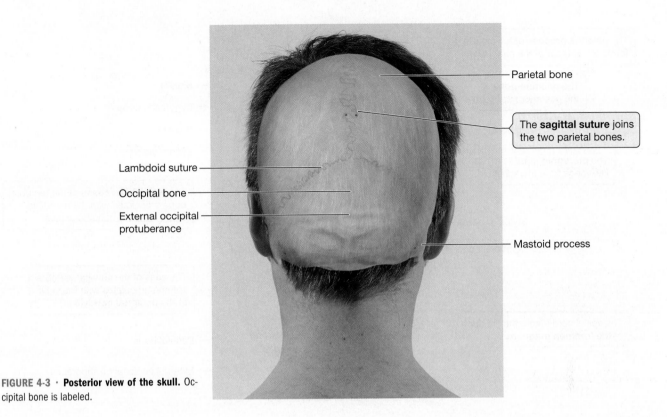

FIGURE 4-3 · Posterior view of the skull. Occipital bone is labeled.

The temporal bones articulate with the parietal, sphenoid, occipital, and zygomatic bones via sutures and with the mandible at the temporal mandibular joint.

The occipital bone (occiput) forms the floor and back wall of the skull. The foramen magnum is an opening in the occiput through which the spinal cord passes. The occiput also has condyles that rest on the first cervical vertebra (atlas). In addition, the occiput has a bone marking called the external occipital foramen, which is generally palpable in the center of the posterior head. The occipital bone articulates with the parietal, temporal, sphenoid, and ethmoid bones.

Figure 4-3 shows a posterior view of the skull with the occiput labeled.

The sphenoid bone is wedge-shaped. It has a body and greater and lesser wings, which spread laterally from the body. The superior part of the body has a bone marking called the *sella turcica,* as it is shaped like a Turkish saddle, and it houses the pituitary gland. The sphenoid bone houses paranasal sinuses. (The floor of the sella turcica forms the roof of the sinuses.) The sphenoid bone also forms part of the orbits. The sphenoid bone articulates with eight bones: frontal, parietal, temporal, occipital, ethmoid, vomer, zygomatic, and palatine (see Fig. 4-2).

The last cranial bone to mention is the ethmoid bone, an irregularly shaped bone located anterior to the sphenoid bone and posterior to the nasal bones. It forms the roof of the nasal cavity and part of the medial walls of the orbit. The ethmoid bone also houses paranasal sinuses.

Next, we will consider the 14 facial bones (two single bones and six pairs). We have two maxilla bones, which form the upper jaw (the skeleton of the face between the eyes and mouth). The maxilla join with all other facial bones except the mandible. The maxillae house paranasal sinuses and have sizable palatine processes, which form the anterior part of the hard palate of the roof of the mouth. Failure of the palatine processes to fuse or to fuse with the palatine bones (see below) results in cleft palate. The maxillae also have alveoli, or sockets for the upper teeth (see Fig. 4-1).

We have two palatine bones, which form the posterior part of the hard palate. As mentioned above, failure of these bones to fuse together or to fuse with the palatine process of the maxillae results in cleft palate. Figure 4-4 shows an inferior view of the skull, with the maxilla and palatine bones labeled.

There are two zygomatic bones, or "cheek bones." They join with the zygomatic process of the temporal bone and with the greater wings of the sphenoid bone, as well as with the frontal and maxilla bones. The zygomatic bones form part of the lateral walls of the orbit.

We have two lacrimal bones, which are fingernail-size bones that form part of the medial wall of the orbit. The lacrimal bones have grooves for tear ducts.

Both of our small nasal bones come together to form the bridge of the nose (Fig. 4-1).

We have a single vomer bone in the middle of the nasal cavity. It is part of the nasal septum, which divides the nasal cavity into two parts. *Vomer* means plow, describing the bone's shape.

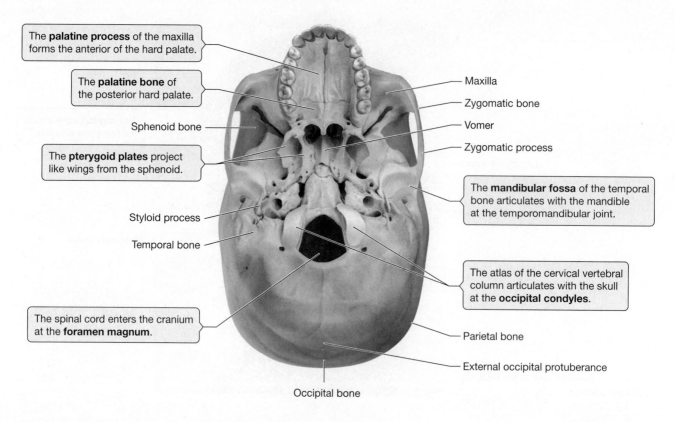

The **palatine process** of the maxilla forms the anterior of the hard palate.

The **palatine bone** of the posterior hard palate.

Sphenoid bone

The **pterygoid plates** project like wings from the sphenoid.

Styloid process

Temporal bone

The spinal cord enters the cranium at the **foramen magnum**.

Maxilla

Zygomatic bone

Vomer

Zygomatic process

The **mandibular fossa** of the temporal bone articulates with the mandible at the temporomandibular joint.

The atlas of the cervical vertebral column articulates with the skull at the **occipital condyles**.

Parietal bone

External occipital protuberance

Occipital bone

FIGURE 4-4 · Inferior view of the skull. Maxilla and palatine bones are labeled.

Our two inferior nasal conchae are thin, curved bones projecting from the walls of the nasal cavity, producing the air passageways through the nose. They are named for their shell-like shape and are also called *turbinates*.

The mandible bone is the lower jaw bone. Our lower teeth are imbedded in the mandible. The mandible is the largest, strongest facial bone. It has a body and two vertical parts called rami. It joins the temporal bone at the temporomandibular joint (Fig. 4-1).

Vertebral Column

We will briefly review the bones and notable bone markings of the spine. This material is covered in greater depth in Chapter 3. The spine is a stack of vertebrae that surrounds and protects the spinal cord. The most superior vertebra is C1, also called the *atlas*. From C1, the spine continues all the way down to the inferior end of the coccyx. There are seven cervical vertebrae, 12 thoracic vertebrae, and five lumbar vertebrae in the spine. In addition, the sacrum contains five fused vertebrae, and the coccyx is made of four fused vertebrae. The spinous processes and transverse processes of the vertebrae are common attachment sites for muscles. Many of the spine- and rib-moving muscles in this chapter will both originate and insert on these processes. Figure 4-5 shows a posterior view of the spine.

Ribs

Recall from Chapter 3 that we have 12 pairs of ribs, simply named rib 1 through rib 12. Rib 1 is the most superior rib and passes from the sternum posterior to the clavicle to the first thoracic vertebra. Ribs 11 and 12, the most inferior ribs, are the shortest and are located entirely posteriorly, as they attach to the eleventh and twelfth thoracic vertebrae. The ribs move upwardly and outwardly when we inhale.

Hyoid

The hyoid bone is located in the anterior neck region. It does not articulate with any other bone but rather is fixed in its place by ligaments and muscles. The hyoid supports the larynx and serves as a muscle attachment site for muscles that move the tongue. Figure 4-6 shows the hyoid bone.

Hip Bone: The Ilium, Ischium, and Pubis

The sacrum articulates with the ilium, one of the three bones that are fused to make each hip bone. The ilium joins with the ischium and the pubis to form a single hip, or innominate bone. Figure 4-7 shows the ilium, ischium, and pubis.

The ilium is the largest and most superior of the three hip bones. The iliac crest is the superior border of the ilium. It runs from the anterior superior iliac spine (ASIS) to the posterior superior iliac spine (PSIS). Just inferior to the ASIS is the anterior

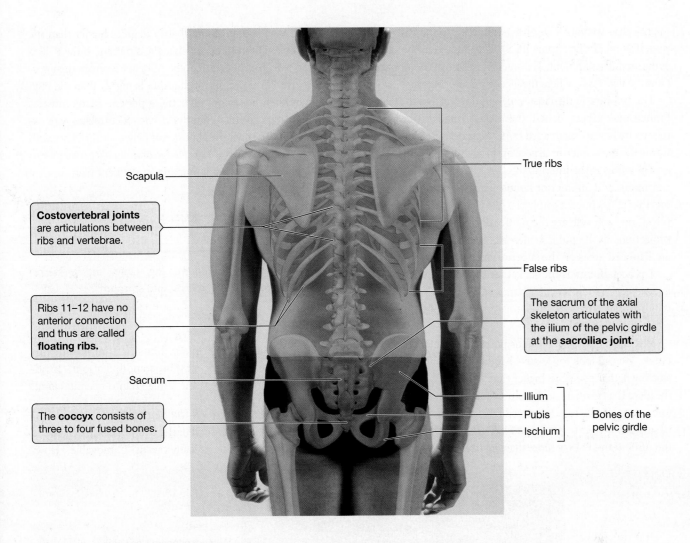

Scapula

Costovertebral joints are articulations between ribs and vertebrae.

Ribs 11–12 have no anterior connection and thus are called **floating ribs.**

Sacrum

The **coccyx** consists of three to four fused bones.

True ribs

False ribs

The sacrum of the axial skeleton articulates with the ilium of the pelvic girdle at the **sacroiliac joint.**

Illium
Pubis — Bones of the
Ischium — pelvic girdle

FIGURE 4-5 · Posterior view of the spine

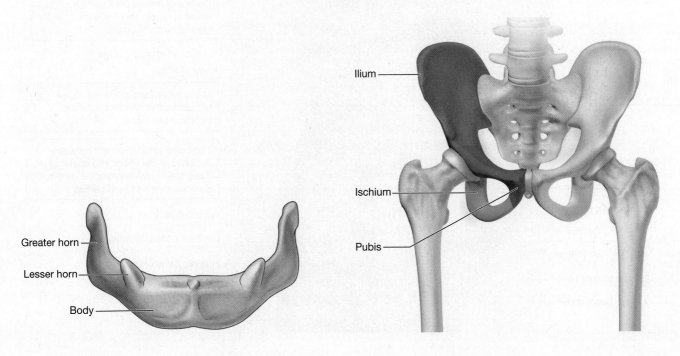

Greater horn

Lesser horn

Body

Ilium

Ischium

Pubis

FIGURE 4-6 · Hyoid bone

FIGURE 4-7 · Ilium, ischium, and pubis

inferior iliac spine (AIIS). And just inferior to the PSIS is the posterior inferior iliac spine (PIIS). The ilium joins the sacrum at the sacroiliac (SI) joint. The anterior surface of the ilium contains the iliac fossa, where the iliacus muscle originates.

The ischium is the posterior, inferior hip bone. It has a branch-like aspect called the *ischial ramus*. The ischial tuberosity (sometimes called the *sit bone* because we sit on it) forms the most inferior aspect of the ischium.

The pubis is the inferior/anterior hip bone. It has a superior ramus and an inferior ramus. The two pubic bones join together at the pubic symphysis. Just lateral to the pubic symphysis on each side are the pubic tubercles, which are small projections in the pubic bones, and the pubic crests, which are flattened areas on the superior, medial pubis.

The acetabulum is the socket for the head of the femur. It is composed of all three hip bones and is thus located where the three hip bones are fused together. Figure 4-8 shows the hip joint with acetabulum.

Massage therapists look at the postural alignment of the hip bones. We can look for relative height of the ilium bones and assess whether one ASIS higher than another. We can look at the tilt of the pelvis. Typical posture for a woman is for the PSIS to be positioned 5 to 10 degrees higher than the ASIS. Typical posture for men is to have the PSIS 0 to 5 degrees higher than the ASIS. If the PSIS is more than 10 degrees higher than the

ASIS in a woman, and more than 5 degrees higher than the ASIS in a man, then anterior pelvic tilt is present. If the PSIS is less than 5 degrees higher than the ASIS in a woman, then posterior pelvic tilt is present. If the ASIS is higher than the PSIS in a man, then posterior pelvic tilt is present. Many muscles contribute to pelvic tilts. Anterior pelvic tilt correlates with exaggerated lumbar curve, and posterior pelvic tilt correlates with a flattened lumbar curve. Knowledge of a client's pelvic tilt can assist a massage therapist in making a treatment plan.

JOINTS, LIGAMENTS, AND BURSAE OF THE REGION

Here, we will consider the joints, ligaments, and bursae related to the skull, vertebrae, ribs, and sternum.

Skull

The skull contains two primary joints or joint groups: the synarthrotic joints and the temporomandibular joint. In addition, the skull joins the spine at the atlanto-occipital joint.

Synarthrotic Joints Between the Skull Bones

The joints between almost all of the skull bones are classified as synarthrotic, which technically means "immovable." How-

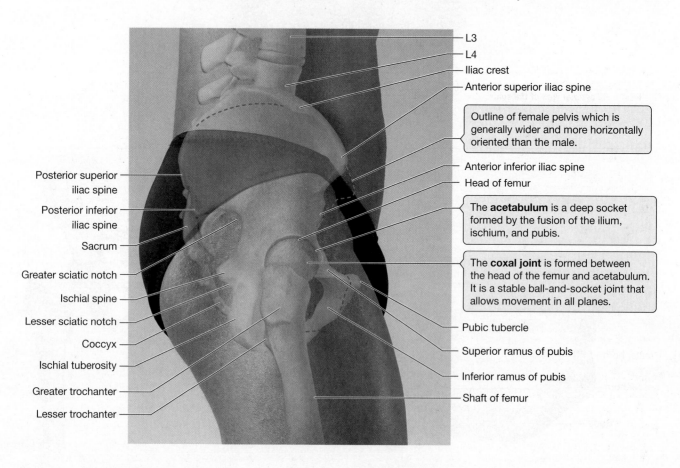

FIGURE 4-8 · Hip joint with acetabulum

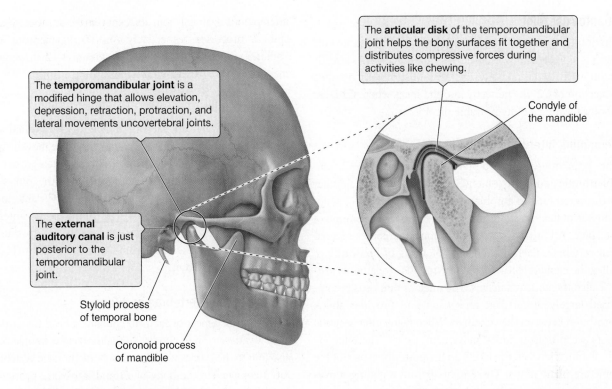

The **articular disk** of the temporomandibular joint helps the bony surfaces fit together and distributes compressive forces during activities like chewing.

The **temporomandibular joint** is a modified hinge that allows elevation, depression, retraction, protraction, and lateral movements uncovertebral joints.

Condyle of the mandible

The **external auditory canal** is just posterior to the temporomandibular joint.

Styloid process of temporal bone

Coronoid process of mandible

FIGURE 4-9 · **Temporomandibular joint**

ever, research has indicated that a small amount of movement is possible between the skull bones. The bodywork modality of craniosacral therapy is based on minute movements between the skull bones.

Temporomandibular Joint

One pair of joints within the skull is not classified as synarthrotic. The joints between the temporal bones and the mandible are classified as freely movable. The condyles on either side of the mandible articulate with mandibular fossas of the temporal bones. A fibrocartilaginous disc lies between the two articular surfaces that create the joint. The temporomandibular joints (TMJ) are classified as modified hinge synovial joints, which permit elevation, depression, protraction, retraction, and a side-to-side movement called *excursion*. Figure 4-9 illustrates the TMJ.

The lateral ligament, also called the temporal mandibular ligament, joins the zygomatic process of the temporal bone to the articular tubercle of the mandible, helping to reinforce the joint.

Atlanto-Occipital Joint

The occiput articulates with the atlas, our most superior vertebrae. C1 is called the *atlas* because it holds the head as the Greek god, Atlas, held the world in his hand. The condyles on the inferior aspect of the occiput fit perfectly into two indentations in the superior aspect of C1. The atlanto-occipital joint is a condyloid or ellipsoidal joint, allowing flexion, extension, and lateral flexion between C1 and the occiput. Figure 4-10 shows the atlanto-occipital joint.

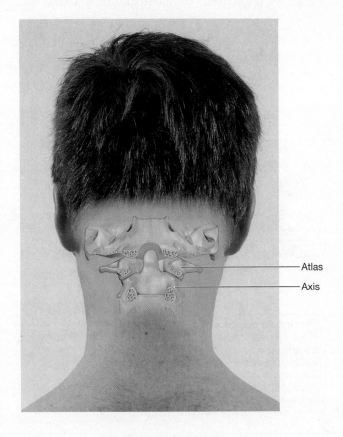

Atlas

Axis

FIGURE 4-10 · **Atlanto-occipital joint**

Atlantoaxial Joint

The joint between C1 and C2, known as the atlantoaxial joint, is a pivot joint, which allows much rotation As already mentioned, C1 has no body. The dens, or superiorly oriented projection of C2, fits perfectly into the space where C1 lacks a body, forming a quite movable pivot joint.

Remaining Intervertebral Joints

The remaining intervertebral joints include both amphiarthrotic and plane joints. The joints between the bodies of the vertebrae are amphiarthrotic, each permitting slight amounts of flexion, extension, lateral flexion, and rotation of the spine. A fibrocartilaginous disc joins the bodies of adjacent vertebrae. Each disc consists of a ring of fibrocartilage called the *annulus fibrosis*, which surrounds a gelatinous center called the *nucleus pulposus*. The nucleus pulposus is composed largely of cartilage and water and provides shock absorption between the vertebrae. When many intervertebral joints act in unison, much movement occurs. The intervertebral joints between the facets on the posterior aspect of the spine are plane joints. These joints permit a gliding movement between the vertebrae when the spine moves. Figure 4-11 shows an anterior view of an intervertebral joint.

The intervertebral joints are stabilized by many ligaments. The anterior longitudinal and posterior longitudinal ligaments join the bodies and discs of adjacent vertebrae anteriorly and posteriorly, respectively. The intertransverse ligaments and interspinous ligaments join adjacent transverse processes and spinous processes, respectively. And the ligamentum flava (yellow) join the adjacent laminae. Figure 4-12 shows ligaments that stabilize the intervertebral joints.

Sacroiliac Joint

The joint between the sacrum and ilium is classified as a plane type of synovial joint, although very little movement is permitted at this joint. The surfaces of both bones are curved and nestle together, limiting the movement of the joint. Several strong ligaments add stability to the joint. The anterior SI ligament joins the medial, anterior ilium to the anterior sacrum. The posterior SI ligament and the interosseus SI ligament join the posterior sacrum to the medial ilium. Figure 4-13 shows the SI joint.

Joints Between Vertebrae and Ribs

The posterior aspect of each rib contains a head that articulates with facets on the bodies of the thoracic vertebrae. Ribs also join to the transverse processes of the thoracic vertebrae. Rib 1 connects to the body of T1 and transverse process of T1. Rib 2 connects to the bodies of both T1 and T2 and transverse process of T2. Rib 3 connects to the bodies of T2 and T3 and transverse processes of T3. Ribs 4 to 9 follow this same pattern, connecting to two adjacent vertebral bodies and one transverse process. Ribs 10 to 12 generally connect only to one thoracic vertebrae and one transverse process each. The joints between the ribs and vertebrae are classified as plane synovial joints. Figure 4-14 illustrates the posterior connections between ribs and thoracic vertebrae.

Joints Between Ribs and Sternum

Ribs 1–10 articulate with the sternum via costal cartilage. These joints are amphiarthrotic joints, moving whenever we breathe and when our thoracic spine moves. Refer back to Figure 3–2, which shows the ribs and the sternum.

CONNECTIVE TISSUE STRUCTURES OF THE REGION

Several important connective tissue structures serve as muscle attachments in the trunk and low back region. The inguinal ligament joins the ASIS and pubic tubercle. It is an attachment point for abdominal muscles. The linea alba is a line of connective tissue running down the center of the abdomen, from the xiphoid process to the pubic symphysis. It is the point of convergence of the abdominal aponeuroses.

The abdominal aponeurosis is a bilayered, sheet-like tendon covering the anterior aspect of the abdomen. The abdominal aponeuroses are insertion tendons for three of the abdominal muscles. In addition, the fourth abdominal muscle is located between the layers of the abdominal aponeurosis.

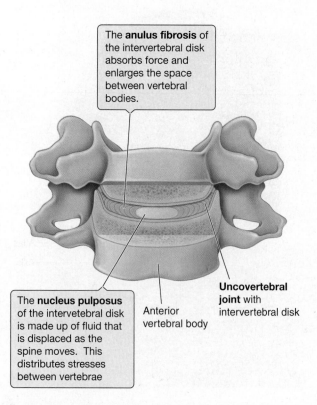

The **anulus fibrosis** of the intervertebral disk absorbs force and enlarges the space between vertebral bodies.

The **nucleus pulposus** of the intervetebral disk is made up of fluid that is displaced as the spine moves. This distributes stresses between vertebrae

Anterior vertebral body

Uncovertebral joint with intervertebral disk

FIGURE 4-11 · **Anterior view of an intervertebral joint**

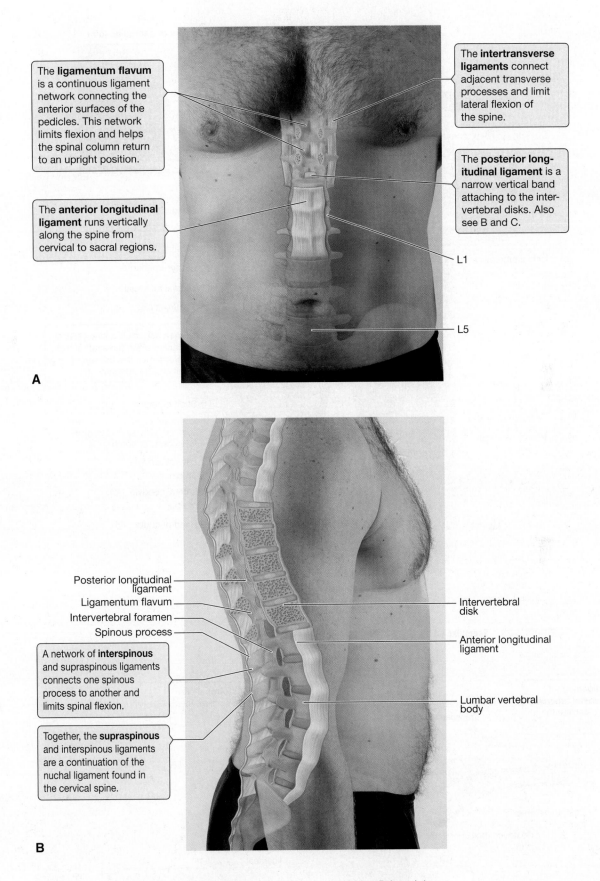

The **ligamentum flavum** is a continuous ligament network connecting the anterior surfaces of the pedicles. This network limits flexion and helps the spinal column return to an upright position.

The **intertransverse ligaments** connect adjacent transverse processes and limit lateral flexion of the spine.

The **posterior long-itudinal ligament** is a narrow vertical band attaching to the inter-vertebral disks. Also see B and C.

The **anterior longitudinal ligament** runs vertically along the spine from cervical to sacral regions.

L1

L5

A

Posterior longitudinal ligament

Ligamentum flavum

Intervertebral foramen

Spinous process

A network of **interspinous** and supraspinous ligaments connects one spinous process to another and limits spinal flexion.

Together, the **supraspinous** and interspinous ligaments are a continuation of the nuchal ligament found in the cervical spine.

Intervertebral disk

Anterior longitudinal ligament

Lumbar vertebral body

B

FIGURE 4-12 · **Ligaments that stabilize the intervertebral joints. A:** Anterior view; **B:** Lateral view.

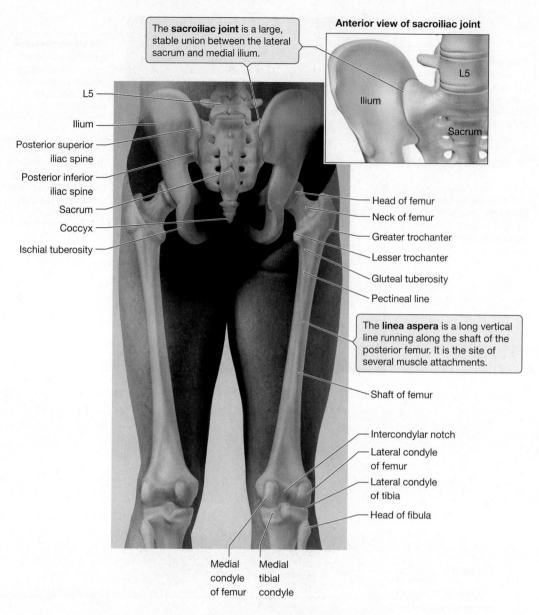

The **sacroiliac joint** is a large, stable union between the lateral sacrum and medial ilium.

Anterior view of sacroiliac joint

L5

Ilium

Sacrum

L5

Ilium

Posterior superior iliac spine

Posterior inferior iliac spine

Sacrum

Coccyx

Ischial tuberosity

Head of femur

Neck of femur

Greater trochanter

Lesser trochanter

Gluteal tuberosity

Pectineal line

The **linea aspera** is a long vertical line running along the shaft of the posterior femur. It is the site of several muscle attachments.

Shaft of femur

Intercondylar notch

Lateral condyle of femur

Lateral condyle of tibia

Head of fibula

Medial condyle of femur

Medial tibial condyle

FIGURE 4-13 · **Sacroiliac joint**

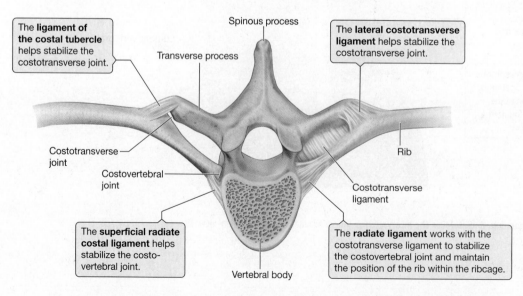

The **ligament of the costal tubercle** helps stabilize the costotransverse joint.

Spinous process

Transverse process

The **lateral costotransverse ligament** helps stabilize the costotransverse joint.

Costotransverse joint

Costovertebral joint

Rib

Costotransverse ligament

The **superficial radiate costal ligament** helps stabilize the costovertebral joint.

The **radiate ligament** works with the costotransverse ligament to stabilize the costovertebral joint and maintain the position of the rib within the ribcage.

Vertebral body

FIGURE 4-14 · **Posterior connections between ribs and thoracic vertebrae**

The linea alba, which literally means "white line," is a rope-like piece of connective tissue that joins the two abdominal aponeuroses, as it runs from the xiphoid process of the sternum to the pubic tubercle. Hormone changes during pregnancy cause the white line to darken and take on the name *linea nigra*, or "black line." Figure 4-15 shows the inguinal ligament, abdominal aponeuroses, and linea alba.

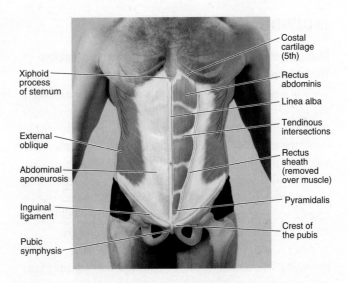

FIGURE 4-15 · **Inguinal ligament, abdominal aponeuroses, and linea alba**

INDIVIDUAL MUSCLES

Muscles Involved in Facial Expression and Muscles That Move the Jaw

We will begin our study of individual muscles by exploring the muscles of facial expression. These muscles tend to be quite small and move the eyes, nose, and lips to allow us to create the vast array of unique facial expressions we use. Massage therapists do not typically address each facial muscle independently but rather massage the face as a whole, seeking to relax these muscles. For that reason, we will not cover the origins and insertions of the muscles, but rather will look at some of their names and a group illustration of them.

After covering the muscles of facial expression, we will move on to the muscles that move our jaw. Movements of the jaw include elevation and depression, protraction and retraction, and side-to-side movements called excursion.

MUSCLES OF FACIAL EXPRESSION

Major muscles of facial expression include the following:

- Occipitofrontalis, which raises the eyebrows and wrinkles the forehead skin upwardly
- Procerus, which wrinkles skin above nose downwardly
- Zygomaticus major and minor, which elevate the upper lip and angle of mouth, as in smiling
- Risorius, which pulls the corners of the mouth backward
- Orbicular oris, which closes the lips
- Levator labii superioris, which raises the upper lip, as in smiling or sneering
- Depressor labii inferioris, which pulls the lower lip down

Figure 4-16 shows an anterior view of many muscles of facial expression.

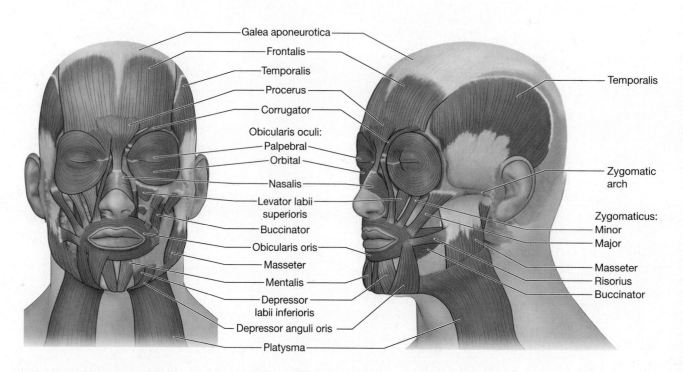

FIGURE 4-16 · Anterior view of muscles of facial expression

MEDIAL PTERYGOID (me-de-al ter-i-goid)

Meaning of Name

Pterygoid means "wing-like," describing the shape of the muscle. In addition, the medial pterygoid attaches to the medial aspect of the lateral pterygoid plate of the sphenoid bone.

Location

This muscle is located deep in the lateral cheek area, along the inner aspect of the ramus of the mandible.

Origin and Insertion

Origin: medial surface of the lateral pterygoid plate of the sphenoid bone
Insertion: medial and inferior aspects of the inner surface of the ramus of the mandible

Actions

Elevates the mandible; can protract the mandible and, when contracting unilaterally, can cause excursion

Explanation of Actions

Medial pterygoid elevates the mandible because the origin is superior to the insertion on the mandible, and thus contraction pulls the mandible upward. Medial pterygoid produces protraction because the origin on the sphenoid is more anterior than the insertion on the mandible, and thus contraction pulls the mandible forward.

Notable Muscle Facts

Muscle tension in medial pterygoid can lead to a sensation of pressure or "fullness" in the ear canal.

Implications of Shortened and/or Lengthened/ Weak Muscle

Shortened: Teeth may be clenched and difficulty in fully depressing the jaw may be experienced. In addition, TMJ pain may be present.
Lengthened: Limited ability to elevate the mandible is noted.

Palpation and Massage

Medial pterygoid is difficult to palpate, as it lies behind or deep to the ramus of the mandible. Trained bodyworkers can

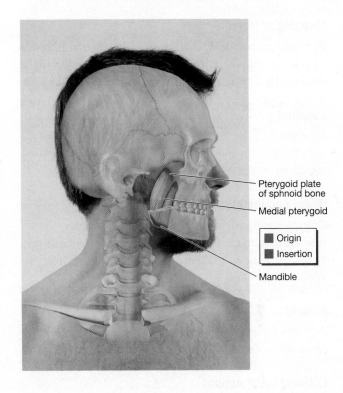

Pterygoid plate of sphenoid bone
Medial pterygoid
■ Origin
■ Insertion
Mandible

FIGURE 4-17 · Medial pterygoid

access this muscle by working in the mouth, pressing the muscle into the inner aspect of the ramus of the mandible.

How to Stretch This Muscle

Depress and retract the mandible.

Synergists

Masseter and temporalis

Antagonists

Platysma and the digastric muscle within the suprahyoid muscle group

Innervation and Arterial Supply

Innervation: cranial nerve V
Arterial supply: maxillary artery

LATERAL PTERYGOID (lat-er-al ter-i-goid)

Meaning of Name

Pterygoid means "wing-like," describing the shape of the muscle. In addition, lateral pterygoid attaches to the lateral aspect of the lateral pterygoid plate of the sphenoid bone.

Location

This muscle is located inferior and deep to the zygomatic arch. Some of the muscle is only possible to access by working inside the mouth.

Origin and Insertion

Origin: lateral surface of the lateral pterygoid bone
Insertion: joint capsule of the TMJ and the articular disc within the joint and the inner surface of the mandible just inferior to the condyle

Actions

Protracts the mandible and, when contracting unilaterally, can produce excursion of the mandible

Explanation of Actions

Lateral pterygoid produces protraction of the mandible because the origin of the muscle is anterior to the insertion; thus, when contracting, the muscle pulls the mandible forward. Unilateral contraction of lateral pterygoid pulls one TMJ capsule medially toward the sphenoid bone, causing excursion.

Notable Muscle Facts

Lateral pterygoid is significant in holding the mandible in place when chewing.

Implications of Shortened and/or Lengthened/ Weak Muscle

Shortened: Difficulty in retracting the mandible may be experienced, and the teeth may be pulled out of line. In addition, TMJ pain and/or dysfunction may be noted.
Lengthened: Limited ability to protract the mandible is noted.

Palpation and Massage

Applying pressure inferiorly as well as superiorly to the zygomatic arch can help the lateral pterygoid to relax. Trained bodyworkers can also apply pressure to the lateral pterygoid by working in the mouth.

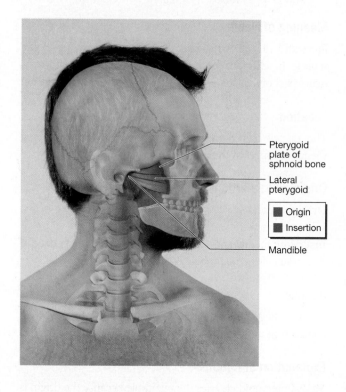

Pterygoid plate of sphnoid bone
Lateral pterygoid
■ Origin
■ Insertion
Mandible

FIGURE 4-18 · **Lateral pterygoid**

How to Stretch This Muscle

Retract the mandible.

Synergists

Masseter and medial pterygoid (protract the mandible)

Antagonists

Temporalis (retracts the mandible)

Innervation and Arterial Supply

Innervation: cranial nerve V
Arterial supply: maxillary artery

MASSETER (mas-a-ter)

Meaning of Name
One who chews.

Location
This muscle is located in the superficial lateral cheek area.

Origin and Insertion
Origin: inferior border of the zygomatic arch
Insertion: lateral external surface of the ramus of the mandible

Actions
Elevates and protracts the mandible

Explanation of Actions
Masseter elevates the mandible because the origin is above the insertion, and thus contraction pulls the mandible upward. Masseter protracts the mandible because the origin is more anterior than the insertion, and contraction pulls the mandible forward.

Notable Muscle Facts
This muscle is designed for strength in mandible elevation, as needed for forceful biting or prolonged chewing. It has been said that the masseter is one of the first muscles to contract upon emotional stress. It is difficult to relax the masseter when one is in an upright position; it is more easily relaxed when one is supine.

Implications of Shortened and/or Lengthened/ Weak Muscle
Shortened: Masseter is a very strong muscle and, if shortened, could cause the teeth to appear clenched. Difficulty in fully depressing the jaw may be noted. In addition, TMJ pain may be present.
Lengthened: Reduced ability to elevate the mandible is noted.

Palpation and Massage
It is easy to palpate and massage the masseter, as it lies superficial to the ramus of the mandible. It is a thick muscle.

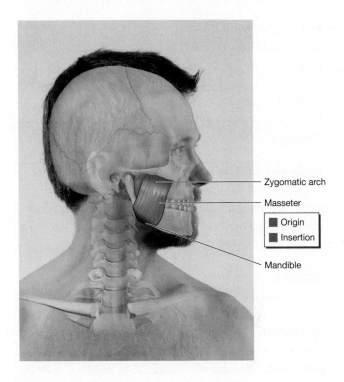

FIGURE 4-19 · **Masseter**

Friction and direct pressure are appropriate and effective strokes to apply to the lateral cheek area.

How to Stretch This Muscle
Depress and retract the mandible.

Synergists
Medial pterygoid and temporalis (elevate the mandible); lateral pterygoid and medial pterygoid (protract the mandible)

Antagonists
Platysma and the digastric muscles (depress the mandible); temporalis (retracts the mandible)

Innervation and Arterial Supply
Innervation: cranial nerve V
Arterial supply: maxillary artery

TEMPORALIS (tem-por-ra-lis)

Meaning of Name

Temple and temporal bone, referring to the location of this muscle.

Location

This muscle covers much of the lateral temporal and parietal bones.

Origin and Insertion

Origin: a large portion of the lateral temporal bone, as well as lateral parts of the parietal, sphenoid, and frontal bones

Insertion: anterior border of the ramus of the mandible, including the coronoid process

Actions

Elevates and retracts the mandible

Explanation of Actions

Temporalis elevates the mandible because the origin is superior to the insertion on the mandible, and thus pulls the mandible up. The posterior/inferior section of temporalis retracts the mandible because the origin is more posterior than the insertion, and thus contraction pulls the mandible back.

Notable Muscle Facts

A forward-head posture may contribute to overuse of temporalis, to counteract the pull of the mandible downward. See digastrics muscle for related information.

Implications of Shortened and/or Lengthened/Weak Muscle

Shortened: Temporomandibular joint pain and/or headaches may be present. In addition, clenched teeth may be noted, and difficulty in fully depressing the mandible may be present.

Lengthened: A reduced ability to elevate the mandible may be noted.

Palpation and Massage

Temporalis is easy to access along the lateral side of the skull. The muscle can be felt shortening when one clenches his or

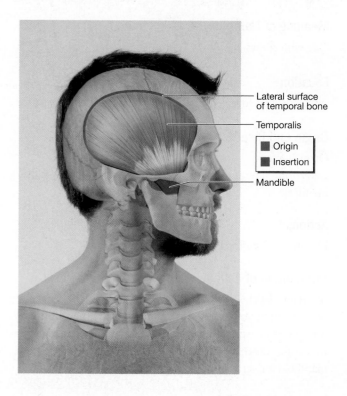

FIGURE 4-20 · Temporalis

her teeth. Direct pressure and friction are appropriate strokes to apply to temporalis.

How to Stretch This Muscle

Depress and protract the mandible.

Synergists

Medial pterygoid and masseter (elevate the mandible)

Antagonists

Platysma and digastric muscles (depress the mandible and masseter); medial pterygoid and lateral pterygoid (protract the mandible)

Innervation and Arterial Supply

Innervation: cranial nerve V

Arterial supply: maxillary artery

PLATYSMA (pla-tiz-ma)

Meaning of Name
Flat plate

Location
This muscle is located within the subcutaneous fascia of the superficial, anterior neck and upper chest region.

Origin and Insertion
Origin: fascia over pectoralis major and anterior deltoid
Insertion: anterior mandible below the lips and surrounding muscles of facial expression

Actions
Depresses the mandible and pulls the lower lip down

Explanation of Actions
Because origin is below insertion on the mandible, platysma pulls the mandible down.

Notable Muscle Facts
Platysma has the ability to pull on the fascia of the anterior neck and upper chest, causing a visible tightening of the superficial soft tissue of the anterior neck.

Implications of Shortened and/or Lengthened/ Weak Muscle
Shortened: Muscle tightness in the superficial, anterior neck is noted.
Lengthened: Reduced strength of mandible depression is noted.

Palpation and Massage
This is a very thin muscle in the superficial anterior neck and upper chest. Pressure must be applied with care in the anterior neck region, thus the more inferior aspects of the muscle are easier to address. Applying direct pressure to the upper anterior chest will address platysma.

How to Stretch This Muscle
It is difficult to stretch the platysma by simply elevating the mandible. Depress the mandible, and then gently press or stretch the muscle tissue inferiorly while elevating the mandible.

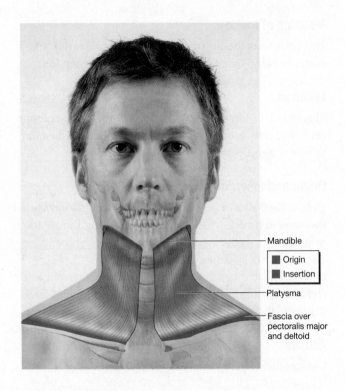

Mandible
Origin
Insertion
Platysma
Fascia over pectoralis major and deltoid

FIGURE 4-21 · Platysma

Synergists
Digastric (depresses the mandible)

Antagonists
Medial pterygoid, masseter, and temporalis (elevate the mandible)

Innervation and Arterial Supply
Innervation: facial nerve
Arterial supply: facial artery

DIGASTRIC (di-gas-trik)

Meaning of Name

Two bellies, as the digastric muscle has an anterior and a posterior belly, joined to each other by a central tendon.

Location

This muscle is located above the hyoid bone in the anterior neck, and thus is one of the *suprahyoid* muscles. The entire muscle is directly deep to the thin platysma muscle.

Origin and Insertion

Origin: the posterior belly of the digastric muscle connects to the mastoid process of the temporal bone, and the anterior belly attaches to the medial, inferior edge of the mandible. The anterior belly is shown in Figure 4-22.
Insertion: hyoid bone, although this attachment is not a direct attachment, but rather occurs through a loop of fascia that surrounds the hyoid bone

Actions

Elevates the hyoid bone and depresses the mandible

Explanation of Actions

Because both origins are superior to the insertion on the hyoid bone, both bellies work together to pull the hyoid bone superiorly. In addition, when the hyoid bone is stable, the anterior portion of digastric pulls the mandible down.

Notable Muscle Facts

A forward-head posture leads to a pull on the digastric muscle, which in turn pulls the mandible in a downward direction.

Implications of Shortened and/or Lengthened/ Weak Muscle

Shortened: Hyoid bone may be pulled superiorly.
Lengthened: Reduced ability to depress the mandible is noted.

Palpation and Massage

This muscle is located in the anterior neck and must be addressed with little pressure to the anterior neck or to the attachments on the mandible and mastoid process.

How to Stretch This Muscle

Protraction of the mandible can stretch the anterior belly of the digastric muscle.

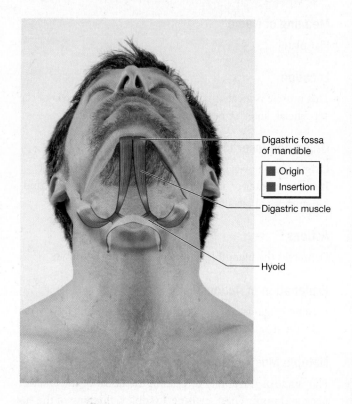

Digastric fossa of mandible
■ Origin
■ Insertion
Digastric muscle
Hyoid

FIGURE 4-22 · Digastric

Synergists

Platysma (depresses the mandible)

Antagonists

Medial pterygoid, masseter, and temporalis (elevate the mandible)

Innervation and Arterial Supply

Innervation: cranial nerves V and VII
Arterial supply: occipital, posteroauricular, and facial arteries

Muscles That Move the Neck

The neck-moving muscles can be divided easily into two groups. One group performs flexion and opposite-side rotation. These muscles are located in the anterolateral neck. The other group of muscles performs extension and same-side rotation and is located in the posterior neck. The anterolateral neck muscles are covered first.

SCALENES: ANTERIOR, MIDDLE, AND POSTERIOR (ska-lens)

Meaning of Name

Uneven

Location

This muscle is located in the lateral neck. The superior portion of anterior scalene lies deep to the SCM, although the inferior portion is superficial and lies posterior to SCM. Middle scalene lies just lateral to anterior scalene, and posterior scalene is quite small and lies lateral, between middle scalene and levator scapula.

Origin and Insertion

Anterior Scalene

Origin: transverse processes of C3–C6
Insertion: anterior aspect of rib 1, more anterior than the origin

Middle Scalene

Origin: transverse processes of C2–C7
Insertion: rib 1, directly inferior to the origin on the cervical transverse processes

Posterior Scalene

Origin: transverse processes of C4–C6
Insertion: rib 2, directly inferior to the origin on the cervical transverse processes

Actions

Scalenes have two unilateral actions, lateral flexion and minimal rotation to the opposite side, and a bilateral action of neck flexion. In addition, scalenes can elevate ribs 1 and 2, to assist in inhalation.

Explanation of Actions

Anterior scalenes perform minimal opposite-side rotation because they pull the origin on the transverse processes forward toward the insertion on rib 1. Pulling the side of the neck forward causes the head and neck to rotate to the opposite side. Because the origin of all three scalenes is above the insertion, in the lateral neck region, the unilateral contraction of scalenes pulls the lateral neck inferiorly, causing lateral flexion. When both right and left scalenes contract simultaneously, the transverse processes on both sides are pulled anteriorly, causing neck flexion. It should be noted that scalenes move the neck by pulling the origin toward the insertion. Elevation of ribs 1 and 2 occurs because the origin is above the insertion on the ribs, thus causing ribs 1 and 2 to rise on contraction.

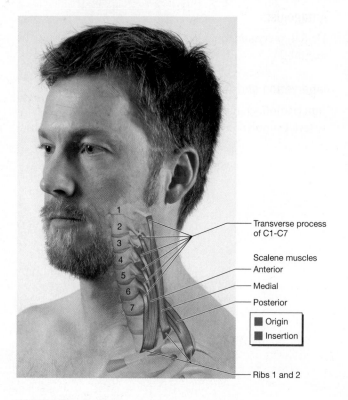

Transverse process of C1-C7

Scalene muscles
Anterior
Medial
Posterior

■ Origin
■ Insertion

Ribs 1 and 2

FIGURE 4-23 · Scalenes

Notable Muscle Facts

Some sources name scalenes as significant muscles of respiration. Their ability to elevate ribs 1 and 2 is the reason for this distinction. In addition, scalenes provide postural support of the cervical spine, limiting unwanted lateral movement.

Implications of Shortened and/or Lengthened/Weak Muscle

Shortened: When scalenes are shortened unilaterally, the head could be minimally rotated to the opposite side. Limited lateral flexion to the opposite side could also be experienced. It is not common to witness a client with his or her neck in a position of lateral flexion simply due to shortened lateral flexors of the neck. This is because the righting reflex alters our posture to compensate for muscle imbalances, to allow our eyes to be level. When scalenes are short bilaterally, one could experience limited ability to extend the neck fully. It is not typical to witness a posture of head and neck flexion, as it is difficult to perform daily activities with the head flexed. Therefore, we are likely to compensate for short neckflexors by adjusting our spine or pelvis. Such compensation can lead to pain in other areas of the spine or in the pelvis. In addition, the brachial plexus passes between anterior and middle scalenes. Thus, when scalenes are short or tight, the muscle can impinge the brachial plexus, causing thoracic outlet syndrome.

Lengthened: Reduced ability to perform the actions of this muscle may be noted.

Palpation and Massage

This muscle can be palpated in the lateral neck.

How to Stretch This Muscle

Laterally flex the neck to the other side.

Synergists

Sternocleidomastoid (performs flexion, lateral flexion, and opposite-side rotation of the neck)

Antagonists

Splenius capitis and splenius cervicis (perform extension of the neck and same-side rotation of the neck)

Innervation and Arterial Supply

Innervation: cervical spinal nerves
Arterial supply: ascending cervical artery and transverse cervical artery

STERNOCLEIDOMASTOID (ster-no-kli-do-mas-toyd)

Meaning of Name

Sternocleidomastoid is named for its attachments. "Sterno" refers to the sternum, "cleido" to the clavicle, and "mastoid" to the mastoid process of the temporal bone.

Location

This muscle is located superficially in the anterolateral neck. The origin is quite anterior, and the fibers pass laterally and superiorly to reach the insertion.

Origin and Insertion

Origin: superior aspect of the sternum and the medial clavicle
Insertion: mastoid process of the temporal bone

Actions

Unilateral actions: lateral flexion and rotation to the opposite side
Bilateral action: neck flexion

Explanation of Actions

The SCM performs rotation to the opposite side because the origin is medial and anterior to the insertion. Pulling the mastoid process anteriorly causes opposite-side rotation. The SCM performs lateral flexion because the origin is inferior to the insertion, and the muscle is located in the lateral neck. Pulling the mastoid process inferiorly causes lateral flexion. The SCM can perform neck flexion because origin is anterior to insertion, and simultaneously pulling both mastoid processes anteriorly causes neck flexion.

Notable Muscle Facts

Sternocleidomastoid is the muscle commonly injured when one experiences whiplash, as the muscle is in position to resist quick, forceful backward movement of the head. Such forceful movement of the head is common when one is in a car that is struck from behind. Whiplash commonly causes tears in the SCM muscle.

Implications of Shortened and/or Lengthened/Weak Muscle

Shortened: If SCM is shortened unilaterally, a common posture is opposite-side rotation of the neck. Functionally, a shortened SCM could cause limited ability to perform lateral flexion to the opposite side. Bilateral shortening of the SCM might result in limited ability to fully extend the neck. Finally, shortening of SCM can lead to headaches felt behind the eyes.
Lengthened: Reduced ability to perform the actions of this muscle is noted.

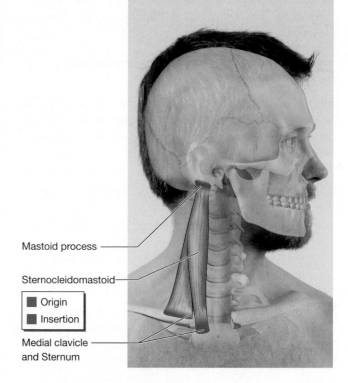

Mastoid process

Sternocleidomastoid

■ Origin
■ Insertion

Medial clavicle and Sternum

FIGURE 4-24 · Sternocleidomastoid

Palpation and Massage

Sternocleidomastoid is easy to palpate in the anterolateral neck, as it is completely superficial. Press your forehead into your hand to make the muscle contract isometrically. Trace it from the superior aspect of the sternum to the mastoid process of the temporal bone. Squeezing the tissue between your fingers and thumb allows you to apply direct pressure, friction, or pétrissage to the muscle. Massage to the SCM can help to relieve frontal headaches.

How to Stretch This Muscle

Laterally flex to the same side while laterally flexing to the opposite side.

Synergists

Scalenes

Antagonists

Splenius capitis and splenius cervicis

Innervation and Arterial Supply

Innervation: spinal accessory nerve
Arterial supply: occipital and posterior auricular arteries

SUBOCCIPITALS (sub-ok-sip-i-tals)

Meaning of Name

Below or inferior to the occiput

Location

This group of eight tiny muscles is located just inferior to the occiput, between the occiput and C2 in the posterior neck.

Origin and Insertion

Origin: spinous process or transverse process of C1 or C2
Insertion: transverse process of C1 or the occiput

Actions

As a group: extend the spine between C1 and the occiput when contracting bilaterally
Unilaterally: laterally flex the atlanto-occipital joint and perform same-side rotation at the atlanto-occipital joint

Explanation of Actions

Obliques capitis inferior is capable of producing same-side rotation by pulling the transverse process of C1 posteriorly toward the origin on the spinous process of C2. Rectus capitis posterior major, rectus capitis posterior minor, and obliques capitis superior produce extension when left and right sides contract simultaneously as they pull the insertion on the posterior occiput posteriorly toward the back of C1 and C2. Finally, a unilateral contraction of rectus capitis posterior major, rectus capitis posterior minor, and obliquus capitis superior produces lateral flexion by pulling one side of the occiput down toward the origin below.

Notable Muscle Facts

There is speculation that restrictions in the suboccipital muscles can disrupt the healthful functioning of the central nervous system. This is likely because the suboccipital's attachment to the occiput can influence its position, and therefore influence the position of the meninges, which connect to the inner surface of the skull bones, including the occiput. Forward head posture can lead to muscle tension in the suboccipital muscles. Forward head posture causes gravity to pull the head into flexion, and the suboccipitals contract to counteract this pull.

Implications of Shortened and/or Lengthened/ Weak Muscle

Shortened: Shortened suboccipitals can lead to headaches felt in the posterior skull and upper neck.

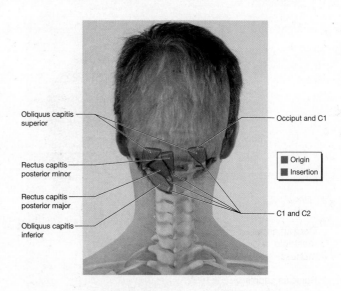

FIGURE 4-25 · **Suboccipitals: Obliquus capitis superior and inferior and rectus capitis posterior major and minor**

Lengthened: Reduced ability to perform the actions of this muscle is noted.

Palpation and Massage

Suboccipitals can be palpated directly inferior to the occiput. They are deep to semispinalis capitis. Friction and direct pressure are useful massage strokes to address these muscles.

How to Stretch This Muscle

Flex the atlanto-occipital joint and perform opposite side-rotation of the atlantoaxial joint.

Synergists

Splenius capitis and splenius cervicis

Antagonists

Sternocleidomastoid and scalenes

Innervation and Arterial Supply

Innervation: suboccipital nerve
Arterial supply: occipital artery

SPLENIUS CAPITIS (sple-ne-us kap-i-tis)

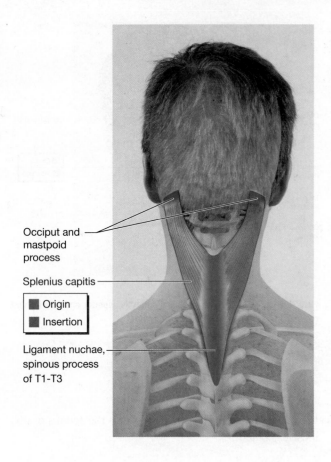

Occiput and mastpoid process

Splenius capitis

- Origin
- Insertion

Ligament nuchae, spinous process of T1-T3

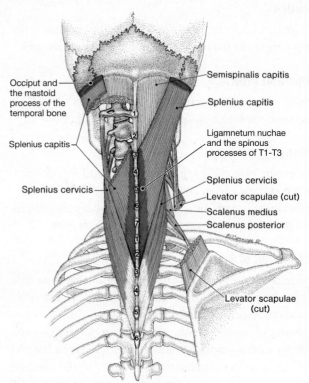

Occiput and the mastoid process of the temporal bone

Splenius capitis

Splenius cervicis

Semispinalis capitis

Splenius capitis

Ligamnetum nuchae and the spinous processes of T1-T3

Splenius cervicis

Levator scapulae (cut)

Scalenus medius

Scalenus posterior

Levator scapulae (cut)

FIGURE 4-26 · Splenius capitis

Meaning of Name

Splenius means "bandage," and capitis refers to the head.

Location

This muscle is located in the posterior neck. It is a midlayer muscle.

Origin and Insertion

Origin: ligamentum nuchae and the spinous processes of C7–T3

Insertion: mastoid process of the temporal bone and the occiput

Actions

Bilateral: extends the head and neck

Unilateral: produces lateral flexion and same-side rotation of the neck

Explanation of Actions

Because origin is inferior to insertion and the muscle crosses many intervertebral joints, as well as the atlanto-occipital joint, from a posterior perspective, this muscle extends the head and neck. Unilateral contraction pulls the mastoid process on the lateral posterior aspect of the skull inferiorly, causing lateral flexion. And because origin is posterior to insertion, contraction pulls the mastoid process posteriorly, resulting in same-side rotation.

Notable Muscle Facts

Forward-head posture can lead to muscle tension on both splenius capitis and splenius cervicis.

Implications of Shortened and/or Lengthened/ Weak Muscle

Shortened: Shortened splenius muscles can cause the head to be turned to the side of the shortened muscle. In addition, shortened splenius muscles can cause difficulty in flexing the neck and difficulty performing lateral flexion to the opposite side. Headaches are also common in those with shortened splenius capitis and cervicis.

Lengthened: Reduced ability to perform the actions of this muscle is noted.

Palpation and Massage

Both splenius muscles are located in the posterior neck, at the midlayer of depth. To palpate splenius capitis, find the mastoid process and move just posterior and inferior. The muscle can be accessed lateral to upper trapezius and partially superficial to levator scapula. In addition, effleurage and petrissage to the posterior neck addresses splenius capitis and splenius cervicis. Friction to the posterior aspect of the mastoid process and along the lateral, posterior occiput is an effective way to massage this muscle.

How to Stretch This Muscle

Laterally flex the neck, combined with rotation of the neck to the same side, to stretch the opposite-side splenius muscles.

Synergists

Splenius capitis, splenius cervicis, and the suboccipital muscles

Antagonists

Sternocleidomastoid and scalenes

Innervation and Arterial Supply

Innervation: dorsal rami of the middle to lower cervical nerves
Arterial supply: occipital artery

SPLENIUS CERVICIS (sple-ne-us ser-vi-sis)

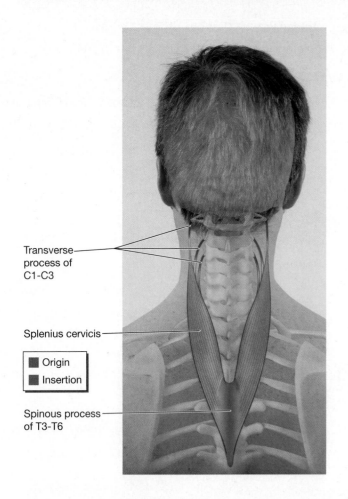

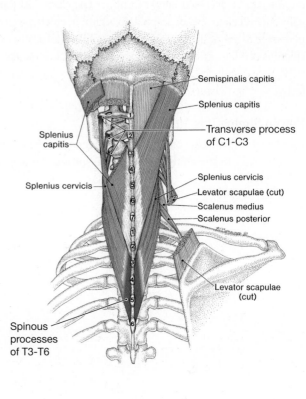

FIGURE 4-27 · **Splenius cervicis**

Meaning of Name

Splenius means "bandage," and capitis refers to the neck.

Location

This muscle is a midlayer muscle of the posterior neck.

Origin and Insertion

Origin: spinous processes of T3–T6
Insertion: transverse processes of C1–C3

Actions

Bilateral: extends the head and neck
Unilateral: produces lateral flexion and same-side rotation of the neck

Explanation of Actions

Splenius cervicis extends the neck when contracting bilaterally because the origin is inferior to the insertion and the muscle is located in the posterior neck. Thus, C1 to C3 are pulled posteriorly toward T3 to T6. Unilaterally, splenius cervicis allows lateral flexion because the muscle pulls the lateral aspects of C1 to C3 inferiorly. Same-side rotation is achieved because the origin of this muscle is more medial and posterior than its insertion. Therefore, the transverse processes of C1 to C3 are pulled posteriorly, causing same-side rotation.

Notable Muscle Facts

Forward-head posture can lead to muscle tension in both splenius capitis and splenius cervicis.

Implications of Shortened and/or Lengthened/Weak Muscle

Shortened: Shortened splenius muscles can cause the head to be turned to the side of the shortened muscle. In addition, shortened splenius muscles can cause difficulty in flexing the neck and difficulty in performing lateral flexion to the opposite side.

Lengthened: Reduced ability to perform the actions of this muscle is noted.

Palpation and Massage

Because these muscles are more flat than belly-like, and because they are located in the midlayer of depth, deep effleurage and friction to the bony attachments are probably the most effective application of Swedish massage in this area. Circular friction around the transverse processes of C1–C3 and around the spinous processes of T3–T6, as well as deep effleurage between these landmarks, is suggested.

How to Stretch This Muscle

Laterally flex the neck while rotating the neck to the same side.

Synergists

Splenius capitis, splenius cervicis, and the suboccipital muscles

Antagonists

Sternocleidomastoid and scalenes

Innervation and Arterial Supply

Innervation: dorsal rami of the lower cervical nerves
Arterial supply: occipital artery

Muscles That Move the Neck, Trunk, and Low Back

The spine-moving muscles located in the back are arranged in a complex pattern, providing thorough stabilization of the spine. These muscles play important roles in maintaining our posture, as well as in providing movement. It is useful to understand the organizational complexity of these intrinsic back muscles, including their locations, the fiber directions of the muscles, and their actions. These deep muscles are typically massaged in groups or sections, rather than as individual muscles.

SEGMENTALS: INTERSPINALIS (seg-men-tal in-ter-spi-na-lis)

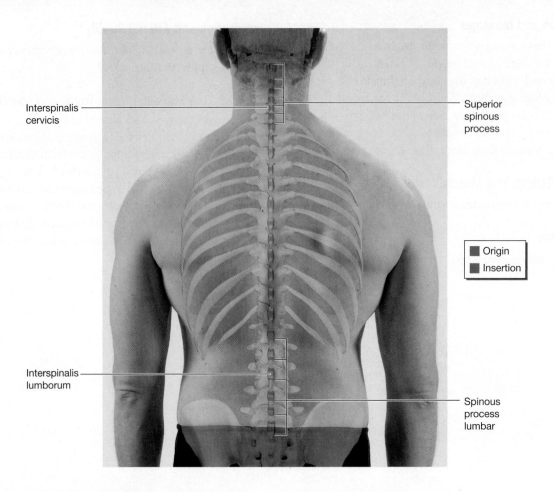

Interspinalis cervicis

Superior spinous process

■ Origin
■ Insertion

Interspinalis lumborum

Spinous process lumbar

FIGURE 4-28 · **Segmentals: interspinalis**

Meaning of Name

Segmentals refers to the fact that these muscles are one segment in length, or that they span only one intervertebral joint. *Interspinalis* means "between the spines" and refers to the fact that these muscles are located between spinous processes.

Location

These short muscles are located between adjacent spinous processes, primarily in the cervical, upper thoracic, and lumbar regions of the spine. Interspinalis muscles are divided into three sections, based on their location: interspinalis cervicis, interspinalis thoracis, and interspinalis lumborum.

Origin and Insertion

Interspinalis Cervicis
Origin: superior surfaces of spinous processes of vertebrae C3–T1

Insertion: inferior aspect of the spinous process of the vertebra right above (C2–C7)

Interspinalis Thoracis
Origin: superior surfaces of vertebrae T2, T3, and T12
Insertion: spinous processes of T1, T2, and T11, respectively.
Note: Interspinalis do not cover all of the thoracic region.

Interspinalis Lumborum
Origin: superior surfaces of vertebrae L2–L5
Insertion: inferior aspects of the spinous processes of L1–L4

Actions

Extends the spine from T2–C2 and from L5–T11

Explanation of Actions

Because origin is inferior to insertion, and the muscles cross the posterior side of intervertebral joints, they pull spinous processes inferiorly, causing extension of the spine.

Notable Muscle Facts

These tiny muscles have postural as well as functional purpose. They assist us in keeping our spines erect.

Implications of Shortened and/or Lengthened/ Weak Muscle

Shortened: Limited flexion of cervical and/or lumbar region of the spine is noted.
Lengthened: Reduced ability to perform the actions of this muscle is noted.

Palpation and Massage

Interspinalis muscles are located deep between the spinous processes in the cervical and lumbar region. Careful application of friction and/or direct pressure to the area can help the muscles to relax.

How to Stretch This Muscle

Flex the neck and lumbar spine.

Synergists

Splenius capitis, splenius cervicis, semispinalis capitis, multifidus, iliocostalis cervicis and lumborum, longissimus cervicis and lumborum, and spinalis cervicis

Antagonists

Sternocleidomastoid, scalenes, and the abdominal muscles that flex the trunk

Innervation and Arterial Supply

Innervation: dorsal branches of spinal nerves
Arterial supply: dorsal branches of the intercostal arteries

SEGMENTALS: INTERTRANSVERSARII (seg-men-tal in-ter-tranz-ver-sa-re-i)

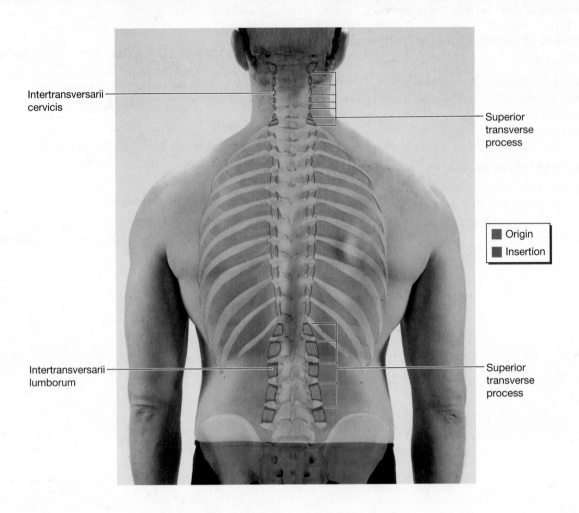

FIGURE 4-29 · **Segmentals: intertransversarii**

Meaning of Name

The group name *segmentals* refers to the fact that these muscles are one segment in length, or that they span only one intervertebral joint. *Intertransversarii* means that these muscles are located between transverse processes.

Location

Between transverse processes, primarily in the cervical and lumbar regions of the spine; these small, paired muscles lie between the transverse processes of adjacent vertebrae. They are divided into sections as follows:

1. Intertransversarii anterior cervicis
2. Intertransversarii posterior cervicis
3. Intertransversarii thoracis
4. Intertransversarii medial lumborum
5. Intertransversarii lateral lumborum

Origin and Insertion

Intertransversarii Anterior Cervicis

Origin: anterior, superior surfaces of the transverse processes of C3–T1

Insertion: inferior, anterior surface of the transverse processes of C2–C7

Intertransversarii Posterior Cervicis

This muscle has a medial and a lateral part, but both connect transverse processes of adjacent vertebrae.

Origin: posterior, superior aspect of the transverse processes of C2–T1

Insertion: posterior, inferior aspects of transverse processes of C1–C7

Intertransversarii Thoracis

This muscle has only three segments.
Origin: transverse processes of T11, T12, and L1
Insertion: transverse processes of T10–T12

Intertransversarii Medial Lumborum

Origin: medial aspect of the transverse processes of L2–L5 and the sacrum (S1)
Insertion: medial aspect of the transverse processes of L1–L5

Intertransversarii Lateral Lumborum

This muscle has two parts, anterior and posterior. Both share the same origin and insertion sites.
Origin: transverse processes of L2–S1
Insertion: transverse processes of L1–L5

Actions

Bilateral: extend the neck and low back
Unilateral: perform lateral flexion of the neck and low back

Explanation of Actions

Because origin is inferior to insertion, and the muscles cross the posterior side of intervertebral joints, intertransversarii extend the spine. Unilaterally, intertransversarii are positioned to pull transverse processes inferior, causing lateral flexion.

Notable Muscle Facts

These tiny muscles have postural as well as functional purpose. They assist us in keeping our spines erect.

Implications of Shortened and/or Lengthened/ Weak Muscle

Shortened: Limited flexion of cervical and/or lumbar region of the spine is noted.
Lengthened: Reduced ability to perform the actions of this muscle is noted.

Palpation and Massage

Intertransversarii muscles are located deep between the transverse processes in the cervical and lumbar region. Careful application of friction and/or direct pressure to the area can help the muscles to relax.

How to Stretch This Muscle

Flex cervical and lumbar regions of the spine.

Synergists

Splenius capitis, splenius cervicis, semispinalis capitis, multifidus, iliocostalis cervicis and lumborum, longissimus cervicis and lumborum, and spinalis cervicis

Antagonists

Sternocleidomastoid, scalenes, and the abdominal muscles that flex the trunk

Innervation and Arterial Supply

Innervation: dorsal branches of spinal nerves
Arterial supply: dorsal branches of the intercostal arteries

TRANSVERSOSPINALIS: ROTATORES (tranz-ver-so-spi-na-lis rot-a-to-rez)

Meaning of Name

Transversospinalis refers to the fact that these muscles originate on a transverse process and insert on a spinous process. *Rotatores* refers to the ability of the muscles to rotate the spine.

Location

These short, paired muscles are located in the lamina groove, joining the transverse process of a vertebra to the spinous process of the vertebra just above. They are divided into groups as follows:

1. Rotatores cervicis
2. Rotatores thoracis
3. Rotatores lumborum

Origin and Insertion

Rotatores Cervicis

Origin: transverse processes of C3–C7
Insertion: spinous processes of C2–C6

Rotatores Thoracis

Origin: transverse processes of T1–T12
Insertion: spinous processes of C7–T11

Rotatores Lumborum

Origin: transverse processes of L1–S1
Insertion: spinous processes of T12–L5

Actions

Unilateral: rotation of the spine to the opposite side
Bilateral: extension of the spine

Explanation of Actions

Because the origin is more lateral than the insertion, the muscle pulls the spinous processes laterally, causing the spine to turn to the opposite side. Of course, this action occurs when the muscle contracts unilaterally. When working bilaterally, rotatores pull the spinous processes inferiorly, causing extension of the spine.

Notable Muscle Facts

These small muscles serve as stabilizers of the intervertebral joints. In addition, they allow small, specific movements between adjacent vertebrae.

Implications of Shortened and/or Lengthened/ Weak Muscle

Shortened: Transversospinalis muscles shortened on one side only can cause the spine to be rotated to the opposite side.

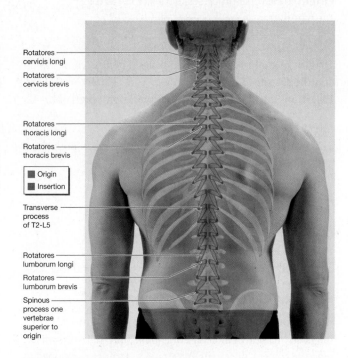

FIGURE 4-30 · **Transversospinalis: rotatores**

Bilaterally shortened transversospinalis muscles can cause difficulty in fully flexing the spine.
Lengthened: Reduced ability to perform the actions of this muscle is noted.

Palpation and Massage

It is generally easy to find the lamina groove. Locate the spinous processes and palpate just laterally to them. Friction and/or direct pressure are appropriate strokes to apply to these muscles.

How to Stretch This Muscle

Perform same-side rotation and flexion of the spine.

Synergists

External obliques (perform opposite-side rotation of the spine)
Erector Spinae Group (perform extension of spine)

Antagonists

Obliques and rectus abdominis (perform flexion of the spine)

Innervation and Arterial Supply

Innervation: dorsal branches of spinal nerves
Arterial supply: dorsal branches of the posterior intercostal arteries

TRANSVERSOSPINALIS: MULTIFIDUS (tranz-ver-so-spi-na-lis mul-tif i-dus)

Meaning of Name

Transversospinalis refers to the fact that these muscles originate on a transverse process and insert on a spinous process. *Multifidus* means "many splits."

Location

This muscle is located in the lamina groove, directly superficial to rotatores. Multifidus joins the transverse process of a vertebra to the spinous process of two to four above it. The multifidus muscle is considered a single muscle group, but it does have cervical, thoracic, lumbar, and sacral areas.

Origin and Insertion

Origin: sacrum, ilium, and transverse processes of lumbar, thoracic, and C4–C7 vertebrae
Insertion: spinous processes of the vertebra two to four vertebrae above the origin

Actions

Bilateral: extends the spine
Unilateral: rotates the spine to the opposite side

Explanation of Actions

Because the origin is more lateral than the insertion, the muscle pulls the spinous processes laterally, causing the spine to turn to the opposite side. Of course, this action occurs when the muscle contracts unilaterally. When working bilaterally, multifidus pulls the spinous processes inferiorly, causing extension of the spine.

Notable Muscle Facts

Multifidus allows small, specific movements between vertebrae. The postural function of this muscle group is important.

Implications of Shortened and/or Lengthened/ Weak Muscle

Shortened: Transversospinalis muscles shortened on one side only can cause the spine to be rotated to the opposite side. Bilaterally shortened transversospinalis muscles can cause one to have difficulty fully flexing the spine.
Lengthened: Reduced ability to perform the actions of this muscle is noted.

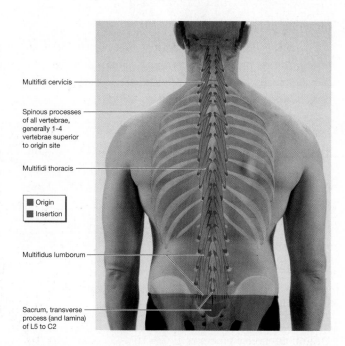

Multifidi cervicis

Spinous processes of all vertebrae, generally 1-4 vertebrae superior to origin site

Multifidi thoracis

■ Origin
■ Insertion

Multifidus lumborum

Sacrum, transverse process (and lamina) of L5 to C2

FIGURE 4-31 · Transversospinalis: multifidus

Palpation and Massage

It is generally easy to find the lamina groove. Locate the spinous processes and palpate just laterally to them. Friction and/or direct pressure are appropriate strokes to apply to these muscles.

How to Stretch This Muscle

Perform same-side rotation and flexion of the spine.

Synergists

External obliques (perform opposite-side rotation of the spine)

Antagonists

Obliques and rectus abdominis (flex the spine)
Erector Spinae Group (perform extension of spine)

Innervation and Arterial Supply

Innervation: dorsal rami of spinal nerves
Arterial supply: dorsal branches of the posterior intercostal arteries

TRANSVERSOSPINALIS: SEMISPINALIS (tranz-ver-so-spi-na-lis sem-e-spin-a-lis)

Meaning of Name

Transversospinalis refers to the fact that these muscles originate on a transverse process and insert on a spinous process. *Semispinalis* means one half, as semispinalis is located in the cervical and thoracic regions only.

Location

This muscle is located in the lamina groove, directly superficial to multifidus. The muscle joins each transverse process from C-4 to T-10 to a spinous process 3–6 vertebrae above. Semispinalis is divided into groups as follows:

1. Semispinalis capitis
2. Semispinalis cervicis
3. Semispinalis thoracis

Origin and Insertion

Semispinalis Capitis
Origin: transverse processes of C4–T6
Insertion: occiput

Semispinalis Cervicis
Origin: transverse processes of T1–T6
Insertion: spinous processes of C2–C6

Semispinalis Thoracis
Origin: transverse processes of T6–T10
Insertion: spinous processes of C6–T6

Actions

Bilateral: extend the spine
Unilateral: rotate the spine to the opposite side

Explanation of Actions

Because the origin is more lateral than the insertion, the muscle pulls the spinous processes laterally, causing the spine to turn to the opposite side. Of course, this action occurs when the muscle contracts unilaterally. When working bilaterally, semispinalis pulls the spinous processes inferiorly, causing extension of the spine.

Notable Muscle Facts

Semispinalis is largest in the cervical region. Because this muscle is the most vertically oriented of the three transversospinalis muscles, it is best suited for extension of the spine and least suited for contralateral rotation of the spine.

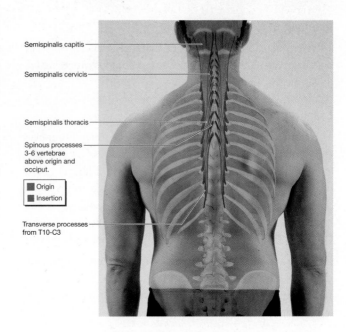

Semispinalis capitis

Semispinalis cervicis

Semispinalis thoracis

Spinous processes
3-6 vertebrae
above origin and
occiput.

■ Origin
■ Insertion

Transverse processes
from T10-C3

FIGURE 4-32 · Transversospinalis: semispinalis

Implications of Shortened and/or Lengthened/ Weak Muscle

Shortened: Transversospinalis muscles shortened on one side can cause the spine to be rotated to the opposite side. Bilaterally shortened transversospinalis muscles can cause difficulty in fully flexing the spine.

Lengthened: Reduced ability to perform the actions of this muscle is noted.

Palpation and Massage

It is generally easy to find the lamina groove. Locate the spinous processes and palpate just laterally to them. Friction and/or direct pressure are appropriate strokes to apply to these muscles.

How to Stretch This Muscle

Perform same-side rotation and flexion of the spine.

Synergists

External obliques (perform opposite-side rotation of the spine)

Antagonists

Obliques and rectus abdominis (flex the spine)

Innervation and Arterial Supply

Innervation: dorsal rami of spinal nerves

Arterial supply: dorsal branches of the posterior intercostal arteries and the occipital artery

ERECTOR SPINAE GROUP: ILIOCOSTALIS (e-rek-tor spi-ne grup: il-e-o-kos-ta-lis)

Meaning of Name

Erector spinae group refers to a group of muscles that keep the spine erect or straight. "Iliocostalis" refers to the fact that this muscle articulates with both the ilium and the ribs.

Location

The erector spinae group contains three vertically oriented bands of muscle, on both sides of the spine. They lie deep to the scapula nad to the rhomboids and serratus posterior muscles. They share an origin on the thoracolumbar aponeurosis, which is attached to the middle and lateral aspects of the sacrum and posterior iliac crest. Iliocostalis is the most lateral band of the erector spinae group. It has three parts:

1. Iliocostalis cervicis
2. Iliocostalis thoracis
3. Iliocostalis lumborum

Origin and Insertion

Iliocostalis Cervicis
Origin: posterior ribs 3 to 6
Insertion: transverse processes of C4–C6

Iliocostalis Thoracis
Origin: posterior ribs 7–12
Insertion: upper six ribs and the transverse process of C7

Iliocostalis Lumborum
Origin: iliac crest and thoracolumbar aponeurosis
Insertion: transverse processes of the lumbar vertebrae and the lower seven ribs

Actions

Bilateral: extends the spine
Unilaterally: laterally flexes the spine

Explanation of Actions

Because origin is below insertion, and because the muscle is located on the back, iliocostalis pulls the ribs and/or upper vertebrae back and down, thus causing extension of the spine. If one side contracts alone, the ribs and/or upper vertebrae are pulled down to the side and the result is lateral flexion of the spine.

Notable Muscle Facts

The erector spinae muscles contract to stabilize the spine when coughing, sneezing, and maintaining an upright position against gravity. In addition, the erector spinae group is designed for use in broad movements of the spine, primarily extension and lateral flexion.

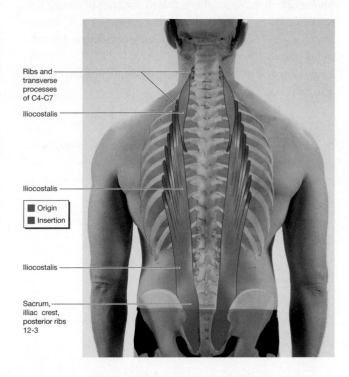

Ribs and transverse processes of C4-C7

Iliocostalis

Iliocostalis

■ Origin
■ Insertion

Iliocostalis

Sacrum, illiac crest, posterior ribs 12-3

FIGURE 4-33 · Erector spinae group member: iliocostalis

Implications of Shortened and/or Lengthened/Weak Muscle

Shortened: If iliocostalis is shortened unilaterally, it may limit the ability to perform lateral flexion to the opposite side. If iliocostalis is shortened bilaterally, limited flexion of the spine is likely.

Lengthened: Reduced ability to perform the actions of this muscle is noted.

Palpation and Massage

Iliocostalis, together with longissimus, is generally palpable as vertical bands that run just lateral to the lamina groove. Friction and direct pressure are appropriate massage strokes to address this muscle.

How to Stretch This Muscle

Laterally flex the spine to the opposite side.

Synergists

Longissimus and spinalis

Antagonists

The external obliques, internal obliques, and rectus abdominis (flex the spine)

Innervation and Arterial Supply

Innervation: dorsal rami of spinal nerves
Arterial supply: posterior intercostal and lumbar

ERECTOR SPINAE GROUP: LONGISSIMUS (e-rek-tor spi-ne grup: lon-jis-i-mus)

Meaning of Name

Longissimus refers to the extensive length of this muscle.

Location

This muscle is located just medial to iliocostalis and just lateral to the lamina groove. The muscle group consists of three sections:

1. Longissimus capitis
2. Longissimus cervicis
3. Longissimus thoracis

Origin and Insertion

Longissimus Capitis

Origin: transverse processes of T1–T4
Insertion: mastoid process of the temporal bone

Longissimus Cervicis

Origin: transverse processes of T1–T5
Insertion: transverse processes of C2–C6

Longissimus Thoracis

Origin: transverse processes of lumbar vertebrae and the thoracolumbar aponeurosis
Insertion: transverse processes of T1–T12 and ribs 2–12

Actions

Bilateral: extends the spine
Unilateral: laterally flexes the spine

Explanation of Actions

Because origin is below insertion, and because the muscle is located on the back, longissimus pulls the vertebrae back and down, thus causing extension of the spine. If one side contracts alone, the vertebrae are pulled down to the side and the result is lateral flexion of the spine.

Notable Muscle Facts

The erector spinae muscles contract to stabilize the spine when coughing, sneezing, and maintaining an upright position against gravity. In addition, the erector spinae group is designed for use in broad movements of the spine, primarily extension and lateral flexion.

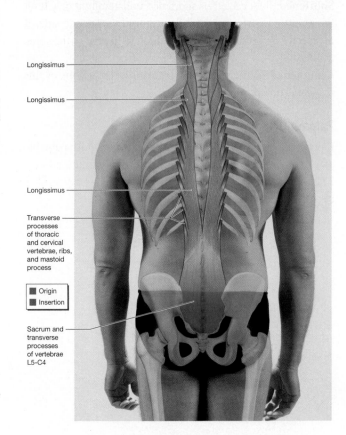

Longissimus

Longissimus

Longissimus

Transverse processes of thoracic and cervical vertebrae, ribs, and mastoid process

■ Origin
■ Insertion

Sacrum and transverse processes of vertebrae L5–C4

FIGURE 4-34 · Erector spinae group member: longissimus

Implications of Shortened and/or Lengthened/Weak Muscle

Shortened: If longissimus is shortened unilaterally, it may limit the ability to perform lateral flexion to the opposite side. If longissimus is shortened bilaterally, limited flexion of the spine may be noted.

Lengthened: Reduced ability to perform the actions of this muscle is noted.

Palpation and Massage

Longissimus, together with iliocostalis, is generally palpable as vertical bands that run just lateral to the lamina groove. Friction and direct pressure are appropriate massage strokes to address this muscle.

How to Stretch This Muscle

Laterally flex the spine to the opposite side.

Synergists

Iliocostalis and spinalis

Antagonists

The external obliques, internal obliques, and rectus abdominis (permit flexion of the spine)

Innervation and Arterial Supply

Innervation: dorsal branches of spinal nerves
Arterial supply: posterior intercostal and lumbar arteries

ERECTOR SPINAE GROUP: SPINALIS (e-rek-tor spi-ne grup: spin-a-lis)

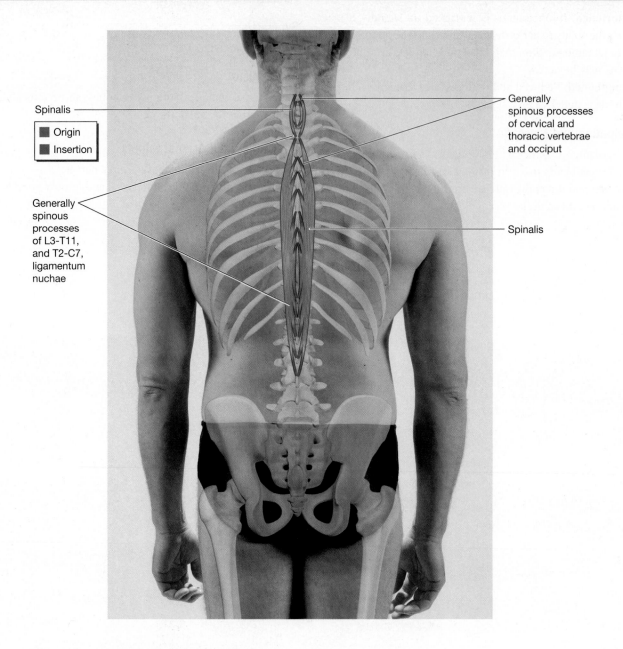

FIGURE 4-35 · Erector spinae group member: spinalis

Meaning of Name

Spinalis refers to the spine, as this muscle is in close proximity to the spine and attaches to spinous processes.

Location

This muscle is the most medial band of the erector spinae group and is located in the lamina groove, superficial to the transversospinalis group. It has three sections:

1. Spinalis capitis
2. Spinalis cervicis
3. Spinalis thoracis

Origin and Insertion

Spinalis Capitis
Origin: spinous processes of C6–T2
Insertion: occiput

Spinalis Cervicis
Origin: spinous processes of C6–T2
Insertion: spinous processes of C2–C4

Spinalis Thoracis
Origin: spinous processes of T11–L2
Insertion: spinous processes of T2–T7

Actions

Bilateral: extends the spine
Unilateral: laterally flexes the spine

Explanation of Actions

Because origin is below insertion, and because the muscle is located on the back, spinalis pulls the vertebrae back and down, thus causing extension of the spine. If one side contracts alone, the vertebrae are pulled down to the side and the result is lateral flexion of the spine.

Notable Muscle Facts

The erector spinae muscles contract to stabilize the spine when coughing, sneezing, and maintaining an upright position against gravity. In addition, the erector spinae group is designed for use in broad movements of the spine, primarily extension and lateral flexion. Spinalis is the weakest of the erector spinae group.

Implications of Shortened and/or Lengthened/Weak Muscle

Shortened: If spinalis is shortened unilaterally, it limits the ability to perform lateral flexion to the opposite side. If spinalis is shortened bilaterally, limited flexion of the spine is noted.
Lengthened: Reduced ability to perform the actions of muscle is noted.

Palpation and Massage

Spinalis lies in the lamina groove, directly superficial to semispinalis. Friction and direct pressure are appropriate massage strokes to address this muscle.

How to Stretch This Muscle

Laterally flex the spine to the opposite side.

Synergists

Iliocostalis and longissimus

Antagonists

The external obliques, internal obliques, and rectus (flexes the spine)

Innervation and Arterial Supply

Innervation: dorsal rami of the spinal nerves
Arterial supply: posterior intercostal and lumbar arteries

Muscles of the Abdominal Wall

The abdomen is located inferior to the thorax and superior to the pelvis. The stomach, intestines, liver, and pancreas are among the important organs that reside in the abdominal cavity. Four muscles comprise much of the abdominal wall that surrounds and protects the viscera. Three of the main abdominal muscles are large, flat muscles located in the anterolateral abdomen. The fourth abdominal muscle is thicker, particularly in its inferior aspect, and lies quite central in the anterior abdomen. These muscles have roles in moving and stabilizing the spine, as well as roles in forced exhalation.

TRANSVERSE ABDOMINIS (trans-vers ab-dom-i-nus)

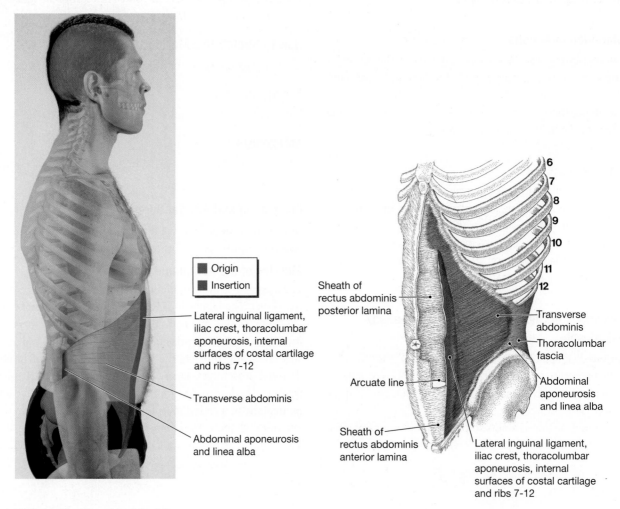

FIGURE 4-36 · Transverse abdominis

Meaning of Name

Transverse indicates a horizontal direction of fibers. *Abdominis* refers to the abdominal region.

Location

This muscle is located deep in the lateral abdominal wall.

Origin and Insertion

Origin: lateral inguinal ligament, the iliac crest, thoracolumbar aponeurosis, internal surfaces of the costal cartilage of ribs 7–10, and the internal surfaces of ribs 7–12
Insertion: abdominal aponeurosis and the linea alba

Actions

Compresses the contents of the abdomen, as is necessary for forced exhalation, coughing, sneezing, vomiting, pushing in childbirth, and forced defecation.

Explanation of Actions

The transverse abdominis muscle forms a wide ring of muscle from the thoracolumbar aponeurosis in back to the abdominal aponeurosis in front. Thus, the muscle's contraction literally squeezes the contents of the abdomen.

Notable Muscle Facts

Isometric contraction of the transverse abdominis helps support the lower thoracic and lumbar spine. When lifting a heavy object or performing other activities that require a forceful contraction of the extensors of the spine, we tighten our abdominal muscles to help stabilize our spine. In fact, most movements requiring balance against gravity begin with contraction of transverse abdominis.

Implications of Shortened and/or Lengthened/ Weak Muscle

Shortened: If the transverse abdominis are shortened, difficulty inhaling deeply is noted.

Lengthened: Reduced ability to perform the actions of this muscle is noted.

Palpation and Massage

This muscle is the deepest abdominal muscle in the antero-lateral wall. The location of the muscle affords us no easy bony surface to push the muscle into, just abdominal organs, thus friction is difficult. It is possible to press the muscle into the lower five ribs and the iliac crest. However, strokes such as deep effleurage and vibration are perhaps easier to use on transverse abdominis than friction.

How to Stretch This Muscle

Inhale fully.

Synergists

Not applicable

Antagonists

Not applicable

Innervation and Arterial Supply

Innervation: anterior rami of the T7–L1
Arterial supply: subcostal and posterior intercostal arteries

INTERNAL OBLIQUE (in-tern-al ob-leek)

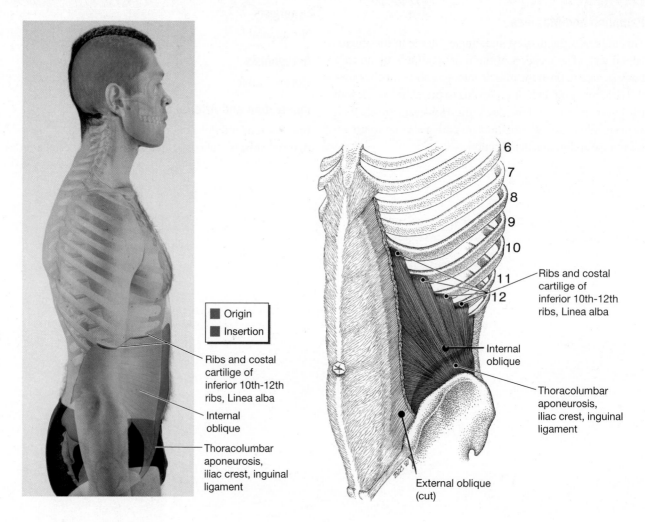

FIGURE 4-37 · Internal obliques

Meaning of Name

Internal refers to the fact that internal obliques are directly deep to external obliques. *Oblique* means diagonal, referring to the direction of fibers of this muscle. The fibers run superiorly as they run medially.

Location

This muscle is located in the anterolateral abdominal wall. It is directly superficial to transverse abdominis and directly deep to external obliques.

Origin and Insertion

Origin: thoracolumbar aponeurosis, anterior iliac crest, and inguinal ligament

Insertion: ribs 10–12 and the linea alba to the abdominal aponeurosis

Actions

Bilateral: flexes the trunk
Unilateral: performs lateral flexion and same-side rotation of the spine

Explanation of Actions

The internal oblique flexes the trunk/spine because its origin is inferior to the insertion, and the muscle crosses the anterior side of the intervertebral joints. Thus, pulling the linea aspera inferiorly causes flexion of the spine.

Unilaterally, internal obliques perform lateral flexion because the linea alba is pulled toward the anterior iliac crest. Unilaterally, internal obliques can produce same-side rotation because pulling the linea alba laterally toward insertion causes rotation.

Notable Muscle Facts

Both internal and external obliques assist in stabilization of the lower spine. The fiber direction of internal obliques correspond to the fiber direction of internal intercostals.

Implications of Shortened and/or Lengthened/ Weak Muscle

Shortened: Shortened internal obliques may cause difficulty in performing lateral flexion to the opposite side and may produce a posterior pelvic tilt.

Lengthened: Reduced ability to perform the actions of this muscle is noted.

Palpation and Massage

This muscle is the midlayer muscle of the three abdominal muscles in the anterolateral wall. Deep effleurage and vibration are two useful strokes to apply to this muscle.

How to Stretch This Muscle

Laterally flex and rotate the trunk to the opposite side.

Synergists

External oblique and rectus abdominis (flex the trunk)

Antagonists

External oblique (performs opposite-side rotation of the trunk)

Innervation and Arterial Supply

Innervation: anterior rami of the T7–L1

Arterial supply: subcostal and posterior intercostal arteries

EXTERNAL OBLIQUE (eks-tern-al ob-leek)

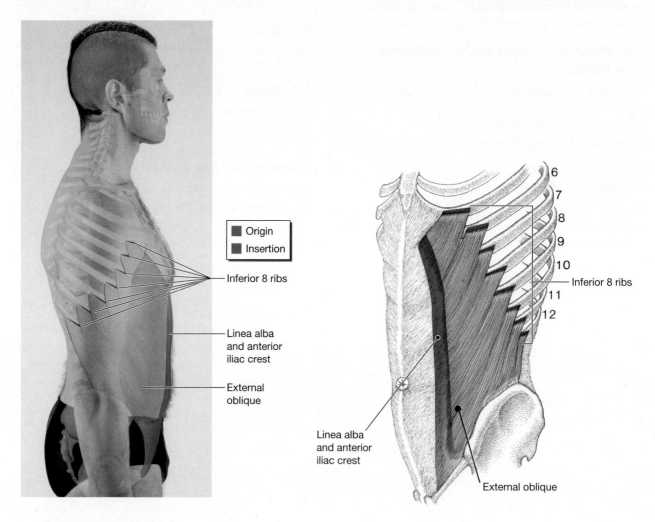

Origin
Insertion

Inferior 8 ribs

Linea alba
and anterior
iliac crest

External
oblique

6
7
8
9
10
11
12

Inferior 8 ribs

Linea alba
and anterior
iliac crest

External oblique

FIGURE 4-38 · External obliques

Meaning of Name

External means superficial, referring to the fact that external obliques are superficial to internal obliques. *Oblique* means diagonal, referring to the orientation of fibers of this muscle. The fibers run inferiorly as they run medially.

Location

This muscle is located in the anterolateral abdominal wall. It is the most superficial of the three muscles located here.

Origin and Insertion

Origin: inferior eight ribs
Insertion: linea alba and the anterior iliac crest

Actions

Bilateral: flexes the trunk
Unilateral: lateral flexion and opposite-side rotation of the spine

Explanation of Actions

In the case of this muscle, the actions occur when the origin moves toward the insertion. Bilaterally, pulling the ribs toward the iliac crest and the lower linea alba causes flexion of the trunk. Unilaterally, pulling the ribs toward the iliac crest produces lateral flexion. Pulling the lateral ribs toward a medial and anterior linea alba causes rotation to the opposite side.

Notable Muscle Facts

Both internal and external obliques assist in stabilization of the lower spine. The fiber direction of external obliques corresponds to the fiber direction of external intercostals.

Implications of Shortened and/or Lengthened/ Weak Muscle

Shortened: Shortened external obliques may cause difficulty in performing lateral flexion to the opposite side, and may produce a posterior pelvic tilt.

Lengthened: Reduced ability to perform the actions of this muscle is noted.

Palpation and Massage

Effleurage to the anterolateral trunk is appropriate for addressing external obliques.

How to Stretch This Muscle

Perform lateral flexion and rotation of the trunk to the same side.

Synergists

External oblique and rectus abdominis (flex the trunk)

Antagonists

External oblique (performs opposite-side rotation of the trunk)

Innervation and Arterial Supply

Innervation: anterior rami of the T7–L1
Arterial supply: subcostal and posterior intercostal arteries

RECTUS ABDOMINIS (rek-tus ab-dom-i-nis)

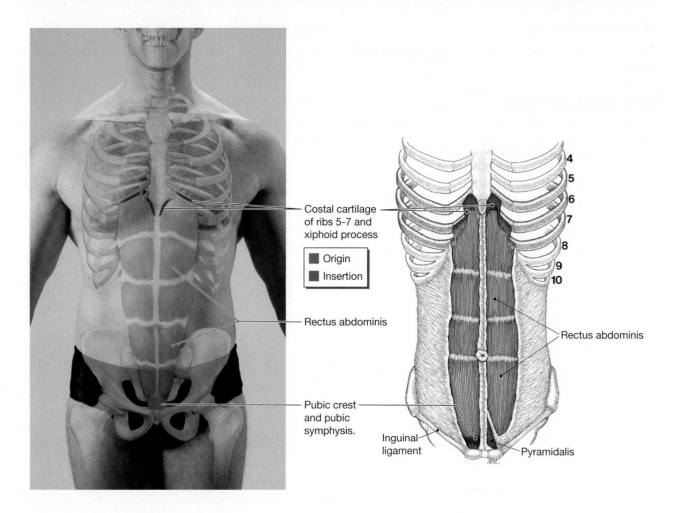

Costal cartilage
of ribs 5-7 and
xiphoid process

■ Origin
■ Insertion

Rectus abdominis

Pubic crest
and pubic
symphysis.

Rectus abdominis

Inguinal
ligament

Pyramidalis

FIGURE 4-39 · Rectus abdominis

Meaning of Name

Rectus means straight, implying a vertical direction of the muscle fibers. *Abdominis* refers to the abdominal region.

Location

This muscle is located in the medial, anterior abdominal wall between the two layers of the abdominal aponeurosis. It has transversely oriented tendinous lines, passing through the muscle, which give the muscle added strength and its noted "six-pack" or "eight-pack" shape.

Origin and Insertion

Origin: pubic crest and pubic symphysis
Insertion: costal cartilage of ribs 5–7 and the xiphoid process of the sternum

Actions

Flexes the trunk

Explanation of Actions

Because its origin is directly inferior to the insertion and the muscle crosses intervertebral joints anteriorly, the muscle pulls the xiphoid process toward the pubic symphysis, causing trunk flexion.

Notable Muscle Facts

Rectus abdominis works with the three other abdominal muscles to stabilize the spine.

Implications of Shortened and/or Lengthened/ Weak Muscle

Shortened: A shortened rectus abdominis contributes to a posterior pelvic tilt.
Lengthened: Reduced ability to perform the actions of this muscle is noted.

Palpation and Massage

Effleurage is perhaps the easiest stroke to apply to rectus abdominis, as the muscle is located superficially in the anterior abdomen. Friction to the superior attachment areas of the muscle is certainly an option as well.

How to Stretch This Muscle

Extend the trunk.

Synergists

The internal and external obliques (flex the trunk)

Antagonists

The erector spinae group and the transversospinalis muscles (extend the spine)

Innervation and Arterial Supply

Innervation: anterior rami of the T7–T12
Arterial supply: superior epigastric artery

QUADRATUS LUMBORUM (kwah-drat-us lum-bo-rum)

Meaning of Name

Quadratus refers to the four-sided, square shape of this muscle. *Lumborum* refers to the lumbar area where the muscle is located.

Location

This muscle is located in the deep low back, so deep in fact, that it is within the posterior abdominal wall.

Origin and Insertion

Origin: posterior iliac crest
Insertion: twelfth rib and the transverse processes of L1–L5

Actions

Unilateral: lateral flexion of the lumbar spine and "hip hiking"
Bilateral: extends the lumbar spine
Role in breathing: contracts isometrically when the diaphragm contracts to hold the twelfth rib down, thus contributing to the expansion of the thoracic cavity

Explanation of Actions

Quadratus lumborum (QL) can produce lateral flexion by pulling one twelfth rib toward the iliac crest. Hip hiking occurs when the twelfth rib is held fixed and the ilium is raised. When both left and right quadratus lumborum muscles contract simultaneously and both twelfth ribs are pulled posteriorly, extension of the lumbar area occurs.

Notable Muscle Facts

Quadratus lumborum helps to maintain the position of the twelfth rib during inhalation. As the diaphragm contracts, it exerts an upward pull on the twelfth rib. The QL counteracts this pull by exerting a downward pull on the twelfth rib, thus stabilizing its position and providing the diaphragm with a more stable origin. Greater stability of a muscle's origin enhances the efficiency of its contraction.

Implications of Shortened and/or Lengthened/ Weak Muscle

Shortened: Shortened QL muscles can cause anterior pelvic tilt by raising the iliac crest superiorly, increasing the lumbar curve and tipping the pelvis forward. Shortened QL muscles can also cause limited lateral flexion to the opposite side.
Lengthened: Reduced ability to perform the actions of this muscle is noted.

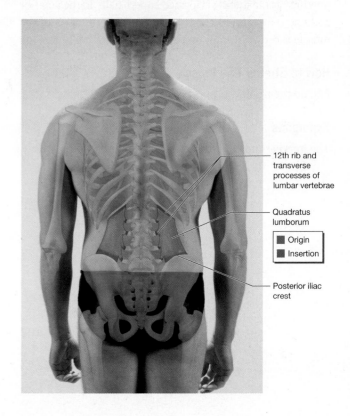

12th rib and transverse processes of lumbar vertebrae

Quadratus lumborum

■ Origin
■ Insertion

Posterior iliac crest

FIGURE 4-40 · Quadratus lumborum

Palpation and Massage

Deep pressure and friction into the low back region are effective in addressing this muscle.

How to Stretch This Muscle

Laterally flex to the opposite side.

Synergists

The lumbar erector spinae muscles (extend the lumbar spine)

Antagonists

The obliques and rectus abdominis (flex the lumbar spine)

Innervation and Arterial Supply

Innervation: ventral rami of T12–L4
Arterial supply: subcostal and lumbar arteries

Muscles of Respiration

The muscles of respiration work together to alter the size of the thoracic cavity. Enlarging the thoracic cavity reduces the pressure within the cavity, thus reducing the pressure within our lungs. When the pressure in our lungs falls below the pressure in the atmosphere, air rushes into the lungs to balance the pressure. We inhale simply by using muscles to enlarge our thoracic cavities, creating reduced pressure, which acts like a vacuum to pull air into our lungs. Gentle exhalation is typically passive and does not require the use of our muscles. The elastic nature of the lungs causes them to recoil and push air out. However, when we want to force the air out of our lungs, as in blowing into a musical instrument, blowing out a candle, or exercising aerobically, we do use musculature. We use muscles to reduce the size of the thoracic cavity, which increases pressure in the lungs and forces air out.

DIAPHRAGM (di-a-fram)

Meaning of Name

Diaphragm means partition.

Location

The name of this muscle is appropriate, given that it separates the thoracic and abdominal cavities.

Origin and Insertion

Origin: bodies of lumbar vertebrae 1–3, the internal surfaces of the inferior six ribs and their costal cartilage, and the posterior aspect of the xiphoid process of the sternum
Insertion: central tendon, an aponeurotic sheet of fascia, forming a dome-like shape for the superior part of the diaphragm

Actions

Expands the thoracic cavity, allowing inspiration

Explanation of Actions

When the muscular portion of the diaphragm contracts, the central tendon is flattened or pulled down, thus enlarging the volume of the thoracic cavity. In response to the increased volume, the pressure in the lungs is reduced, drawing air into them. The diaphragm is the chief muscle of inspiration.

Notable Muscle Facts

The diaphragm is a thin, musculotendinous structure, creating the roof of the abdominopelvic cavity and the floor of the thoracic cavity. There are openings in the diaphragm for the esophagus, aorta, and inferior vena cava to pass through. Relaxed breathing can be accomplished by the diaphragm alone, but deeper or more forced inhalation requires additional muscles. The diaphragm can be considered both a voluntary and an involuntary muscle, as we have some conscious control over our rate of breathing, yet the diaphragm responds to cues from the central nervous system, as well.

Implications of Shortened and/or Lengthened/ Weak Muscle

Shortened: A shortened diaphragm limits full and easy breathing.
Lengthened: Because the respiratory diaphragm has no direct antagonist, the typical muscle imbalance between shortened and lengthened skeletal muscles does not apply here. Perhaps an underused, lengthened diaphragm would lead to reduced ability to fully inhale. However, such a condition would not be the result of an inhibition caused by excessive contraction of antagonists.

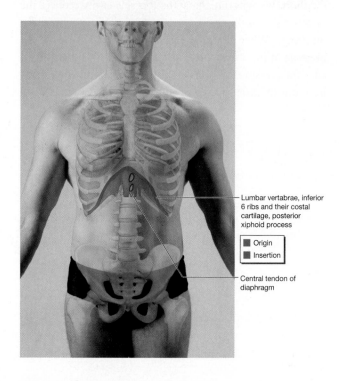

Lumbar vertabrae, inferior 6 ribs and their costal cartilage, posterior xiphoid process

■ Origin
■ Insertion

Central tendon of diaphragm

FIGURE 4-41 · **Diaphragm**

Palpation and Massage

It is possible to palpate the portion of the diaphragm that attaches to the inner surfaces of the ribs by pressing your fingers gently around the most inferior aspect of the anterolateral rib cage and pushing gently upward into the muscle.

How to Stretch This Muscle

Breathe deeply, with focus on full exhalation to help relax the diaphragm.

Synergists

External intercostals and serratus posterior superior

Antagonists

Although no muscle elevates the central tendon of the diaphragm, the internal intercostals, serratus posterior inferior, and transverse abdominis can be considered antagonists as they are muscles used in forced exhalation.

Innervation and Arterial Supply

Innervation: phrenic nerve
Arterial supply: branches of the aorta and the internal thoracic artery

EXTERNAL INTERCOSTALS (eks-tern-al in-ter-kos-tals)

Meaning of Name

External refers to the fact that this muscle is superficial (more on the outside) of the internal intercostals. *Intercostal* means "between ribs."

Location

This muscle is located between the ribs. The external intercostals do not fill the space between the costal cartilages of the ribs.

Origin and Insertion

Origin: inferior border of the rib above
Insertion: superior border of the rib below

Actions

Elevate the ribs to assist in enlarging the thoracic cavity

Explanation of Actions

Because the origin is above the insertion, the superior border of the rib below is pulled upward, closer to the rib above. To understand the difference between the actions of external intercostals and internal intercostals, it is important to recognize that all areas on the ribs are not equal in terms of stability and mobility. The portion of the ribs closest to the thoracic vertebrae is most stable, and the lateral and anterior aspects of the ribs are more mobile.

In general, the oblique direction of the fibers of the external intercostals provides an arrangement in which the origin is located at a more stable area (closer to the vertebral connection) of the ribs than is the insertion. The more stable origin is on the rib above, and the more moveable insertion is on the rib below. Thus, contraction of the external intercostals results in elevation of the ribs.

However, there are times when the lower ribs are stabilized, most likely by the contraction of other muscles, and thus the rib above is more mobile. In these instances, the external intercostals can depress the ribs to assist in forced exhalation.

Notable Muscle Facts

The upper two to four pairs of external intercostals are most important for inhalation, with the middle and lower external intercostals muscles engaging only in exertive or forced inhalation. The external intercostals have the same direction of fibers as do the external obliques. The external intercostals are thicker than the internal intercostals.

Implications of Shortened and/or Lengthened/Weak Muscle

Shortened: If the external intercostal muscles are shortened, difficulty exhaling fully is noted.
Lengthened: Reduced ability to elevate the ribs is noted.

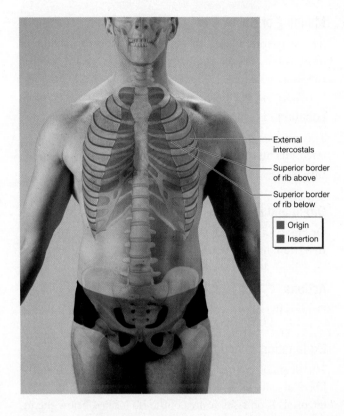

External intercostals

Superior border of rib above

Superior border of rib below

■ Origin
■ Insertion

FIGURE 4-42 · **External intercostals**

Palpation and Massage

Direct pressure and friction between the ribs is an effective way to address the intercostals. These muscles are common trigger point sites, so communicate well with your client about any potential discomfort.

How to Stretch This Muscle

Perform any movement that elongates the spaces between the ribs. Breathe deeply.

Synergists

Diaphragm and serratus posterior superior

Antagonists

Internal intercostals, serratus posterior inferior, and transverse abdominis (forced exhalation)

Innervation and Arterial Supply

Innervation: intercostal nerves
Arterial supply: anterior intercostal arteries

INTERNAL INTERCOSTALS (in-tern-al in-ter-kos-tals)

Meaning of Name

Internal refers to the fact that this muscle is deep (more on the inside) of the external intercostals. *Intercostal* means between ribs.

Location

This muscle is located between the ribs. The internal intercostals fill the space between the costal cartilages of the ribs.

Origin and Insertion

Origin: superior border of the rib below
Insertion: inferior border of the rib above

Actions

Depress the ribs to assist with forced exhalation

Explanation of Actions

The fibers of internal intercostals run perpendicular to the fibers of external intercostals. The origin of the internal intercostals is on a stable area of the rib located below the insertion. The insertion is on a more movable part of the ribs above the origin. Thus, contraction of the external intercostals results in depression of the ribs.

However, there are times when the upper rib of attachment is stabilized by the contraction of other muscles, and thus the lower attachment rib is more mobile. In these instances, the internal intercostals can elevate the ribs to assist in inhalation.

Notable Muscle Facts

Internal intercostals are not as thick as the external intercostals. There is another layer of intercostals muscles, deep to internal intercostals, called the *innermost intercostals*. These muscles have the same direction of fibers as the internal intercostals. The internal intercostals have the same direction of fibers as the internal obliques.

Implications of Shortened and/or Lengthened/ Weak Muscle

Shortened: If the internal intercostal muscles are shortened, difficulty inhaling fully is noted.
Lengthened: Reduced ability to depress the ribs is noted.

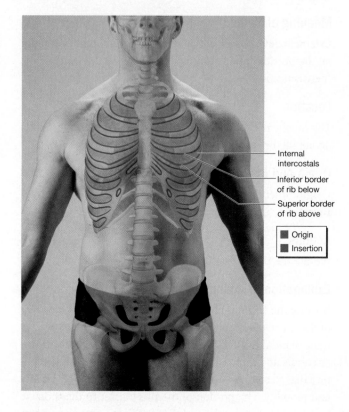

Internal
intercostals

Inferior border
of rib below

Superior border
of rib above

■ Origin
■ Insertion

FIGURE 4-43 · Internal intercostals

Palpation and Massage

Direct pressure and friction between the ribs are effective ways to address the intercostals. These muscles are common trigger point sites, so communicate well with your client about any potential discomfort.

How to Stretch This Muscle

Perform any movement that elongates the spaces between the ribs. Breathe deeply.

Synergists

Serratus posterior inferior and transverse abdominis

Antagonists

The diaphragm, external intercostals, and serratus posterior superior

Innervation and Arterial Supply

Innervation: intercostal nerves
Arterial supply: anterior intercostal arteries

SERRATUS POSTERIOR SUPERIOR (ser-a-tus pos-ter-e-or su-per-e-or)

Meaning of Name

Serratus means jagged, such as a serrated knife. The word *posterior* in this muscle name tells us that the serratus posterior muscles are located posterior to the serratus anterior muscle. The word *superior* in this muscle indicates that serratus posterior superior is above serratus posterior inferior.

Location

This muscle is located in the upper back. It is deep to upper trapezius and rhomboids and is superficial to the erector spinae group in that region.

Origin and Insertion

Origin: inferior part of the ligamentum nuchae and the spinous processes of C7–T3
Insertion: superior border of ribs 2–5

Actions

Elevates ribs 2–5, assisting in enlarging the thoracic cavity as needed for inhalation

Explanation of Actions

Because origin is located above the insertion on the ribs, a shortening of the muscle results in raising the ribs.

Notable Muscle Facts

The fiber direction of serratus posterior superior is comparable to the fiber direction of rhomboids.

Implications of Shortened and/or Lengthened/ Weak Muscle

Shortened: Shortened serratus posterior superior muscles may limit ability to exhale fully.
Lengthened: Reduced ability to elevate the ribs is noted.

Palpation and Massage

Serratus posterior superior is a thin, flat muscle that can be difficult to distinguish from the rhomboids when palpating and massaging. Locate the spinous process of C7–T3 and palpate and/or massage laterally and inferiorly to ribs 2–5. Deep effleurage is an appropriate stroke for this muscle.

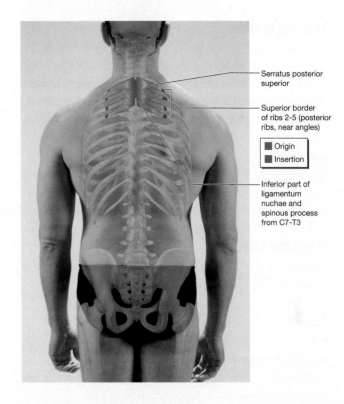

Serratus posterior superior

Superior border of ribs 2-5 (posterior ribs, near angles)

■ Origin
■ Insertion

Inferior part of ligamentum nuchae and spinous process from C7-T3

FIGURE 4-44 · Serratus posterior superior

How to Stretch This Muscle

Breathe deeply.

Synergists

Diaphragm and the external intercostals

Antagonists

Internal intercostals, serratus posterior inferior, and transverse abdominis

Innervation and Arterial Supply

Innervation: intercostal nerves
Arterial supply: dorsal branches of the posterior intercostal arteries

SERRATUS POSTERIOR INFERIOR (ser-a-tus pos-ter-e-or in-fer-e-or)

Meaning of Name

Serratus means jagged, such as a serrated knife. The word *posterior* in this muscle name tells us that the serratus posterior muscles are located posterior to the serratus anterior muscle. The word *inferior* in this muscle indicates that serratus posterior inferior is below serratus posterior superior.

Location

This muscle is a midlayer muscle, located in the mid to low back. It is deep to latissimus dorsi, yet superficial to the erector spinae group.

Origin and Insertion

Origin: spinous processes of T11–L3
Insertion: ribs 9–12

Actions

Serratus anterior depresses ribs 9–12, assisting in forced exhalation. Some sources claim that this muscle has a stabilization role, which assists in inhalation. When contracting isometrically, or without movement, serratus posterior inferior can keep the lower ribs in position when the diaphragm contracts, preventing them from moving upward. Such stabilization assists the efficiency of the diaphragm in inhalation.

Explanation of Actions

The origin of serratus posterior inferior is inferior to the insertion; therefore, the muscle is in position to pull the ribs downward, thus causing depression of ribs 9–12.

Notable Muscle Facts

Some sources suggest that serratus posterior inferior is more important as an ipsilateral trunk rotator and spine extensor than it is as a muscle of respiration.

Implications of Shortened and/or Lengthened/ Weak Muscle

Shortened: Shortened serratus posterior inferior muscles may limit ability to inhale fully.
Lengthened: Reduced ability to depress the ribs is noted.

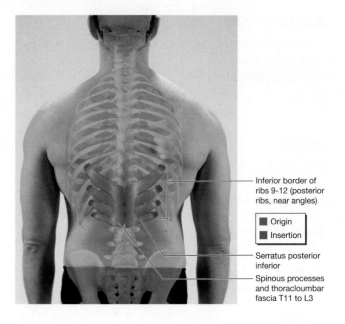

Inferior border of ribs 9-12 (posterior ribs, near angles)

■ Origin
■ Insertion

Serratus posterior inferior

Spinous processes and thoracloumbar fascia T11 to L3

FIGURE 4-45 · Serratus posterior inferior

Palpation and Massage

Find the spinous processes of T11–L3 and palpate and/or massage laterally and superiorly toward ribs 9–12. Deep effleurage is an appropriate stroke for this muscle.

How to Stretch This Muscle

Flex the trunk. Breathe deeply.

Synergists

Internal intercostals and transverse abdominis

Antagonists

Diaphragm, external intercostals, and serratus posterior superior

Innervation and Arterial Supply

Innervation: subcostal and intercostal nerves
Arterial supply: dorsal branches of the posterior intercostal arteries

Regional Illustrations of Muscles

Figure 4-46 shows a regional picture of the neck.

Figure 4-47 shows a regional picture of the intrinsic back muscles.

Figure 4-48 shows a posterior view of midlayer back muscles.

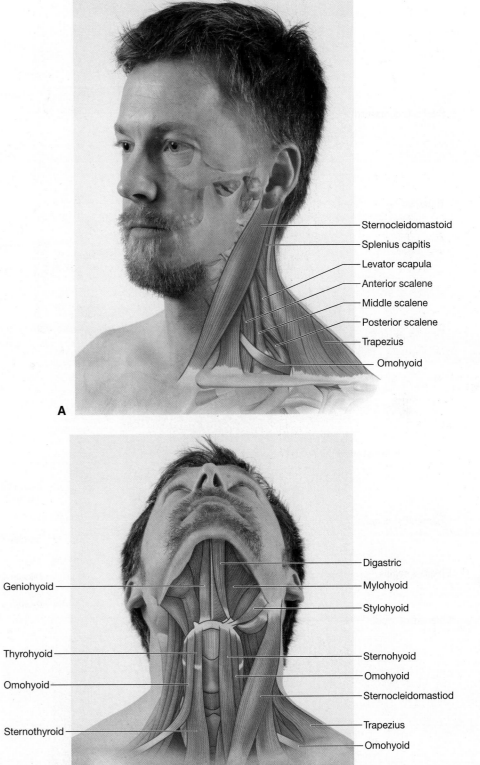

A

— Sternocleidomastoid

— Splenius capitis

— Levator scapula

— Anterior scalene

— Middle scalene

— Posterior scalene

— Trapezius

— Omohyoid

Geniohyoid —

Thyrohyoid —

Omohyoid —

Sternothyroid —

— Digastric

— Mylohyoid

— Stylohyoid

— Sternohyoid

— Omohyoid

— Sternocleidomastiod

— Trapezius

— Omohyoid

B

FIGURE 4-46 · Regional illustration of the neck. A: Anterolateral view; **B:** Anterior view (*continued*)

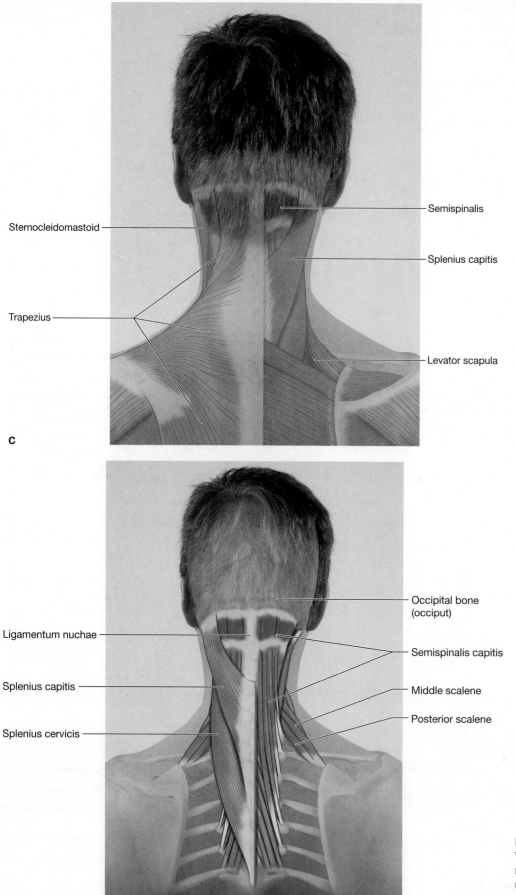

Sternocleidomastoid

Trapezius

Semispinalis

Splenius capitis

Levator scapula

C

Ligamentum nuchae

Splenius capitis

Splenius cervicis

Occipital bone (occiput)

Semispinalis capitis

Middle scalene

Posterior scalene

D

FIGURE 4-46 (*Continued*) **C:** View of superficial and midlayer posterior neck muscles; **D:** View of deeper and midlayer posterior neck muscles.

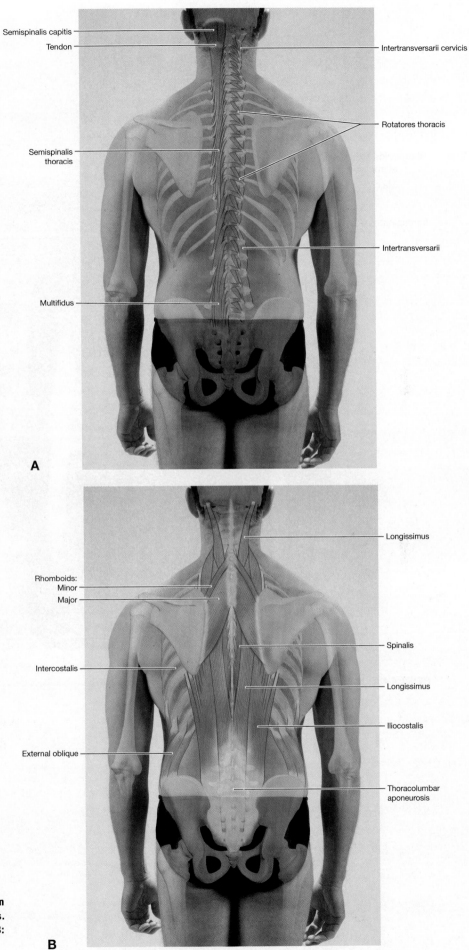

Semispinalis capitis

Tendon

Semispinalis thoracis

Multifidus

Intertransversarii cervicis

Rotatores thoracis

Intertransversarii

A

Rhomboids:
Minor
Major

Intercostalis

External oblique

Longissimus

Spinalis

Longissimus

Iliocostalis

Thoracolumbar aponeurosis

B

FIGURE 4-47 · Regional illustration of the intrinsic back muscles. A: Transversospinalis group; **B:** Erector Spinae Group.

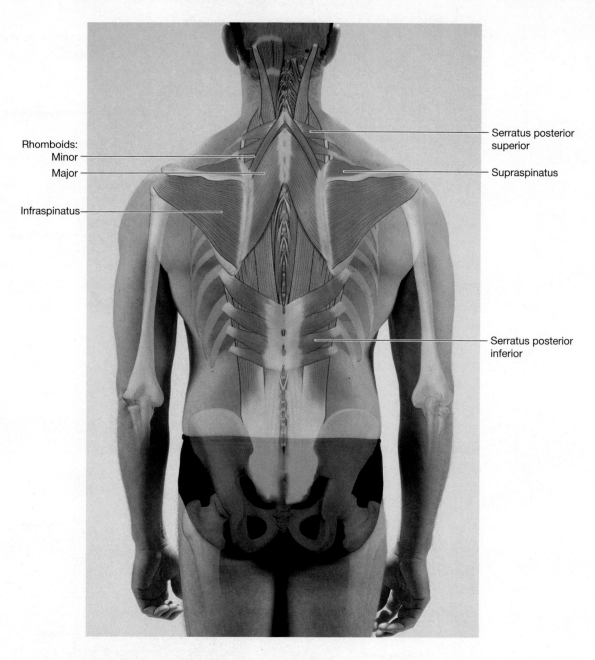

Rhomboids:
Minor
Major

Infraspinatus

Serratus posterior
superior

Supraspinatus

Serratus posterior
inferior

FIGURE 4-48 · Posterior view of midlayer back muscles

■ CHAPTER SUMMARY

This chapter has covered the basic anatomy of the head, trunk, abdomen, and back. Although it is true that these regions are complex, with a multitude of bones and many intricate muscles, it is also true that a thorough understanding of the muscles in these regions is important for the practice of massage therapy. Headaches, TMJ dysfunction, neck pain, and low back pain are among the most common reasons clients seek massage therapy. The knowledge presented in this chapter will help you address these common complaints.

■ WORKBOOK

Muscle Drawing Exercises

MEDIAL PTERYGOID

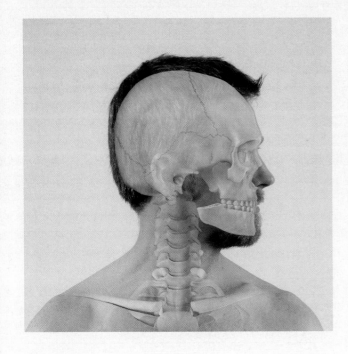

ORIGIN: _____

INSERTION: _____

ACTION(S): _____

NERVE: _____

ARTERIAL SUPPLY: _____

LOCATION AND/OR HOW TO PALPATE:

_____
_____
_____

WHEN MUSCLE IS SHORTENED:

_____
_____
_____

WHEN MUSCLE IS LENGTHENED:

_____
_____
_____

HOW TO STRETCH THIS MUSCLE:

_____
_____

SYNERGIST(S):

_____
_____

ANTAGONIST(S):

_____
_____
_____

NOTES: _____

_____
_____

LATERAL PTERYGOID

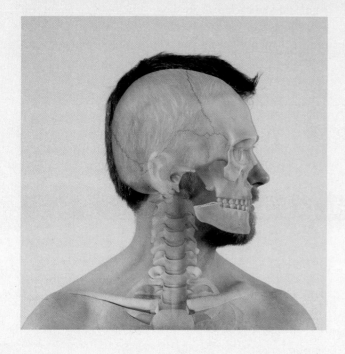

ORIGIN: _____

INSERTION: _____

ACTION(S): _____

NERVE: _____

ARTERIAL SUPPLY: _____

LOCATION AND/OR HOW TO PALPATE:
_____
_____
_____
_____
_____

WHEN MUSCLE IS SHORTENED:
_____
_____
_____
_____

WHEN MUSCLE IS LENGTHENED:
_____
_____
_____
_____

HOW TO STRETCH THIS MUSCLE:
_____
_____

SYNERGIST(S):
_____
_____

ANTAGONIST(S):
_____
_____
_____
_____

NOTES: _____
_____
_____
_____
_____
_____

MASSETER

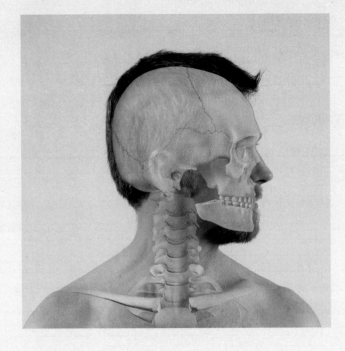

ORIGIN: _____

INSERTION: _____

ACTION(S): _____

NERVE: _____

ARTERIAL SUPPLY: _____

LOCATION AND/OR HOW TO PALPATE:
_____
_____
_____
_____
_____

WHEN MUSCLE IS SHORTENED:
_____
_____
_____
_____

WHEN MUSCLE IS LENGTHENED:
_____
_____
_____
_____

HOW TO STRETCH THIS MUSCLE:
_____
_____

SYNERGIST(S):
_____
_____

ANTAGONIST(S):
_____
_____
_____

NOTES: _____
_____
_____
_____
_____
_____
_____

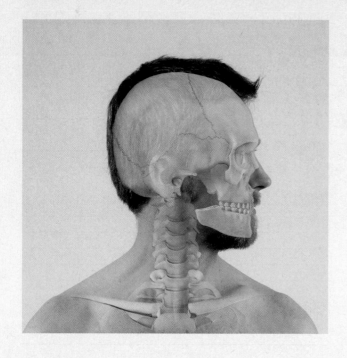

ORIGIN: _____

INSERTION: _____

ACTION(S): _____

NERVE: _____

ARTERIAL SUPPLY: _____

LOCATION AND/OR HOW TO PALPATE:

_____
_____
_____
_____
_____

WHEN MUSCLE IS SHORTENED:

_____
_____
_____
_____

WHEN MUSCLE IS LENGTHENED:

_____
_____
_____
_____

HOW TO STRETCH THIS MUSCLE:

_____
_____

SYNERGIST(S):

_____
_____

ANTAGONIST(S):

_____
_____
_____
_____

NOTES: _____
_____
_____
_____
_____
_____
_____

PLATYSMA

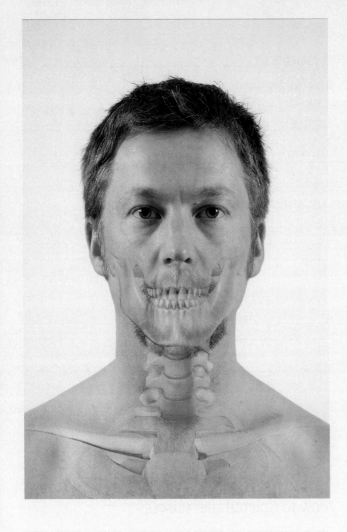

ORIGIN: _____

INSERTION: _____

ACTION(S): _____

NERVE: _____

ARTERIAL SUPPLY: _____

LOCATION AND/OR HOW TO PALPATE:
_____
_____
_____
_____
_____

WHEN MUSCLE IS SHORTENED:
_____
_____
_____
_____

WHEN MUSCLE IS LENGTHENED:
_____
_____
_____
_____

HOW TO STRETCH THIS MUSCLE:
_____
_____

SYNERGIST(S):
_____
_____

ANTAGONIST(S):
_____
_____
_____
_____

NOTES: _____
_____
_____
_____
_____
_____

DIGASTRIC

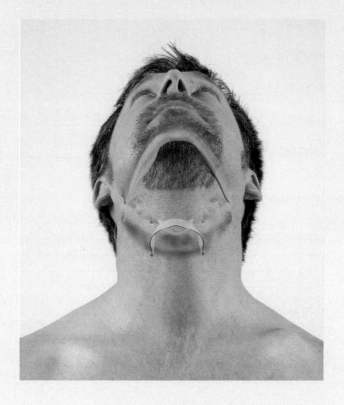

ORIGIN: _____

INSERTION: _____

ACTION(S): _____

NERVE: _____

ARTERIAL SUPPLY: _____

LOCATION AND/OR HOW TO PALPATE:
_____
_____
_____
_____

WHEN MUSCLE IS SHORTENED:
_____
_____
_____
_____

WHEN MUSCLE IS LENGTHENED:
_____
_____
_____
_____

HOW TO STRETCH THIS MUSCLE:
_____
_____

SYNERGIST(S):
_____
_____

ANTAGONIST(S):
_____
_____
_____

NOTES: _____
_____
_____
_____
_____
_____

SCALENES

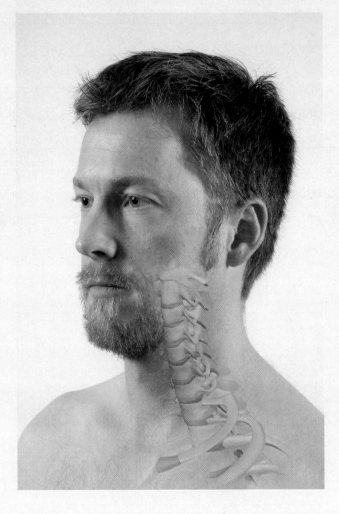

ORIGIN: _____

INSERTION: _____

ACTION(S): _____

NERVE: _____

ARTERIAL SUPPLY: _____

LOCATION AND/OR HOW TO PALPATE:
_____
_____
_____
_____

WHEN MUSCLE IS SHORTENED:
_____
_____
_____
_____

WHEN MUSCLE IS LENGTHENED:
_____
_____
_____
_____

HOW TO STRETCH THIS MUSCLE:
_____
_____

SYNERGIST(S):
_____
_____

ANTAGONIST(S):
_____
_____
_____
_____

NOTES: _____
_____
_____
_____
_____
_____

STERNOCLEIDOMASTOID (SCM)

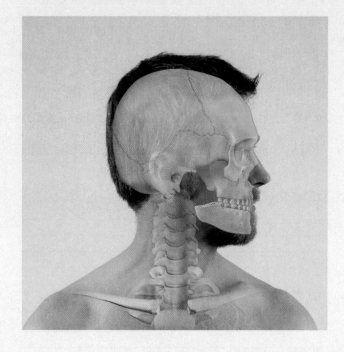

ORIGIN: _____

INSERTION: _____

ACTION(S): _____

NERVE: _____

ARTERIAL SUPPLY: _____

LOCATION AND/OR HOW TO PALPATE:
_____
_____
_____
_____

WHEN MUSCLE IS SHORTENED:
_____
_____
_____
_____

WHEN MUSCLE IS LENGTHENED:
_____
_____
_____
_____

HOW TO STRETCH THIS MUSCLE:
_____
_____

SYNERGIST(S):
_____
_____

ANTAGONIST(S):
_____
_____
_____
_____

NOTES: _____
_____
_____
_____
_____
_____

SUBOCCIPITALS

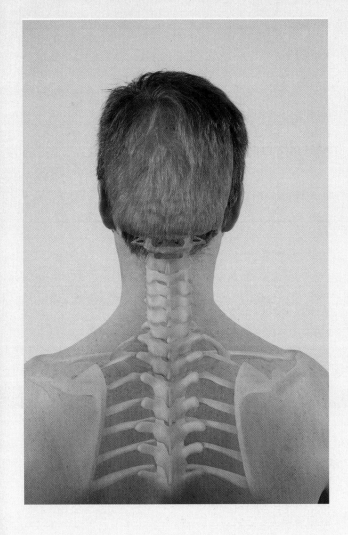

ORIGIN: _____

INSERTION: _____

ACTION(S): _____

NERVE: _____

ARTERIAL SUPPLY: _____

LOCATION AND/OR HOW TO PALPATE:
_____
_____
_____
_____

WHEN MUSCLE IS SHORTENED:
_____
_____
_____
_____

WHEN MUSCLE IS LENGTHENED:
_____
_____
_____
_____

HOW TO STRETCH THIS MUSCLE:
_____
_____

SYNERGIST(S):
_____
_____

ANTAGONIST(S):
_____
_____
_____
_____

NOTES: _____
_____
_____
_____
_____
_____

SPLENIUS CAPITIS

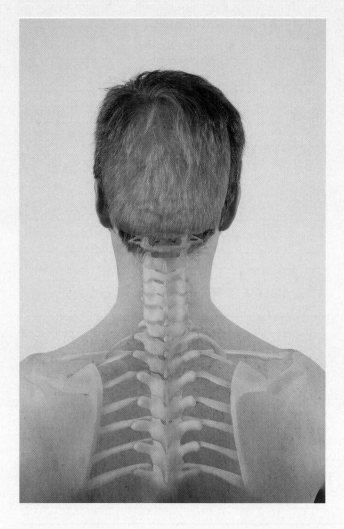

ORIGIN: _____

INSERTION: _____

ACTION(S): _____

NERVE: _____

ARTERIAL SUPPLY: _____

LOCATION AND/OR HOW TO PALPATE:
_____
_____
_____
_____
_____

WHEN MUSCLE IS SHORTENED:
_____
_____
_____
_____

WHEN MUSCLE IS LENGTHENED:
_____
_____
_____
_____

HOW TO STRETCH THIS MUSCLE:
_____
_____

SYNERGIST(S):
_____
_____

ANTAGONIST(S):
_____
_____
_____

NOTES: _____
_____
_____
_____
_____
_____
_____

SPLENIUS CERVICIS

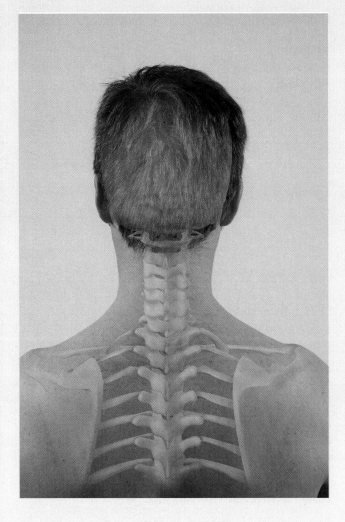

ORIGIN: _____

INSERTION: _____

ACTION(S): _____

NERVE: _____

ARTERIAL SUPPLY: _____

LOCATION AND/OR HOW TO PALPATE:
_____
_____
_____
_____
_____

WHEN MUSCLE IS SHORTENED:
_____
_____
_____
_____

WHEN MUSCLE IS LENGTHENED:
_____
_____
_____
_____

HOW TO STRETCH THIS MUSCLE:
_____
_____

SYNERGIST(S):
_____
_____

ANTAGONIST(S):
_____
_____
_____
_____

NOTES: _____
_____
_____
_____
_____
_____

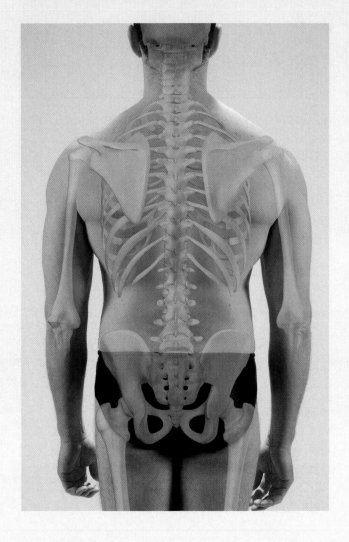

ORIGIN: _____

INSERTION: _____

ACTION(S): _____

NERVE: _____

ARTERIAL SUPPLY: _____

LOCATION AND/OR HOW TO PALPATE:
_____
_____
_____
_____
_____

WHEN MUSCLE IS SHORTENED:
_____
_____
_____
_____

WHEN MUSCLE IS LENGTHENED:
_____
_____
_____
_____

HOW TO STRETCH THIS MUSCLE:
_____
_____

SYNERGIST(S):
_____
_____

ANTAGONIST(S):
_____
_____
_____

NOTES: _____
_____
_____
_____
_____
_____

SEGMENTALS: INTERTRANSVERSARII

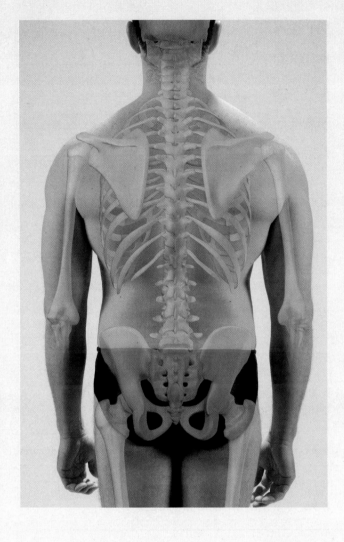

ORIGIN: _____

INSERTION: _____

ACTION(S): _____

NERVE: _____

ARTERIAL SUPPLY: _____

LOCATION AND/OR HOW TO PALPATE:

_____
_____
_____
_____
_____

WHEN MUSCLE IS SHORTENED:

_____
_____
_____
_____

WHEN MUSCLE IS LENGTHENED:

_____
_____
_____
_____

HOW TO STRETCH THIS MUSCLE:

_____
_____

SYNERGIST(S):

_____
_____

ANTAGONIST(S):

_____
_____
_____
_____

NOTES: _____

_____
_____
_____
_____
_____
_____

TRANSVERSOSPINALIS: ROTATORES

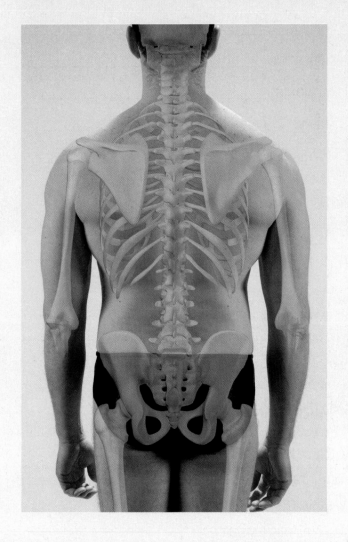

ORIGIN: _____

INSERTION: _____

ACTION(S): _____

NERVE: _____

ARTERIAL SUPPLY: _____

LOCATION AND/OR HOW TO PALPATE:
_____
_____
_____
_____
_____

WHEN MUSCLE IS SHORTENED:
_____
_____
_____
_____

WHEN MUSCLE IS LENGTHENED:
_____
_____
_____
_____

HOW TO STRETCH THIS MUSCLE:
_____
_____

SYNERGIST(S):
_____
_____

ANTAGONIST(S):
_____
_____
_____

NOTES: _____
_____
_____
_____
_____
_____

TRANSVERSOSPINALIS: MULTIFIDUS

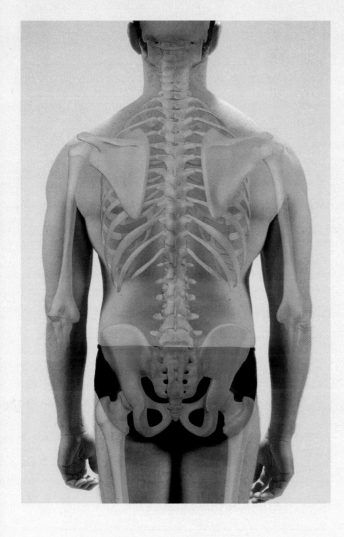

ORIGIN: _____

INSERTION: _____

ACTION(S): _____

NERVE: _____

ARTERIAL SUPPLY: _____

LOCATION AND/OR HOW TO PALPATE:
_____
_____
_____
_____
_____

WHEN MUSCLE IS SHORTENED:
_____
_____
_____
_____

WHEN MUSCLE IS LENGTHENED:
_____
_____
_____
_____

HOW TO STRETCH THIS MUSCLE:
_____
_____

SYNERGIST(S):
_____
_____

ANTAGONIST(S):
_____
_____
_____
_____

NOTES: _____
_____
_____
_____
_____
_____

TRANSVERSOSPINALIS: SEMISPINALIS

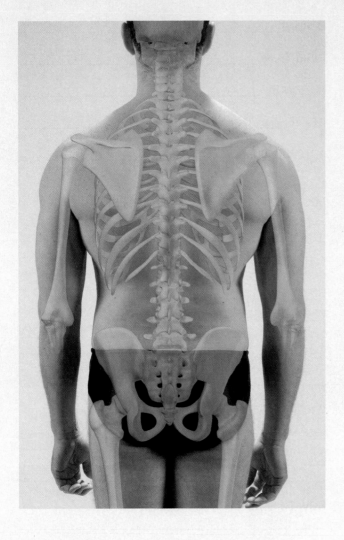

ORIGIN: _____

INSERTION: _____

ACTION(S): _____

NERVE: _____

ARTERIAL SUPPLY: _____

LOCATION AND/OR HOW TO PALPATE:
_____
_____
_____
_____
_____

WHEN MUSCLE IS SHORTENED:
_____
_____
_____
_____

WHEN MUSCLE IS LENGTHENED:
_____
_____
_____
_____

HOW TO STRETCH THIS MUSCLE:
_____
_____

SYNERGIST(S):
_____
_____

ANTAGONIST(S):
_____
_____
_____
_____

NOTES: _____
_____
_____
_____
_____
_____
_____

ERECTOR SPINAE GROUP: ILIOCOSTALIS

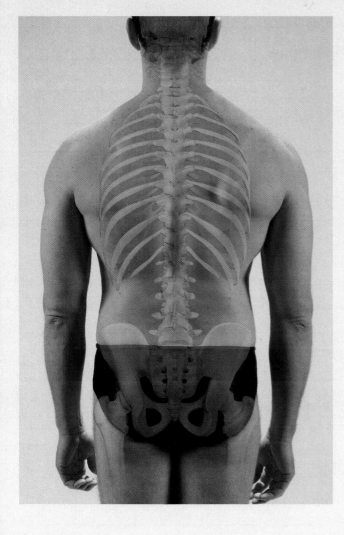

ORIGIN: _____

INSERTION: _____

ACTION(S): _____

NERVE: _____

ARTERIAL SUPPLY: _____

LOCATION AND/OR HOW TO PALPATE:
_____
_____
_____
_____
_____

WHEN MUSCLE IS SHORTENED:
_____
_____
_____
_____

WHEN MUSCLE IS LENGTHENED:
_____
_____
_____
_____

HOW TO STRETCH THIS MUSCLE:
_____
_____

SYNERGIST(S):
_____
_____

ANTAGONIST(S):
_____
_____
_____

NOTES: _____
_____
_____
_____
_____
_____

ERECTOR SPINAE GROUP: LONGISSIMUS

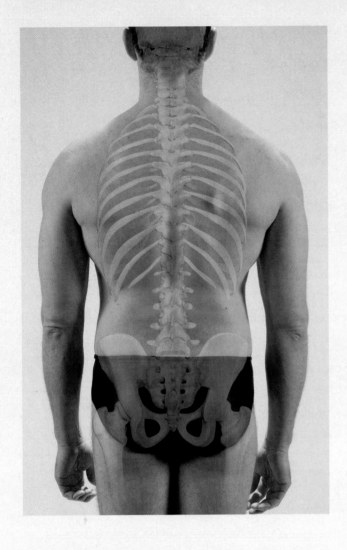

ORIGIN: _____

INSERTION: _____

ACTION(S): _____

NERVE: _____

ARTERIAL SUPPLY: _____

LOCATION AND/OR HOW TO PALPATE:
_____
_____
_____
_____
_____

WHEN MUSCLE IS SHORTENED:
_____
_____
_____
_____

WHEN MUSCLE IS LENGTHENED:
_____
_____
_____
_____

HOW TO STRETCH THIS MUSCLE:
_____
_____

SYNERGIST(S):
_____
_____

ANTAGONIST(S):
_____
_____
_____
_____

NOTES: _____
_____
_____
_____
_____
_____

ERECTOR SPINAE GROUP: SPINALIS

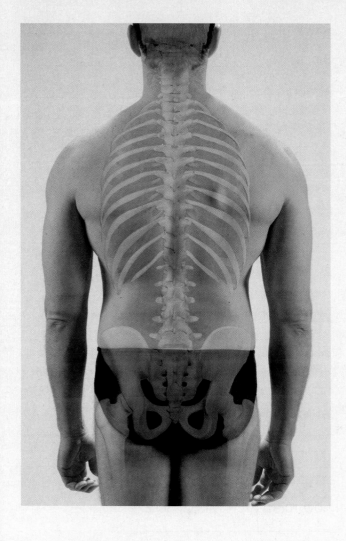

ORIGIN: _____

INSERTION: _____

ACTION(S): _____

NERVE: _____

ARTERIAL SUPPLY: _____

LOCATION AND/OR HOW TO PALPATE:
_____
_____
_____
_____
_____

WHEN MUSCLE IS SHORTENED:
_____
_____
_____
_____

WHEN MUSCLE IS LENGTHENED:
_____
_____
_____
_____

HOW TO STRETCH THIS MUSCLE:
_____
_____

SYNERGIST(S):
_____
_____

ANTAGONIST(S):
_____
_____
_____
_____

NOTES: _____
_____
_____
_____
_____
_____

TRANSVERSE ABDOMINIS

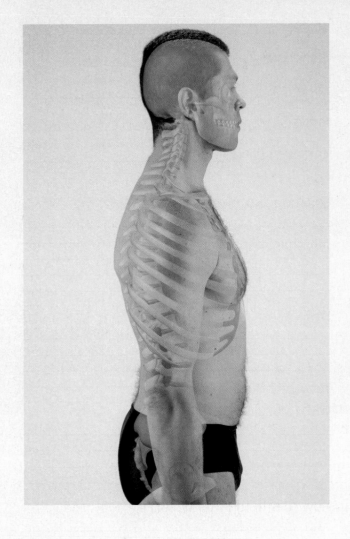

ORIGIN: _____

INSERTION: _____

ACTION(S): _____

NERVE: _____

ARTERIAL SUPPLY: _____

LOCATION AND/OR HOW TO PALPATE:
_____
_____
_____
_____
_____

WHEN MUSCLE IS SHORTENED:
_____
_____
_____
_____

WHEN MUSCLE IS LENGTHENED:
_____
_____
_____
_____

HOW TO STRETCH THIS MUSCLE:
_____
_____

SYNERGIST(S):
_____

ANTAGONIST(S):
_____
_____
_____

NOTES: _____
_____
_____
_____
_____
_____

INTERNAL OBLIQUE

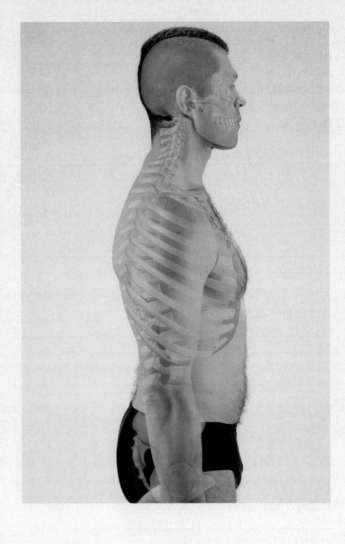

ORIGIN: _____

INSERTION: _____

ACTION(S): _____

NERVE: _____

ARTERIAL SUPPLY: _____

LOCATION AND/OR HOW TO PALPATE:
_____
_____
_____
_____
_____

WHEN MUSCLE IS SHORTENED:
_____
_____
_____
_____

WHEN MUSCLE IS LENGTHENED:
_____
_____
_____
_____

HOW TO STRETCH THIS MUSCLE:
_____
_____
_____

SYNERGIST(S):
_____
_____

ANTAGONIST(S):
_____
_____
_____
_____

NOTES: _____
_____
_____
_____
_____
_____

EXTERNAL OBLIQUE

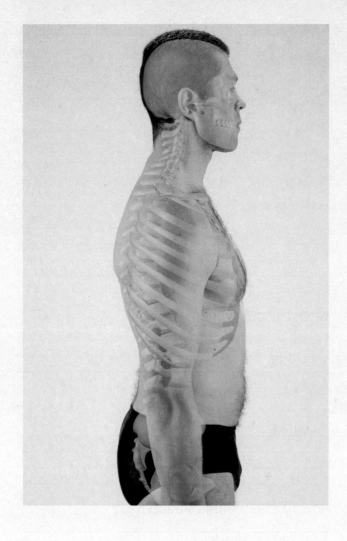

ORIGIN: _____

INSERTION: _____

ACTION(S): _____

NERVE: _____

ARTERIAL SUPPLY: _____

LOCATION AND/OR HOW TO PALPATE:
_____
_____
_____
_____
_____

WHEN MUSCLE IS SHORTENED:
_____
_____
_____
_____

WHEN MUSCLE IS LENGTHENED:
_____
_____
_____
_____

HOW TO STRETCH THIS MUSCLE:
_____
_____

SYNERGIST(S):
_____
_____

ANTAGONIST(S):
_____
_____
_____
_____

NOTES: _____
_____
_____
_____
_____
_____

RECTUS ABDOMINIS

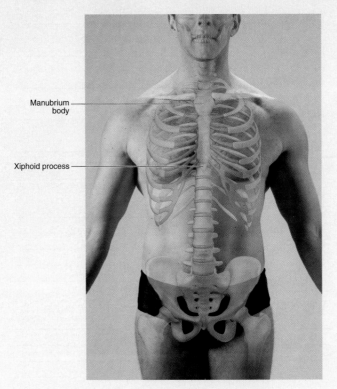

Manubrium body

Xiphoid process

ORIGIN: _____

INSERTION: _____

ACTION(S): _____

NERVE: _____

ARTERIAL SUPPLY: _____

LOCATION AND/OR HOW TO PALPATE:

_____
_____
_____
_____
_____

WHEN MUSCLE IS SHORTENED:

_____
_____
_____
_____

WHEN MUSCLE IS LENGTHENED:

_____
_____
_____
_____

HOW TO STRETCH THIS MUSCLE:

_____
_____

SYNERGIST(S):

_____
_____

ANTAGONIST(S):

_____
_____
_____
_____

NOTES: _____
_____
_____
_____
_____
_____

QUADRATUS LUMBORUM (QL)

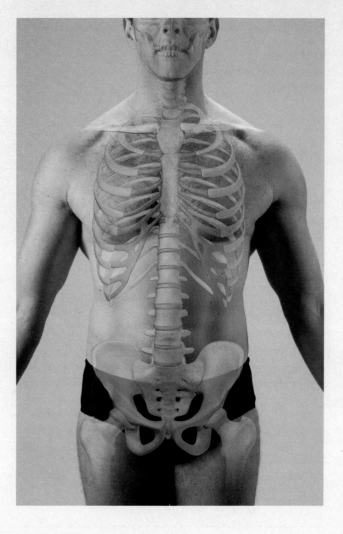

ORIGIN: _____

INSERTION: _____

ACTION(S): _____

NERVE: _____

ARTERIAL SUPPLY: _____

LOCATION AND/OR HOW TO PALPATE:
_____
_____
_____
_____
_____

WHEN MUSCLE IS SHORTENED:
_____
_____
_____
_____

WHEN MUSCLE IS LENGTHENED:
_____
_____
_____
_____

HOW TO STRETCH THIS MUSCLE:
_____
_____

SYNERGIST(S):
_____
_____

ANTAGONIST(S):
_____
_____
_____
_____

NOTES: _____
_____
_____
_____
_____
_____

DIAPHRAGM

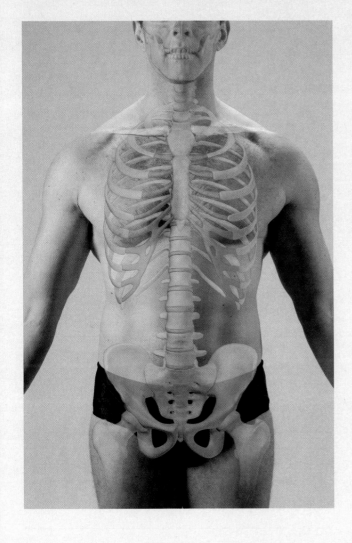

ORIGIN: _____

INSERTION: _____

ACTION(S): _____

NERVE: _____

ARTERIAL SUPPLY: _____

LOCATION AND/OR HOW TO PALPATE:
_____
_____
_____
_____
_____

WHEN MUSCLE IS SHORTENED:
_____
_____
_____
_____

WHEN MUSCLE IS LENGTHENED:
_____
_____
_____
_____

HOW TO STRETCH THIS MUSCLE:
_____
_____

SYNERGIST(S):
_____
_____

ANTAGONIST(S):
_____
_____
_____
_____

NOTES: _____
_____
_____
_____
_____
_____

INTERCOSTALS (External and Internal)

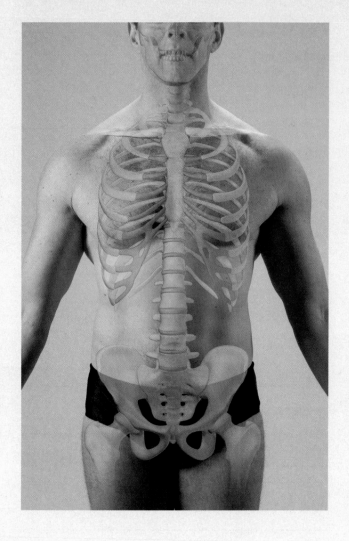

ORIGIN: _____

INSERTION: _____

ACTION(S): _____

NERVE: _____

ARTERIAL SUPPLY: _____

LOCATION AND/OR HOW TO PALPATE:
_____
_____
_____
_____
_____

WHEN MUSCLE IS SHORTENED:
_____
_____
_____
_____

WHEN MUSCLE IS LENGTHENED:
_____
_____
_____
_____

HOW TO STRETCH THIS MUSCLE:
_____
_____

SYNERGIST(S):
_____
_____

ANTAGONIST(S):
_____
_____
_____
_____

NOTES: _____
_____
_____
_____
_____
_____

SERRATUS POSTERIOR SUPERIOR

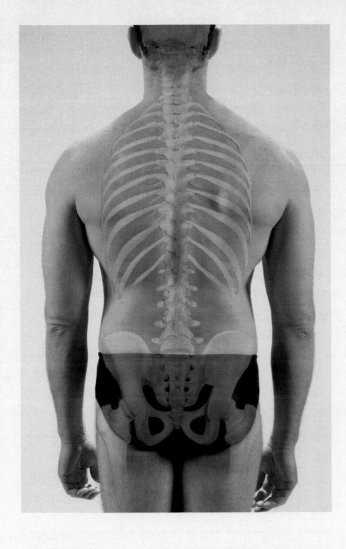

ORIGIN: _____

INSERTION: _____

ACTION(S): _____

NERVE: _____

ARTERIAL SUPPLY: _____

LOCATION AND/OR HOW TO PALPATE:
_____
_____
_____
_____
_____

WHEN MUSCLE IS SHORTENED:
_____
_____
_____
_____

WHEN MUSCLE IS LENGTHENED:
_____
_____
_____
_____

HOW TO STRETCH THIS MUSCLE:
_____
_____

SYNERGIST(S):
_____
_____

ANTAGONIST(S):
_____
_____
_____
_____

NOTES: _____
_____
_____
_____
_____
_____
_____

SERRATUS POSTERIOR INFERIOR

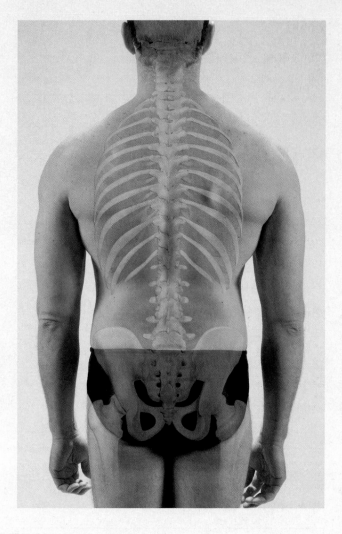

ORIGIN: _____

INSERTION: _____

ACTION(S): _____

NERVE: _____

ARTERIAL SUPPLY: _____

LOCATION AND/OR HOW TO PALPATE:
_____
_____
_____
_____
_____

WHEN MUSCLE IS SHORTENED:
_____
_____
_____
_____

WHEN MUSCLE IS LENGTHENED:
_____
_____
_____
_____

HOW TO STRETCH THIS MUSCLE:
_____
_____

SYNERGIST(S):
_____
_____

ANTAGONIST(S):
_____
_____
_____
_____

NOTES: _____
_____
_____
_____
_____
_____

Palpation Exercises

Palpation of the muscles is important to reinforce their locations and to prepare for the application of muscle knowledge to massage therapy settings.

Palpation Exercise #1

This palpation exercise will require you to locate the following muscles: masseter, temporalis, platysma, SCM, scalenes, suboccipitals, splenius capitis, and splenius cervicis.

Bones/Bony Landmarks

1. **Zygomatic arch:** Locate the prominent ridge of bone in the lateral cheek area, just anterior to the external auditory meatus (opening to the ear canal).
2. **Mastoid process of the temporal bone:** Locate the mastoid process of the temporal bone by finding the bony process just below the ear lobe.

Muscles

1. **Temporalis:** This muscle covers the superior portion of each temporal bone and some of the parietal bones. Palpate the lateral temples. Remember that this muscle passes behind the zygomatic arch to insert on the rami of the mandible.
2. **Masseter:** Palpate the masseter, superficial to the rami of the mandible. Have your partner clench his or her teeth to feel fibers contract.
3. **Platysma:** Palpate the superficial anterior and lateral neck and superficial neck.
4. **Scalenes:** Palpate the insertion of the scalenes on the transverse processes of cervical vertebrae 2–7. Trace the muscle anteriorly and inferiorly to its insertion on ribs 1 and 2. It is necessary to press down (aim for partner's feet) behind the clavicle to access the insertion. A small portion of scalenes is superficial, located between the SCM and upper trapezius. If you press just lateral to SCM's attachment on the clavicle and inferior to levator scapula, you will find scalenes. Palpate carefully, as the brachial plexus runs between the anterior and middle scalenes. However, if you press right on the brachial plexus, it will likely be very uncomfortable for your partner, and he or she should let you know.
5. **Sternocleidomastoid:** Palpate the origin at the superior, lateral sternum and medial clavicle. Trace to the insertion at the mastoid process of the temporal bone. You can place your hand on your partner's forehead and ask him or her to push into your hand. This is equivalent to providing resistance while your partner attempts to flex the neck, thus engaging SCM. The muscle fibers should contract, and it is likely you will even see the muscle tighten. You can squeeze the SCM between your fingers to massage it. Remember that a tight SCM can cause headaches above the eyes and is frequently involved in whiplash.
6. **Splenius capitis/splenius cervicis:** These are both posterior neck muscles. Palpate splenius capitis from the ligamentum nuchae and spinous processes of T1–T3 to the occiput and mastoid process. Palpate splenius cervicis from the spinous processes of T3–T6 to the transverse processes of C1–C3. Remind yourself of the actions of these muscles.

7. **Suboccipitals:** These are four pairs of very small muscles joining the atlas and axis to each other and joining the atlas to the occiput and the axis to the occiput. These muscles include the obliquus capitis superior and inferior and rectus capitis posterior major and minor. Palpate these suboccipitals just inferior to the occiput and between the occiput and C2.

Palpation Exercise #2

This palpation exercise will require you to locate the intrinsic back muscles: segmentals (interspinalis and intertransversarii) and erector spinae group.

Bones/Bony Landmarks

1. Locate the spinous processes of the spine. Begin with C1 and count as you palpate all the way down the center of the spine to L5.
2. Locate the transverse processes in the cervical and lumbar region. In the cervical region, palpate directly into the lateral neck. Feel through the musculature for the dense knobs of bone that make up the transverse processes. It can be challenging to find transverse processes in the lumbar area, due to the musculature that covers them. Palpate with care into the posterolateral lumbar region, a few inches lateral to the spinous processes. Press directly into the tissue first, then angle your pressure medially.

Muscles

1. **Segmental, interspinalis:** Place your fingers between the spinous processes in the cervical and lumbar regions. Use intention, as well as gentle pressure, to help relax these muscles.
2. **Segmental, intertransversarii:** Press gently between the transverse processes in the cervical and lumbar regions.
3. **Transversospinalis group (rotatores, multifidus, and semispinalis):** Press into the lamina groove to access all three of these. What are their actions?
4. **Erector spinae group:** Can you distinguish the three bands that combine to create the erectors? Most medial is spinalis, in the lamina groove. Just lateral to the transverse processes is where you will find longissimus, and most lateral is iliocostalis. To seek out iliocostalis, begin at the sacrum and medial iliac crest. Feel for the band of muscles running vertically over the posterior ribs. Iliocostalis is broader and flatter in the lumbar and upper thoracic regions. It is more narrow in the lower thoracic region.

Palpation Exercise #3

This palpation exercise will require you to palpate the muscles of the abdominal wall.

Bones/Bony Landmarks

1. Gently palpate the xiphoid process of the sternum.
2. Palpate the posterior iliac crest. Note the articulation between the sacrum and the ilium.
3. Palpate the twelfth rib. Sweep upward from the posterior iliac crest, feeling for the inferior border of the twelfth rib.

Muscles

1. **Transverse abdominis, internal obliques, and external obliques:** Place your hands in the anterolateral abdominal area. Recall that these three thin, flat muscles create a wall around our abdominal organs. The deepest muscle is transverse abdominis, the midlayer muscle is internal oblique, and the most superficial of the three is external oblique. Position your hands to reflect the three different fiber directions of these three muscles.

2. **Rectus abdominis:** Locate the insertion on the xiphoid process of the sternum and the ribs and costal cartilage just lateral to the xiphoid process. Press gently and superiorly into the ribs on either side of the xiphoid process. From this point, the muscle runs inferiorly, spanning 2 to 3 inches on either side of the midline. The muscle's origin on the pubic symphysis and pubic crest is generally not appropriate to palpate as it is so close to the genital area. It is important to have clear communication with one's client about the intent of working the inferior aspect of this muscle, as well as assurance to the client that the genital area will not be touched.

3. **Quadratus lumborum:** Find the twelfth rib and press up gently into the inferior border of the rib. Locate the posterior iliac crest. You have found the borders of QL. Palpate and apply direct pressure to this deep, square-shaped muscle that lies between the posterior iliac crest and rib 12.

Palpation Exercise #4

This palpation exercise will require you to palpate the muscles of respiration.

Bones/Bony Landmarks and Muscles

1. **Diaphragm:** Locate the ribs just lateral to the xiphoid process of the sternum. As your partner exhales, gently press up into the tissue posterior to the rib cage.

2. **Intercostals:** Apply pressure into the intercostal spaces. Remember that the intercostals take up the entire space between the ribs, from the sternum to the spine. Recall as well that these muscles frequently contain trigger points and thus may be tender to the touch.

3. **Serratus posterior superior:** Locate the spinous process of C7 and the inferior ligamentum nuchae just above it. Count down the spinous processes to T3. You have found the origin of the muscle. Palpate laterally and inferiorly from the origin to ribs 2–5. This thin, flat muscle runs beneath the scapula as it approaches the ribs, thus much of the muscle is not accessible. The accessible portion of the muscle is deep to rhomboids.

4. **Serratus posterior inferior:** Locate the lower rib cage. Trace the muscle inferiorly and medially to the spinous processes of T11–L3. This thin, flat muscle lies deep to latissimus dorsi.

Clay Work Exercises

These exercises help reinforce the names and locations of muscles. They require the use of small plastic skeletons and clay. In each exercise below, create each of the listed muscles out of clay, one at a time, and attach it to the plastic skeleton where appropriate. Also, list the origin, insertion, and action of each muscle in the spaces provided. Share your understanding of the muscles with your partner as you build them.

Clay Work Exercise #1: Muscles That Move the Jaw

Muscle Name	Origin	Insertion	Location	Action(s)
1. Medial Pterygoid				
2. Lateral Pterygoid				
3. Masseter				
4. Temporalis				
5. Platysma				

Clay Work Exercise #2: Intrinsic Spine Muscles

Muscle Name	Origin	Insertion	Location	Action(s)
1. Segmental: Interspinalis				
2. Segmental: Intertransversarii				
3. Transversospinalis: Rotatores				
4. Transversospinalis: Multifidus				
5. Transversospinalis: Semispinalis				

(Continued)

Muscle Name	Origin	Insertion	Location	Action(s)
6. Erector Spinae Group: Iliocostalis				
7. Erector Spinae Group: Longissimus				
8. Erector Spinae Group: Spinalis				

Clay Work Exercise #3: Abdominal Wall Muscles

Muscle Name	Origin	Insertion	Location	Action(s)
1. Transverse Abdominis				
2. Internal Oblique				
3. External Oblique				
4. Rectus Abdominis				
5. Quadratus Lumborum				

Clay Work Exercise #4: Muscles of Respiration

Muscle Name	Origin	Insertion	Location	Action(s)
1. Diaphragm				
2. Internal Intercostals				
3. External Intercostals				
4. Serratus Posterior Superior				
5. Serratus Posterior Inferior				

Case Study Exercises

Case Study #1

A client cannot fully open her jaw.

List three muscles that would likely be shortened and contributing to this problem:

_____

_____

List two muscles that would likely be lengthened: _____

_____

_____

Case Study #2

A client comes to your office, and you notice that her head is turned to the right.

List five muscles that could be shortened and contributing to this problem.

Please note if the muscles are shortened on the right or left side:

_____

_____

_____

_____

_____

List five muscles that could be lengthened and contributing to this problem.

Please note if the muscles are lengthened on the right or left side:

_____

_____

_____

_____

_____

_____

Describe where you would focus your massage to assist this client in improving her posture.

_____

_____

_____

Case Study #3

Your client cannot fully extend his neck.

List two muscles that could be shortened (bilaterally) and contributing to this problem.

Please note if the muscles are shortened on the right or left side:

_____

_____

_____

_____

_____

List three muscles that could be lengthened (bilaterally) and contributing to this problem:

Please note if the muscles are lengthened on the right or left side:

_____

_____

_____

Describe where you would focus your massage to assist this client in improving the range of motion in his neck.

_____

_____

_____

Case Study #4

A client comes in who cannot fully tilt his head to the left.

List five muscles that could be shortened (unilaterally) and contributing to this problem.

Please note if the muscle is short on the right or left side:

_____

_____

_____

_____

_____

List five muscles that could be lengthened (unilaterally) and contributing to this problem.

Please note if the muscles are lengthened on the right or left side:

_____

_____

_____

_____

Describe where you would focus your massage to assist this client in improving the range of motion in his neck.

_____

_____

_____

Case Study #5

A client's trunk is turned to the left.

List five muscles that could be shortened and contributing to this problem.

Please note if the muscles are shortened on the right or left side:

_____

_____

_____

_____

List five muscles that could be lengthened and contributing to this problem.

Please note if the muscles are lengthened on the right or left side:

_____
_____
_____

Case Study #6

A client is unable to turn his trunk to the left.

List five muscles that could be shortened and contributing to this problem.

Please note if the muscles are shortened on the right or left side:

_____
_____
_____
_____

List five muscles that could be lengthened and contributing to this problem.

Please note if the muscles are lengthened on the right or left side:

_____
_____

Case Study #7

A client is unable to fully flex her spine.

List five muscles that could be shortened and contributing to this problem.

Please note if the muscles are shortened on the right or left side:

_____
_____
_____
_____
_____

List five muscles that could be lengthened and contributing to this problem.

Please note if the muscles are lengthened on the right or left side:

_____
_____
_____

Case Study #8

A client is unable to inhale fully.

List three muscles that could be shortened and contributing to this problem:

_____
_____
_____

List three muscles that could be lengthened and contributing to this problem:

_____
_____
_____

Review Exercises

These review exercises help you to recall what you have learned in this chapter and reinforce your learning.

Review Charts to Study

Origin, Insertion, Location, and Action Chart of Jaw-Moving Muscles

Muscle Name	Origin	Insertion	Location	Action(s)
Medial Pterygoid	Medial side of the lateral pterygoid plate of the sphenoid bone	Mandible	Deep, lateral cheek	Elevate and protract mandible
Lateral Pterygoid	Lateral side of the lateral pterygoid plate of the sphenoid bone	Mandible	Deep, lateral cheek	Protract mandible
Temporalis	Lateral temporal bone	Mandible	Covers lateral temporal bone	Elevate mandible
Masseter	Zygomatic arch	Ramus of mandible	Superficial cheek	Elevate mandible
Platysma	Fascia over pectoralis major and anterior deltoid	Mandible and lower lip	Superficial, anterior neck and upper chest	Depress mandible

Origin, Insertion, Location, and Action Chart of Neck-Moving Muscles

Muscle Name	Origin	Insertion	Location	Action(s)
Scalenes	Transverse processes of C2–C7	Ribs 1 and 2	Anterolateral neck	Unilateral actions: lateral flexion and opposite-side rotation of the neck; Bilateral action: flexion of the neck
Sternocleidomastoid	Sternum and medial clavicle	Mastoid process of the temporal bone	Anterolateral neck	Unilateral actions: lateral flexion and opposite-side rotation of the neck; Bilateral action: flexion of neck
Suboccipitals	C1 and C2	C1 and the occiput	Deep, posterior neck, just below occiput	Unilateral actions: lateral flexion and same-side rotation of the neck; Bilateral action: extension of the neck (between C1 and the occiput)

(continued)

Origin, Insertion, Location, and Action Chart of Neck-Moving Muscles (*Continued*)

Muscle Name	Origin	Insertion	Location	Action(s)
Splenius Capitis	Ligamentum nuchae and spinous processes of T1–T3	Occiput and mastoid process	Midlayer, posterior neck	Unilateral actions: lateral flexion and same-side rotation of the neck; Bilateral action: extension of the neck (between C1 and the occiput)
Splenius Cervicis	Spinous processes of T3–T6	Transverse processes of T1–T3	Midlayer, posterior neck	Unilateral actions: lateral flexion and same-side rotation of the neck Bilateral action: extension of the neck (between C1 and the occiput)

Origin, Insertion, Location, and Action Chart of Intrinsic Back Muscles

Muscle Name	Origin	Insertion	Location	Action
Segmentals: Interspinalis	Spinous process of C3–T1 and T12–L5	Spinous process of vertebra directly above origin	Between spinous process in cervical and lumbar regions	Extend spine
Segmentals: Intertransversarii	Transverse process of C3–T1 and T11–L5 and the sacrum	Transverse process of vertebra directly above origin	Between transverse process in cervical and lumbar regions	Extend spine and laterally flex spine
Transversospinalis: Rotatores	Transverse process of T2–L5	Spinous process of vertebra above	Lamina groove	Extend spine and rotate spine to the opposite side
Transversospinalis: Multifidus	Transverse processes of C2–L5 and the sacrum	Spinous processes of vertebrae 2–4, vertebrae above origin	Lamina groove	Extend spine and rotate spine to the opposite side
Transversospinalis: Semispinalis	Transverse processes of vertebrae T2–L5	Spinous processes of vertebrae 3–6 vertebrae above origin	Lamina groove	Extend spine and rotate spine to the opposite side
Erector Spinae Group: Iliocostalis	Sacrum posterior iliac crest, posterior ribs 3–12	Ribs and transverse processes of C4–C7	Lateral band, ilium to ribs	All three extend and laterally flex spine
Erector Spinae Group: Longissimus	Transverse processes of C4–L5 and the sacrum	Transverse processes of cervical and thoracic vertebrae, ribs, and the mastoid process	Middle band, lateral to transverse processes	All three extend and laterally flex spine
Erector Spinae Group: Spinalis	Ligamentum nuchae, spinous processes of C7–T2 and T11–L3	Spinous processes of cervical and thoracic vertebrae and occiput	Medial band, in lamina groove	All three extend and laterally flex spine

Origin, Insertion, Location, and Action Chart of Abdominal Wall Muscles

Muscle Name	Origin	Insertion	Location	Action(s)
Transverse Abdominis	Lateral inguinal ligament, iliac crest, thoracolumbar aponeurosis, internal costal cartilages, and ribs 7–12	Abdominal aponeurosis and linea alba	Deep anterolateral trunk	Compress contents of abdomen
Internal Oblique	Thoracolumbar aponeurosis, iliac crest, and inguinal ligament	Ribs and costal cartilage of ribs 9–12, linea alba	Midlayer, anterolateral trunk	Unilateral actions: lateral flexion and same-side rotation of trunk; Bilateral action: flex trunk
External Oblique	Ribs 5–12	Linea alba and anterior iliac crest	Superficial anterolateral trunk	Unilateral actions: lateral flexion and opposite-side rotation of trunk; Bilateral action: flex trunk
Rectus Abdominis	Pubic crest and pubic symphysis	Xiphoid process and costal cartilage of ribs 5–7	Superficial anterior trunk	Flexion of trunk
Quadratus Lumborum	Posterior iliac crest	Transverse processes of lumbar vertebrae and twelfth rib	Deep, low back	Unilateral actions: lateral flexion of lumbar spine and hip hiking; Bilateral action: extension of lumbar spine

Origin, Insertion, Location, and Action Chart of Respiration Muscles

Muscle Name	Origin	Insertion	Location	Action(s)
Diaphragm	Lumbar vertebrae, inferior 6 ribs and their costal cartilage, posterior xiphoid process	Central tendon	Between thoracic and abdominopelvic cavities	Chief muscle of inspiration
Internal Intercostals	Superior border of rib below	Inferior border of rib above	Between ribs	Depress ribs in forced exhalation
External Intercostals	Inferior border of rib above	Superior border of rib below	Between ribs	Elevate ribs in inhalation
Serratus Posterior Superior	Inferior portion of ligamentum nuchae, spinous processes of C7–T3	Ribs 2–5	Midlayer mid to upper back	Elevate ribs in inhalation
Serratus Posterior Inferior	Spinous processes of T11–L3	Ribs 9–12	Midlayer low back	Depress ribs in forced exhalation

Review Charts to Fill in

Chart #1: Muscles That Move the Jaw

Muscle Name	Origin	Insertion	Location	Action(s)
Medial Pterygoid				
Lateral Pterygoid				
Masseter				
Temporalis				
Platysma				
Digastric				

Chart #2: Muscles That Move the Neck

Muscle Name	Origin	Insertion	Location	Action(s)
Scalenes				
Sternocleidomastoid (SCM)				
Suboccipitals				
Splenius Capitis				
Splenius Cervicis				

Chart #3: Muscles That Move the Neck, Trunk, and Low Back

Muscle Name	Origin	Insertion	Location	Action(s)
Segmentals: Interspinalis				
Segmentals: Intertransversarii				
Transversospinalis: Rotatores				
Transversospinalis: Multifidus				
Transversospinalis: Semispinalis				
Erector Spinae Group: Iliocostalis				
Erector Spinae Group: Longissimus				
Erector Spinae Group: Spinalis				

Chart #4: Muscles of the Abdominal Wall

Muscle Name	Origin	Insertion	Location	Action(s)
Transverse Abdominis				
Internal Obliques				
External Obliques				
Rectus Abdominis				
Quadratus Lumborum				

Table #5: Muscles of Respiration

Muscle Name	Origin	Insertion	Location	Action(s)
Diaphragm				
External Intercostals				
Internal Intercostals				
Serratus Posterior Superior				
Serratus Posterior Inferior				

Fill in the Blank

Fill in the appropriate muscle in the space provided.

Jaw/mandible elevators:

1. _____ is a lateral cheek muscle, deep to ramus of mandible.

2. _____ is a superficial lateral cheek muscle and a "chewing muscle."

3. _____ is a muscle that is located on the lateral temporal bone.

Jaw/mandible depressors:

1. _____ is a superficial anterior neck and upper chest muscle.

2. _____ joins the hyoid bone to the mandible.

Muscles that perform flexion, lateral flexion, and opposite-side rotation of the neck:

1. _____ is a lateral neck muscle, has anterior, middle, and posterior sections, and can cause thoracic outlet syndrome when shortened.

2. _____ is a superficial, anterolateral neck muscle, named for its attachments.

Muscles that perform extension, lateral flexion, and same-side rotation of the neck:

1. _____ consists of four pairs of deep muscles, located inferior to the occiput.

2. _____ is a midlayer posterior neck muscle that attaches to the ligamentum nuchae and the occiput.

3. _____ is a midlayer, posterior neck muscle that attaches to transverse processes and spinous processes.

Spine extensors:

1. _____ is a segmental group member that joins spinous process to spinous process, located primarily in the cervical and lumbar regions, and extends neck and low back.

2. _____ is a segmental group member that joins transverse process to transverse process, is located primarily in the cervical and lumbar regions, and extends and laterally flexes the neck and low back.

3. _____ is a transversospinalis member that joins transverse processes to spinous processes one vertebrae above, extends and rotates the spine to opposite side, and is located in the lamina groove.

4. _____ is a transversospinalis member that joins transverse processes to spinous processes two to four vertebrae above, extends and rotates the spine to opposite side, and is located in the lamina groove.

5. _____ is a transversospinalis member that joins transverse processes to spinous processes three to six vertebrae above, extends and rotates the spine to opposite side, and is located in the lamina groove.

6. _____ is an erector spinae group member that is located most laterally of the three erectors and performs lateral flexion and extension of the spine.

7. _____ is an erector spinae group member that is the central band of the three erectors and performs lateral flexion and extension of the spine.

8. _____ is an erector spinae group member that is located most medially of the three erectors and performs lateral flexion and extension of the spine.

Muscles of the abdominal wall:

1. _____ is the deepest lateral abdominal wall muscle and performs compression of the contents of the abdomen.

2. _____ is a midlayer lateral abdominal wall muscle that performs flexion, lateral flexion, and same-side rotation of the trunk.

3. _____ is a superficial lateral abdominal wall muscle that performs flexion, lateral flexion, and opposite-side rotation of the trunk.

4. _____ is an anterior abdominal wall muscle that is divided into segments and performs flexion of the trunk.

5. _____ is the deepest posterior abdominal wall muscle, attaches to the posterior iliac crest, the lumbar vertebrae, and the twelfth rib, and performs lateral flexion and extension of the lumbar spine.

Muscles of respiration:

1. _____ is the chief muscle of respiration and pulls the central tendon down to enlarge the volume of the thoracic cavity, causing pressure reduction on the thoracic cavity and causing air to enter the lungs.

2. _____ is a muscle located between the ribs and is generally said to assist in inhalation.

3. _____ is a muscle located between the ribs and is generally said to assist in exhalation.

4. _____ is a muscle located in the midlayer upper back, elevates ribs 2–5, and is generally thought to assist in inhalation.

5. _____ is a muscle located in the midlayer of the low back and is generally said to assist in exhalation, although it may have a role in stabilizing the lower ribs, which can help the diaphragm function more efficiently.

5

Lower Limb

■ CHAPTER OUTLINE

(Continued)

OVERVIEW OF THE REGION

The lower limb is designed for weight-bearing, balance, and mobility. The bones and muscles of the lower limb are larger and stronger than those of the upper limb, which is necessary for the functions of weight-bearing and balance. Our lower limbs carry us, allow us to push forward, and also keep us standing still. Our sense of steadiness and strength often comes from our lower limbs.

The muscles of the thigh are thick and strong and can tolerate greater pressure during massage than the smaller muscles of the arm. Pétrissage is generally welcome and easy to perform in the thigh. The muscles of the posterior leg are also thick and strong, as they propel us forward. The anterior leg is less muscular and more suited to friction or deep effleurage.

The foot is our anchor, grounding us to the earth. Although composed of a complex structure of bones, joints, and muscles, the foot is also our steady connection to the ground.

BONES AND BONE MARKINGS OF THE REGION

The bones of the lower limb include the pelvic girdle, femur, patella, tibia, fibula, and bones of the foot. These are discussed below.

Pelvic Girdle

The pelvic girdle contains the hip bone and the sacrum. As already noted, the hip bone contains the ilium, ischium, and pubis (see Chapter 4). Recall that the iliac crest contains the anterior superior iliac spine (ASIS) and the posterior superior iliac spine (PSIS). The iliac spine contains the entire iliac crest and extends inferiorly in the front and back to include the anterior inferior iliac spine (AIIS) and posterior inferior iliac spine (PIIS), as well. The anterior aspect of the ilium is broad and curved, like a fossa. It is called the *iliac fossa*.

Recall that the ischium has a significant bone marking in the ischial tuberosity. The hamstring muscles connect to the -

ischial tuberosity. In addition, the ischium contains a spine, which separates the greater sciatic notch from the lesser sciatic notch.

Remember that the pubis contains two rami, the superior pubic ramus and the inferior pubic ramus. The thigh adductors originate on the pubis.

Recall that the acetabulum is the name of the socket that articulates with the head of the femur to form the hip joint. The acetabulum is where the ilium, ischium, and pubis join together. Figure 5-1 shows bones and bone markings of the pelvis.

Femur

The femur, or thigh bone, is the longest and strongest bone in the body. Its rounded head, located on the proximal, medial aspect of the femur, fits beautifully in the acetabulum to form the hip joint. The greater trochanter is a sizable bone marking on the lateral aspect of the proximal femur. The lesser trochanter is smaller and is located distal and slightly posterior to the head of the femur on the medial aspect of the bone. Rounded medial and lateral condyles are located on the distal end of the femur and articulate with the tibia. A rough line called the *linea aspera* runs almost the full length of the posterior femur. The gluteal tuberosity is located on the proximal, posterior femur, very close to the proximal linea aspera. The pectineal line is located proximal and medial on the posterior femur, just inferior to the lesser trochanter. Figure 5-2 illustrates the femur and its bone markings, as well as the patella.

Patella

The patella or knee cap is a sesamoid bone that lies anterior to the junction of the femur and tibia. The patella is cartilaginous at birth and ossifies between 3 and 6 years of age. The patella is embedded in the quadriceps tendon and causes the tendon to be positioned more anteriorly, thus enhancing the leverage of the quadriceps tendon as it pulls on the tibial tuberosity to extend the knee. The patella slides up and

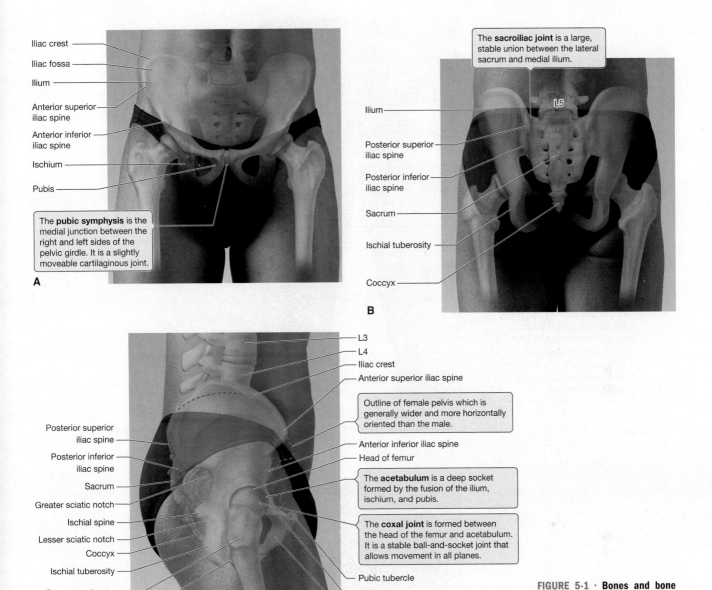

Iliac crest
Iliac fossa
Ilium
Anterior superior iliac spine
Anterior inferior iliac spine
Ischium
Pubis

The **pubic symphysis** is the medial junction between the right and left sides of the pelvic girdle. It is a slightly moveable cartilaginous joint.

A

The **sacroiliac joint** is a large, stable union between the lateral sacrum and medial ilium.

L5

Ilium
Posterior superior iliac spine
Posterior inferior iliac spine
Sacrum
Ischial tuberosity
Coccyx

B

L3
L4
Iliac crest
Anterior superior iliac spine

Outline of female pelvis which is generally wider and more horizontally oriented than the male.

Anterior inferior iliac spine
Head of femur

The **acetabulum** is a deep socket formed by the fusion of the ilium, ischium, and pubis.

The **coxal joint** is formed between the head of the femur and acetabulum. It is a stable ball-and-socket joint that allows movement in all planes.

Posterior superior iliac spine
Posterior inferior iliac spine
Sacrum
Greater sciatic notch
Ischial spine
Lesser sciatic notch
Coccyx
Ischial tuberosity
Greater trochanter
Lesser trochanter

Pubic tubercle
Superior ramus of pubis
Inferior ramus of pubis
Shaft of femur

C

FIGURE 5-1 · Bones and bone markings of the pelvis A: Anterior view; **B:** Posterior view; **C:** Lateral view

down as we flex and extend the leg. Cartilage on the posterior aspect of the patella provides cushioning between the patella and the femur (see Fig. 5-2).

Tibia and Fibula

The tibia and fibula are the bones of the leg. The tibia is much the larger and is located medial to the fibula. The tibia is the weight-bearing bone and is part of the knee joint. Several important bone markings exist on the tibia and fibula. The proximal end of the tibia contains two condyles, a medial condyle and a lateral condyle. The tibial tuberosity is located on the proximal anterior aspect of the tibia, just inferior to the patella. As already noted, it serves as the insertion site for the quadriceps tendon. Pes anserinus, which

means "goose foot," is the name given to a flat area on the proximal, anterior, medial tibia, just medial to the tibial tuberosity. Three muscles insert at pes anserinus, and the triplet of tendons looks somewhat like the three toes of a goose's foot. On the distal medial side of the tibia is the medial malleolus, which is commonly referred to the "inner ankle bone" in lay terms.

The fibula contains some important bone markings, as well. The head of the fibula is the bone's most proximal aspect. Two important muscles connect to this bone marking. Distally, the fibula has a lateral, rounded projection called the *medial malleolus* in anatomical language and called the "outer ankle bone" in common, everyday language. Figure 5-3 illustrates the bones and bone markings of the leg.

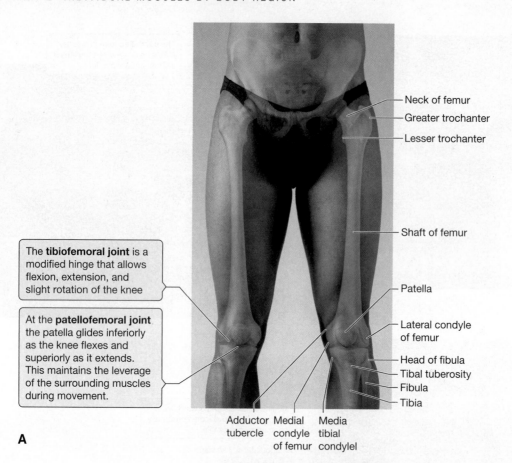

The **tibiofemoral joint** is a modified hinge that allows flexion, extension, and slight rotation of the knee

At the **patellofemoral joint**, the patella glides inferiorly as the knee flexes and superiorly as it extends. This maintains the leverage of the surrounding muscles during movement.

Neck of femur
Greater trochanter
Lesser trochanter

Shaft of femur

Patella

Lateral condyle of femur

Head of fibula
Tibal tuberosity
Fibula
Tibia

Adductor tubercle
Medial condyle of femur
Media tibial condylel

A

Head of femur
Neck of femur
Greater trochanter
Lesser trochanter
Gluteal tuberosity
Pectineal line

The **linea aspera** is a long vertical line running along the shaft of the posterior femur. It is the site of several muscle attachments.

Shaft of femur

Intercondylar notch

Lateral condyle of femur

Lateral condyle of tibia
Head of fibula

Medial condyle of femur
Medial tibial condyle

B

FIGURE 5-2 · **Femur, femoral bone markings, and the patella. A:** Anterior view; **B:** Posterior view

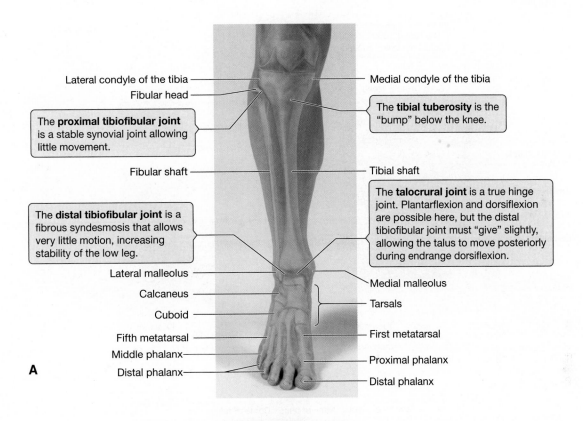

Lateral condyle of the tibia

Fibular head

The **proximal tibiofibular joint** is a stable synovial joint allowing little movement.

Fibular shaft

The **distal tibiofibular joint** is a fibrous syndesmosis that allows very little motion, increasing stability of the low leg.

Lateral malleolus

Calcaneus

Cuboid

Fifth metatarsal

Middle phalanx

Distal phalanx

A

Medial condyle of the tibia

The **tibial tuberosity** is the "bump" below the knee.

Tibial shaft

The **talocrural joint** is a true hinge joint. Plantarflexion and dorsiflexion are possible here, but the distal tibiofibular joint must "give" slightly, allowing the talus to move posteriorly during endrange dorsiflexion.

Medial malleolus

Tarsals

First metatarsal

Proximal phalanx

Distal phalanx

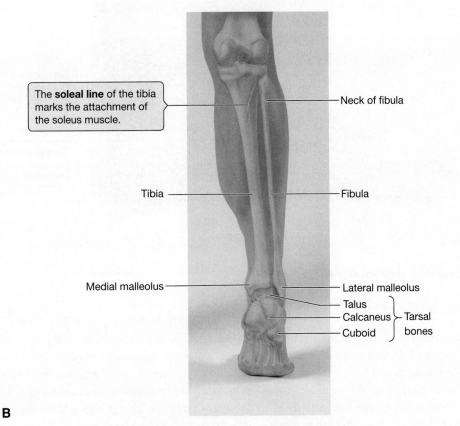

The **soleal line** of the tibia marks the attachment of the soleus muscle.

Tibia

Medial malleolus

B

Neck of fibula

Fibula

Lateral malleolus

Talus

Calcaneus — Tarsal

Cuboid — bones

FIGURE 5-3 · **Bones and bone markings of the leg. A:** Anterior view; **B:** Posterior view

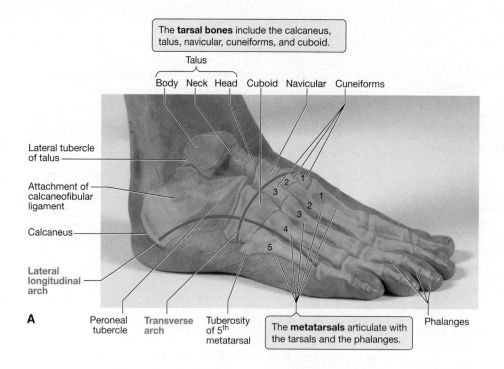

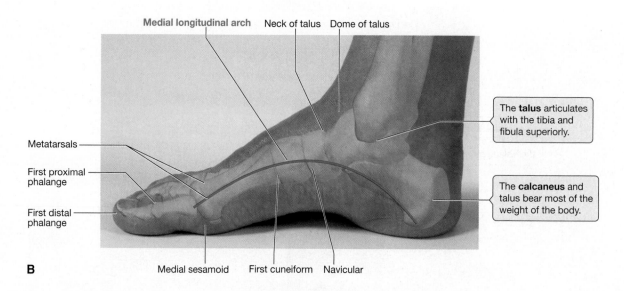

FIGURE 5-4 · Bones and arches of the foot. A: Lateral view; **B:** Medial view

Bones of the Foot

The bones of the foot are organized in a somewhat similar fashion to the bones of the hand. However, a major difference is that the tarsals do not lie in two fairly neat, distinguishable rows of four bones each, as do the carpals of the proximal hand. We have seven tarsals in each foot, a group of three and then a row of four distal to the group of three. The calcaneus is the heel bone and is the largest tarsal bone. The sizable Achilles tendon connects to the posterior aspect of the calcaneus. The calcaneus has a roughened tuberosity on its plantar aspect, where three muscles originate. The talus is superior to the calcaneus and joins with the distal tibia and

distal fibula to form the ankle joint. Anterior to the talus is the navicular. A row of four bones lies distal to the calcaneus and the navicular and includes the medial cuneiform, the middle cuneiform, the lateral cuneiform, and the cuboid. The three cuneiforms are frequently called cuneiform 1, 2, and 3, with the first cuneiform always the medial one and the third cuneiform always the lateral one.

Our metatarsals are located distal to the tarsal bones, one metatarsal per digit, thus matching the hand's metacarpals. The proximal aspect of each metatarsal is called the *base*, and the rounded, distal end of each metatarsal is called a *head*. Distal to the metatarsals are our phalanges, arranged in rows. Each of the four lateral toes has a proximal, middle, and distal phalanx. Digit 1, or the big toe, has only two phalanges, a proximal and a distal. Figure 5-4 illustrates the bones and arches of the foot.

The shapes of our foot bones and their relative position to each other cause the foot to have both longitudinal and transverse arches. We have a longitudinal arch, which runs from the calcaneus to the heads of the metatarsals. The longitudinal arch is often separated into a medial longitudinal and a lateral longitudinal arch. We also have a transverse arch, which runs medially to laterally across the cuneiforms and cuboid. The wedge shape of many of our tarsal bones creates these arches. In addition, ligaments and the intrinsic foot muscles help to maintain our arches.

Our arches enhance our mobility and balance, and assist in the transfer of weight from one part of the foot to another. In addition, the arches serve as shock absorbers. *Pes planus*, or flat feet, occurs when our arches are flattened. This condition can be painful and limit mobility. Because pes planus can shift gait, it can cause muscular issues in the leg or thigh. Massage therapy may help address such muscular issues.

JOINTS, LIGAMENTS, AND BURSAE OF THE REGION

Joints of the lower limb include the sacroiliac joint, hip joint, knee joint, tibiofibular joints, ankle joints, joints that permit inversion and eversion, and other joints within the foot. These are discussed below.

Sacroiliac Joint

The sacrum articulates with the ilium at two sacroiliac (SI) joints. The articulating surfaces of the sacrum and ilium nestle against each other, so that the joints allow very little movement. Many strong ligaments support the SI joints. The anterior SI ligament joins the iliac fossa to the anterior sacrum. The posterior SI ligament joins the PSIS to the sacrum. The sacrotuberous ligament joins the ischial tuberosity to the sacrum. The sacrospinous ligament joins the ischial spine to the sacrum. Figure 5-5 shows the ligaments that support the SI joint.

Hip Joint

The hip joint is a ball-and-socket joint designed to have the stability needed for a weight-bearing joint. A strong ring of fibrocartilage, called the *acetabular labrum*, connects to the edge of the acetabulum, giving the socket greater depth and helping to hold the head of the femur in the socket. Many ligaments help support the hip joint. The ischiofemoral ligament, the iliofemoral ligament, and the pubofemoral ligament join each of the hip bones to the femur. In addition, the ligament of the head of the femur joins the head of the femur to the acetabulum.

Several bursae lie between structures in the area of the hip joint. The ischial bursa prevents friction between the gluteus maximus muscle and the ischial tuberosity. The iliopectineal bursa separates the anterior hip joint capsule from the iliopsoas muscle. And the trochanteric bursa prevents friction between the greater trochanter and the gluteus maximus muscle.

The hip joint permits flexion, extension, abduction, adduction, as well as internal (medial) and external (lateral) rotation.

Knee Joint

The knee joint is the articulation between the proximal tibia and distal femur. The rounded condyles of the distal femur fit into concave condyles of the proximal tibia. The knee joint is classified as a hinge joint and permits a wide range of flexion and extension. The knee joint also allows a small amount of medial and lateral rotation, due to the difference in sizes between the medial and lateral condyles of the femur. The medial condyle of the femur is longer (from front to back) than the lateral condyle of the femur. Thus, as we extend our leg toward full extension, the lateral condyles of femur and tibia touch, forming a pivot around which a small amount of rotation occurs. When we bring our knee into full extension, the tibia rotates laterally to cause a perfect fit and "lock" to the knee joint. When flexing our knee from a fully extended position, the tibia must rotate a bit medially to allow flexion to begin. Rotation of the tibia is possible only when the tibia is free to move. When our weight is on a single leg, and the tibia is thus fixed, the femur rotates laterally to unlock the knee, or the femur rotates medially to "lock" the knee.

Many important muscles and ligaments stabilize the knee. The large quadriceps group and the large hamstring muscles provide stability to the joint. In addition, four ligaments play a major role in knee stabilization. The anterior cruciate ligament (ACL) joins the anterior aspect on the medial tibia to the medial side of the lateral condyle of the femur. The posterior cruciate ligament (PCL) joins the posterior medial tibia to the lateral side of the medial condyle of the femur. Cruciate means "cross," which is an appropriate name, as these two ligaments cross over each other as they pass from the tibia to the femur. The cruciate ligaments prevent the femur from sliding off of the tibia anteriorly or posteriorly. The ACL is susceptible to injury when the knee is hit from the lateral side. A weakened or torn ACL leaves the knee joint lacking stability.

We have two ligaments that run vertically along the sides of the knee joint. The lateral or fibular collateral ligament joins the lateral epicondyle of the femur to the head of the fibula. The medial or tibial collateral ligament joins the medial epicondyle of the femur to the lateral aspect of the proximal tibia. The medial collateral ligament is more susceptible to injury than is the lateral collateral ligament, due to its vulnerability when a force pushes into the lateral side of the knee.

The patellar ligament completes the knee ligaments. This ligament runs from the patella to the tibial tuberosity and is a portion of the quadriceps tendon of insertion. The patellar ligament provides additional stability across the anterior aspect of the knee joint. Figure 5-6 shows the ligaments that stabilize the knee.

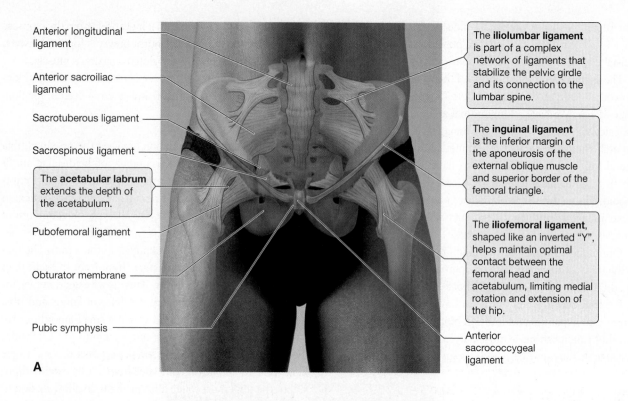

Anterior longitudinal ligament

Anterior sacroiliac ligament

Sacrotuberous ligament

Sacrospinous ligament

The **acetabular labrum** extends the depth of the acetabulum.

Pubofemoral ligament

Obturator membrane

Pubic symphysis

The **iliolumbar ligament** is part of a complex network of ligaments that stabilize the pelvic girdle and its connection to the lumbar spine.

The **inguinal ligament** is the inferior margin of the aponeurosis of the external oblique muscle and superior border of the femoral triangle.

The **iliofemoral ligament**, shaped like an inverted "Y", helps maintain optimal contact between the femoral head and acetabulum, limiting medial rotation and extension of the hip.

Anterior sacrococcygeal ligament

A

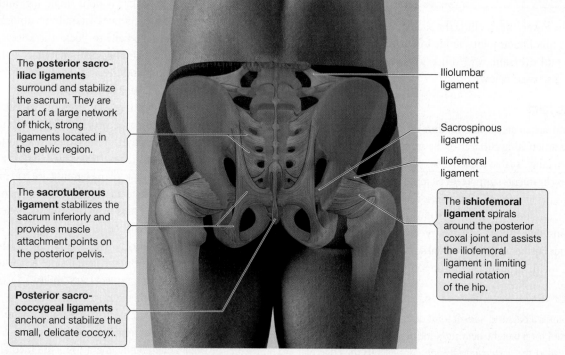

The **posterior sacro-iliac ligaments** surround and stabilize the sacrum. They are part of a large network of thick, strong ligaments located in the pelvic region.

The **sacrotuberous ligament** stabilizes the sacrum inferiorly and provides muscle attachment points on the posterior pelvis.

Posterior sacro-coccygeal ligaments anchor and stabilize the small, delicate coccyx.

Iliolumbar ligament

Sacrospinous ligament

Iliofemoral ligament

The **ishiofemoral ligament** spirals around the posterior coxal joint and assists the iliofemoral ligament in limiting medial rotation of the hip.

B

FIGURE 5-5 · **Ligaments that support the sacroiliac joint. A:** Anterior view; **B:** Posterior view

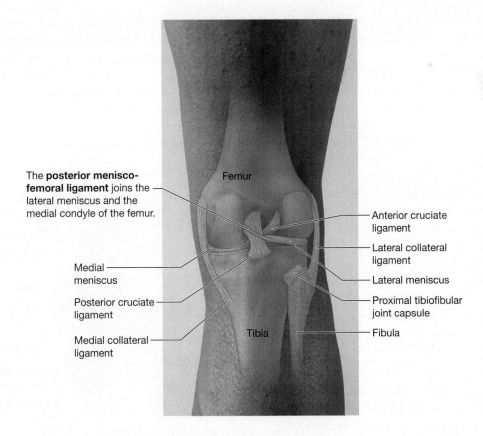

The posterior articular surface of the patella sits in the **femoral groove**. The patellofemoral joint must slide up and down as the knee extends and flexes.

The **lateral meniscus** is circular shaped cartilage that cushions the tibiofemoral joint and increases joint continuity.

The **lateral collateral ligament** connects the lateral femoral condyle to the head of the fibula. It prevents lateral opening of the tibiofemoral joint (varus deformity).

The **patellar tendon** (cut) connects the quadriceps muscles to the tibia. It is sometimes called the patellar ligament because it connects the patella to the tibia.

The **posterior cruciate ligament** connects posteriorly to the tibia and anteriorly to the medial condyle of the femur. Stronger than the anterior cruciate ligament, it prevents the tibia from sliding posteriorly and the femur from sliding anteriorly.

The **anterior cruciate ligament** connects anteriorly to the tibia and posteriorly to the lateral condyle of the femur. It prevents the tibia from sliding anteriorly and the femur from sliding posteriorly.

The **medial meniscus** is a crescent-shaped cartilage that cushions the tibiofemoral joint. It has a direct connection to the medial collateral ligament.

The **medial collateral ligament** connects the medial femoral and tibial condyles. It prevents medial opening of the knee (valgus deformity).

Femur

Patella

Proximal tibiofibular ligament

Fibula

Tibia

A

The **posterior menisco-femoral ligament** joins the lateral meniscus and the medial condyle of the femur.

Femur

Anterior cruciate ligament

Lateral collateral ligament

Lateral meniscus

Proximal tibiofibular joint capsule

Fibula

Medial meniscus

Posterior cruciate ligament

Medial collateral ligament

Tibia

B

FIGURE 5-6 · Ligaments that stabilize the knee. A: Anterior view; **B:** Posterior view

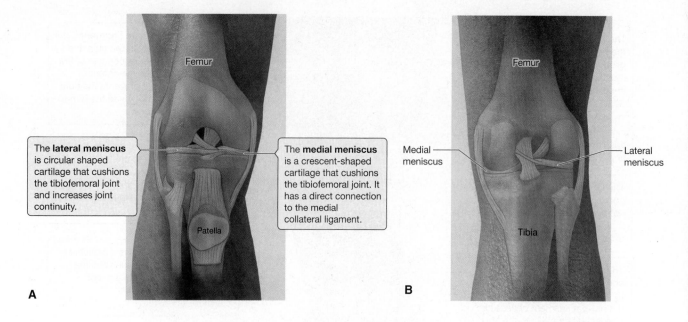

The **lateral meniscus** is circular shaped cartilage that cushions the tibiofemoral joint and increases joint continuity.

The **medial meniscus** is a crescent-shaped cartilage that cushions the tibiofemoral joint. It has a direct connection to the medial collateral ligament.

A

B

FIGURE 5-7 · Medial and lateral menisci of the knee

Two rings of fibrocartilage, called *menisci*, lie between the femur and the tibia and provide cushioning between these two bones. The lateral meniscus forms an almost complete ring, whereas the medial meniscus is more C-shaped. The menisci are susceptible to tears and do not self-repair easily. Figure 5-7 shows the medial and lateral menisci of the knee.

Several bursae help to prevent friction between structures close to the knee joint. The subcutaneous infrapatellar bursa facilitates movement of the skin over the tibial tuberosity as the knee joint moves. The suprapatellar bursa prevents friction between the patella and femur. The gastrocnemius bursa allows the proximal gastrocnemius muscle to move against the posterior femur. Irritation or inflammation of these bursae can be painful and produce swelling. Such bursitis is commonly caused by trauma to the area or overuse of the knee joint. Figure 5-8 shows several bursea of the knee joint.

Massage therapy can help prevent knee injuries by contributing to the health and flexibility of the muscles that help stabilize the knee. In addition, massage therapy can help the process of recovery from a knee injury by assisting in the reduction of adhesions and scar tissue.

Tibiofibular Joints

We have two joints between the tibia and fibula. The proximal tibiofibular joint is a plane joint and permits minimal gliding. The distal tibiofibular joint is an amphiarthrotic joint and permits almost no movement at all. An interosseus membrane adds further stability between the two bones of the leg (see Fig. 5-3).

Ankle Joints

The ankle joint is composed of the distal end of the tibia, the distal end of the fibula, and the talus. The distal ends of the tibia and fibula form a shape that is similar to three sides of a box. This structure fits perfectly with the talus, especially when the ankle is in a dorsiflexed position. When dorsiflexed, the portion of the talus that articulates with the distal tibia and fibula is wider, and thus the three bones fit snugly together. Figure 5-9 shows the ankle joint.

The ankle most resembles a hinge type of synovial joint, and it permits dorsiflexion and plantarflexion. A small amount of abduction, adduction, and rotation are possible, as well.

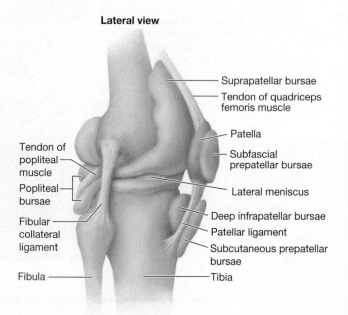

Lateral view

Suprapatellar bursae

Tendon of quadriceps femoris muscle

Patella

Subfascial prepatellar bursae

Lateral meniscus

Deep infrapatellar bursae

Patellar ligament

Subcutaneous prepatellar bursae

Tibia

Tendon of popliteal muscle

Popliteal bursae

Fibular collateral ligament

Fibula

FIGURE 5-8 · Bursae of the knee joint

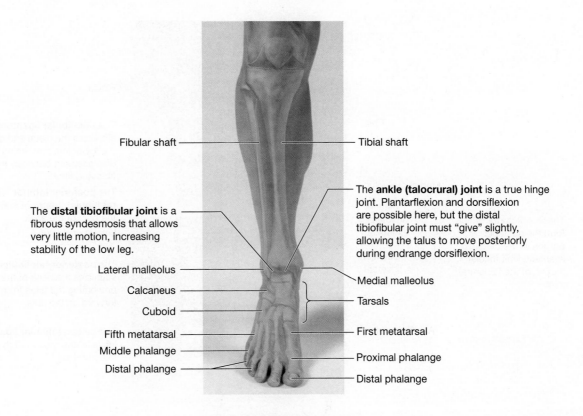

A

Fibular shaft — — Tibial shaft

The **distal tibiofibular joint** is a fibrous syndesmosis that allows very little motion, increasing stability of the low leg.

The **ankle (talocrural) joint** is a true hinge joint. Plantarflexion and dorsiflexion are possible here, but the distal tibiofibular joint must "give" slightly, allowing the talus to move posteriorly during endrange dorsiflexion.

Lateral malleolus — — Medial malleolus
Calcaneus — — Tarsals
Cuboid —
Fifth metatarsal — — First metatarsal
Middle phalange — — Proximal phalange
Distal phalange — — Distal phalange

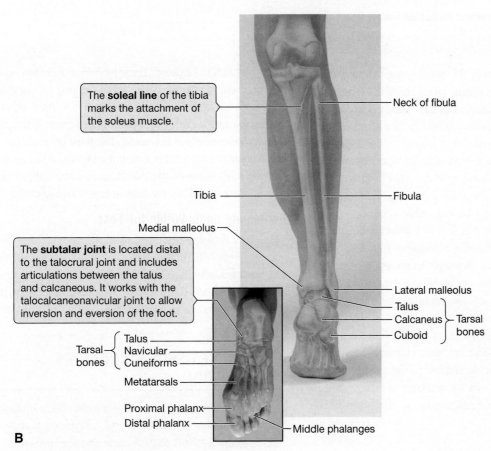

B

The **soleal line** of the tibia marks the attachment of the soleus muscle.

Neck of fibula

Tibia — — Fibula

Medial malleolus —

The **subtalar joint** is located distal to the talocrural joint and includes articulations between the talus and calcaneous. It works with the talocalcaneonavicular joint to allow inversion and eversion of the foot.

Lateral malleolus
Talus
Calcaneus — Tarsal bones
Cuboid

Tarsal bones { Talus
Navicular
Cuneiforms
Metatarsals
Proximal phalanx
Distal phalanx — Middle phalanges

FIGURE 5-9 · Ankle joint. A: Anterior view; **B:** Posterior view

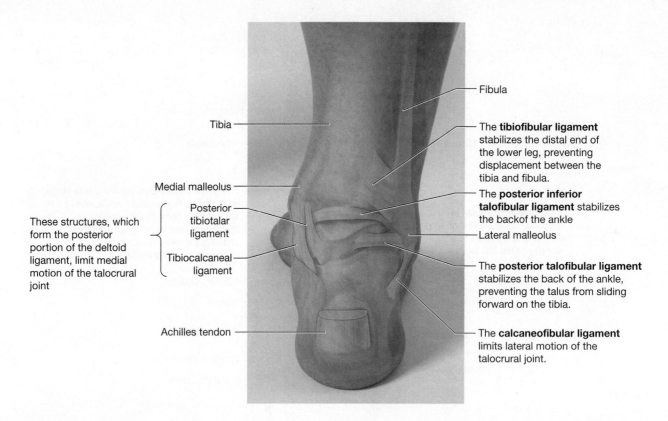

Tibia

Medial malleolus

Posterior tibiotalar ligament

These structures, which form the posterior portion of the deltoid ligament, limit medial motion of the talocrural joint

Tibiocalcaneal ligament

Achilles tendon

Fibula

The **tibiofibular ligament** stabilizes the distal end of the lower leg, preventing displacement between the tibia and fibula.

The **posterior inferior talofibular ligament** stabilizes the backof the ankle

Lateral malleolus

The **posterior talofibular ligament** stabilizes the back of the ankle, preventing the talus from sliding forward on the tibia.

The **calcaneofibular ligament** limits lateral motion of the talocrural joint.

FIGURE 5-10 · Major ligaments of the foot and ankle

Many ligaments support the ankle joint. Among them are the deltoid ligament, a strong, triangular-shaped ligament that joins the medial malleolus to the talus, navicular, and calcaneus. The spring ligament joins the talus to the calcaneus. The posterior talofibular ligament joins the lateral malleolus to the talus. The calcaneofibular ligament joins the lateral malleolus to the calcaneus. Many other ligaments contribute to the stability of the ankle joint. Figure 5-10 shows the major ligaments of the foot and ankle.

Despite the significant number of ligaments helping to stabilize this joint, and despite the shapes of the articular surfaces of the bones that come together so well to form this join, the ankle is the most commonly injured joint in the body. When we lose balance, we put huge amounts of stress on the ligaments that support this joint, often tearing or overstretching them. The ligaments positioned to cross the lateral side of the ankle joint are most vulnerable to injury. Massage therapy can provide benefits to those with chronic ankle weakness and sprains by working to remove adhesions and scar tissue and restoring range of motion to the joint.

Joints That Permit Inversion and Eversion

Recall that *inversion* is the foot movement that results in turning the plantar surface of the foot inward toward the midline. Eversion is the foot movement that causes the plantar surface

of the foot to turn outward. These movements are important in helping us to maintain balance when walking on uneven surfaces or as we shift our weight from one foot to the other.

Several intertarsal joints combine to permit the movements of eversion and inversion. The joint between the talus and calcaneus, the joint between the talus and the navicular, and the joint between the calcaneus and the cuboid are the major joints that allow the foot to invert and to evert.

Remaining Joints Within the Foot

The joints between the tarsals and metatarsals are plane or gliding joints, which permit limited side-to-side movement. The metatarsophalangeal (MP) joints are condyloid joints and allow flexion, extension, abduction, and adduction. The interphalangeal joints are hinge joints and permit flexion and extension only .

CONNECTIVE TISSUE STRUCTURES OF THE REGION

Connective tissue structures of the lower limb include the deep investing fascia, iliotibial band, fascial compartment divisions in the leg, and plantar fascia or aponeurosis.

Deep Investing Fascia and Iliotibial Band

The thigh contains a layer of fascia, which wraps all the muscles of the thigh. This fascia is substantially thicker on the

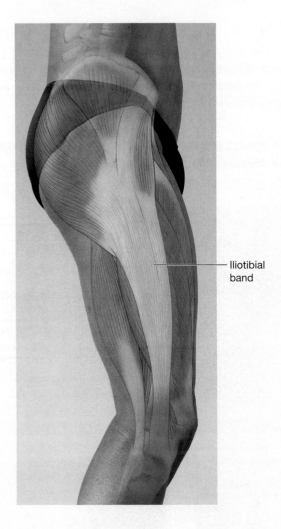

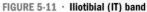

FIGURE 5-11 · **Iliotibial (IT) band**

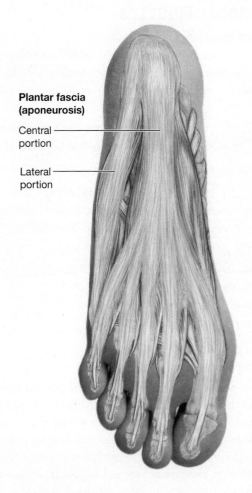

FIGURE 5-12 · **Plantar fascia**

lateral aspect of the thigh, forming the iliotibial (IT) tract. This dense band of connective tissue runs from the ilium to the lateral aspect of the lateral condyle of the tibia. The IT band serves as the tendon of insertion of gluteus maximus and the tensor fascia latae (TFL). The IT band or tract helps to stabilize the knee from a lateral perspective. Figure 5-11 shows the IT band.

Fascial Compartment Divisions in the Leg

The leg muscles are wrapped by investing fascia in a manner similar to the thigh. This crural (leg) fascia joins with inter-muscular sheets of fascia called *septa*, to divide the leg into four rather distinct compartments. Two compartments are located in the posterior leg and are called the *deep posterior leg compartment* and the *superficial posterior leg compartment*. The deep posterior leg compartment contains three muscles. The superficial posterior leg compartment contains two

muscles and the tendon of insertion of a third muscle. The anterior leg compartment lies between the anterior aspects of the tibia and fibula, and includes four muscles. The lateral leg compartment lies along the lateral fibula and houses two muscles. When describing the location of each of the muscles of the leg, the compartment in which each muscle is housed will be named.

Plantar Fascia or Aponeurosis

The plantar fascia runs from the calcaneus to the proximal phalanges of the plantar surface of the foot. Figure 5-12 illustrates the plantar fascia.

This structure provides support to the longitudinal arch of the foot. It can become inflamed, resulting in a condition called *plantar fasciitis*. Massage of the posterior leg muscle may provide symptomatic relief to those dealing with plantar fasciitis.

INDIVIDUAL MUSCLES

Hip Joint Muscles

The muscles that move the hip can be divided into many subgroups. We have a group of deep lateral rotators, located deep in the buttock region. Our hip adductors make up the medial thigh. The hip abductors are located in the lateral hip area. The hip flexors cross the front of the hip joint, and the hip extensors cross the hip joint posteriorly.

PIRIFORMIS AND THE OTHER DEEP LATERAL ROTATORS OF THE HIP

The six deep lateral rotators of the hip include piriformis, gemellus superior, gemellus inferior, obturator internus, obturator externus, and quadratus femoris (Fig. 5-13).

pir-i-form-is
jem-e-lus su-per-e-or
jem-e-lus in-fer-e-or
ob-tu-ra-tor in-tern-us
ob-tu-ra-tor ek-stern-us
kwa-drat-us fem-o-ris

Meaning of Name

Piriformis means "pear-shaped." The name *gemellus superior* indicates that there are two muscles (twins), and one is superior to the other. The name *gemellus inferior* indicates that there are two gemelli (twins) muscles and that this one is inferior to the other. Obturator internus and externus indicate the location of two muscles around the obturator foramen. Quadratus femoris indicates that the shape of the muscle is "square-like" and that it connects to the femur.

Location

All six of the deep lateral rotators of the thigh lie deep in the buttock region. Piriformis lies in the greater sciatic notch and is superficial to the sciatic nerve. Figure 5-14 shows the position of piriformis in relation to the sciatic nerve.

Origin and Insertion

Piriformis
Origin: anterior sacrum
Insertion: greater trochanter

Gemellus Superior
Origin: spine of the ischium
Insertion: greater trochanter

Gemellus Inferior and Quadrates Femoris
Origin: ischial tuberosity
Insertion: greater trochanter

Obturator Internus and Externus
Origin: obturator foramen
Insertion: greater trochanter

Actions

Laterally rotate the thigh

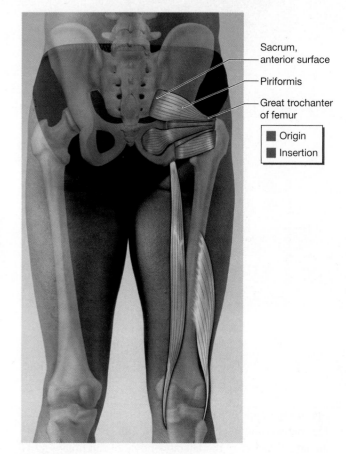

Sacrum, anterior surface
Piriformis
Great trochanter of femur

■ Origin
■ Insertion

FIGURE 5-13 · Six deep lateral rotators of the hip

Explanation of Actions

All of the six deep lateral rotators are positioned to pull the greater trochanter posteriorly, thus causing the femur to rotate laterally.

Notable Muscle Facts

Piriformis is a thick muscle that lies directly superficial to the sciatic nerve. Thus, piriformis is in a position to impinge the sciatic nerve and cause a type of sciatica called *piriformis syndrome.*

Implications of Shortened and/or Lengthened/Weak Muscle

Shortened: The group of lateral rotators can cause a posture in which the toes point out to the sides. A shortened piriformis

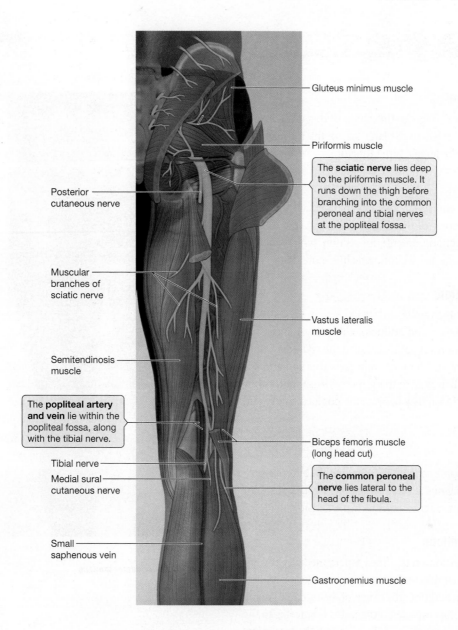

Gluteus minimus muscle

Piriformis muscle

The **sciatic nerve** lies deep to the piriformis muscle. It runs down the thigh before branching into the common peroneal and tibial nerves at the popliteal fossa.

Posterior cutaneous nerve

Muscular branches of sciatic nerve

Vastus lateralis muscle

Semitendinosis muscle

The **popliteal artery and vein** lie within the popliteal fossa, along with the tibial nerve.

Tibial nerve

Medial sural cutaneous nerve

Biceps femoris muscle (long head cut)

The **common peroneal nerve** lies lateral to the head of the fibula.

Small saphenous vein

Gastrocnemius muscle

FIGURE 5-14 · **Position of piriformis in relation to the sciatic nerve**

can cause sciatica, as it lies superficial to the sciatic nerve, and when shortened, can impinge it
Lengthened: Reduced ability to laterally rotate the hip is noted.

Palpation and Massage

It is possible to find piriformis by locating the PSIS and moving an inch or two inferior to this spot. Feel through gluteus maximus for the density of piriformis. The other lateral rotators are not easy to distinguish but can be massaged deep in the buttock region. Friction and direct pressure are the easiest strokes to use.

How to Stretch This Muscle

Medially rotate the hip.

Synergists

Gluteus maximus, iliopsoas, and sartorius (laterally rotate hip/thigh)

Antagonists

Gluteus minimus, gluteus medius, and tensor fascia latae (medially rotate hip/thigh)

Innervation and Arterial Supply

Innervation: lumbosacral plexus, with the exception of obturator externus, which is innervated by the obturator nerve
Arterial supply: obturator artery and superior and inferior gluteal arteries

ADDUCTOR MAGNUS (a-duk-tor mag-nus)

Meaning of Name

The word "adductor" refers to the action of this muscle, and the term "magnus" refers to the large size of the muscle. Adductor magnus is the largest hip adductor.

Location

Adductor magnus comprises much of the medial thigh. It is the largest and deepest of the thigh adductors. This muscle has two distinct sections, an anterior section, which is more proximal, and a posterior section, which is more distal.

Origin and Insertion

Origin: inferior pubic ramus
Insertion: linea aspera and adductor tubercle. A space between these two insertion points is called the *adductor hiatus*. The femoral artery and femoral vein pass through the adductor hiatus on their way to the popliteal fossa. Once they enter the popliteal fossa, they become the popliteal artery and popliteal vein.

Actions

Adducts the hip. Some sources also cite that the anterior portion of adductor magnus allows hip flexion, and the posterior portion of adductor magnus permits hip extension.

Explanation of Actions

By pulling the insertion on the linea aspera medially toward the pubis and ischial tuberosity, the muscle performs adduction of the thigh. In addition, the origin of the more proximal, anterior section of this muscle on the pubis is anterior to the insertion on the linea aspera, and thus can pull the femur forward, causing hip flexion. On the other hand, the origin of the more posterior, distal section of the muscle is posterior to the insertion, and thus contraction pulls the femur posteriorly, resulting in hip extension.

Notable Muscle Facts

Adductor magnus plays a role in stabilization of the pelvis. When the weight is on the limb, contraction of adductor magnus helps to keep the pelvis centered over the foot. In addition, adductor magnus assists during walking by keeping the thigh adducted when our heel strikes the ground and when our lower limb swings forward with each step.

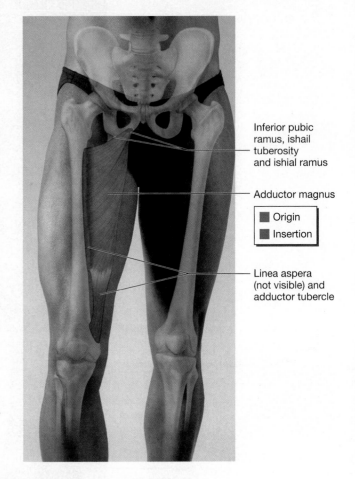

Inferior pubic ramus, ishail tuberosity and ishial ramus

Adductor magnus

■ Origin
■ Insertion

Linea aspera (not visible) and adductor tubercle

FIGURE 5-15 · Adductor magnus

Implications of Shortened and/or Lengthened/ Weak Muscle

Shortened: Limited ability to abduct the thigh and a posture in which the feet are close together is noted. When the hip adductor muscles are shortened, they are more susceptible to tearing, which is a common occurrence when the muscle is overstretched quickly. Such a tear is called a *groin pull*. Chronic groin pulls, or recent groin pulls that have healed to the extent that inflammation is no longer present, can be addressed. Friction to the area of the tear can assist healing, limit scar tissue formation, and reduce the likelihood of repeat injury.

Lengthened: Reduced ability to adduct the hip is noted.

Palpation and Massage

The adductors of the thigh are easy to palpate as a group. They comprise the bulk of the medial thigh. Effleurage and pétrissage are appropriate strokes to apply to the hip adductor muscles. In addition, friction can be applied with care, as the medial thigh can be a tender, vulnerable area. Teaching your client to provide self-massage to the hip adductor muscles can be a useful way to address the more proximal aspect of these muscles.

How to Stretch This Muscle

Abduct the thigh.

Synergists

Adductor longus, adductor brevis, pectineus, and gracilis

Antagonists

Gluteus medius, gluteus minimus, tensor fascia latae, and sartorius

Innervation and Arterial Supply

Innervation: sciatic and obturator nerves
Arterial supply: femoral and obturator arteries

ADDUCTOR LONGUS AND ADDUCTOR BREVIS (a-duk-tor long-gus and a-duk-tor brev-is)

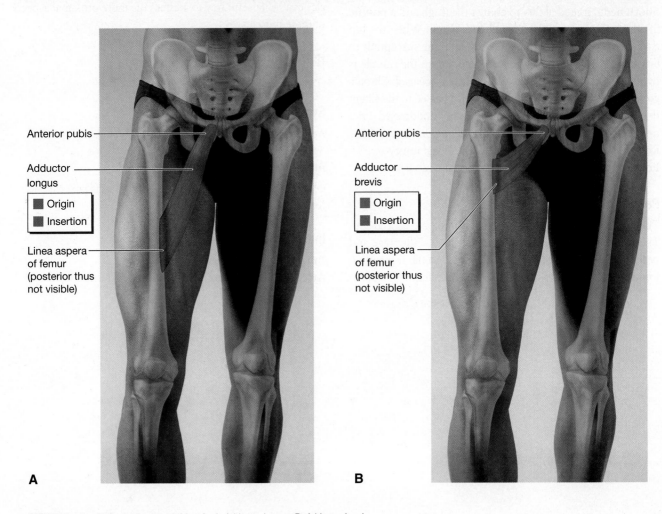

FIGURE 5-16 · **Adductor longus and brevis. A:** Adductor longus; **B:** Adductor brevis

Meaning of Name

Adductor refers to the adduction of hip action. *Longus* means longer than adductor brevis, and *brevis* means shorter than adductor brevis.

Location

Adductor longus and brevis are medial thigh muscles. Adductor longus is the most anterior of the adductor muscles and forms the medial border of the femoral triangle. Figure 5-17 shows the femoral triangle. Adductor brevis is more proximal and deeper than adductor longus.

Origin and Insertion

Origin: anterior pubis
Insertion: linea aspera

Actions

Adduct the thigh; some sources state that adductor longus and adductor brevis assist in hip flexion.

Explanation of Actions

By pulling the insertion on the linea aspera medially toward the pubis, the muscles perform adduction of the thigh. A secondary action of adductor brevis and adductor longus, thigh flexion, is possible due to the fact that the origin on the pubis is anterior to the insertion on the linea aspera, and thus these two muscles can pull the femur forward, causing hip flexion.

Notable Muscle Facts

The thick tendon of the origin of adductor longus makes it the most palpable tendon in the area of the anterior pubis.

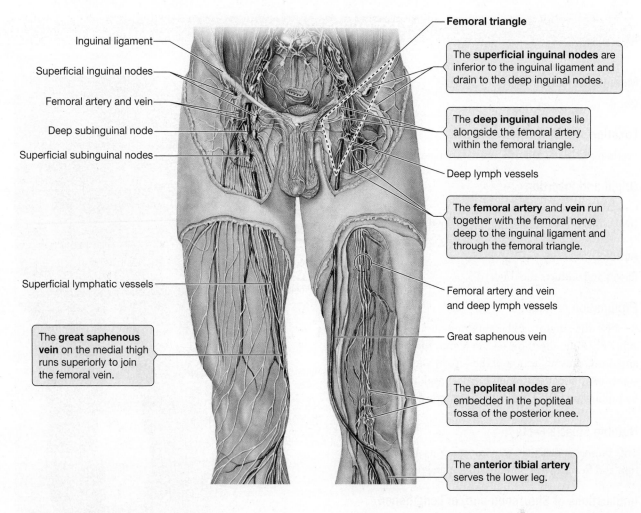

Inguinal ligament

Superficial inguinal nodes

Femoral artery and vein

Deep subinguinal node

Superficial subinguinal nodes

Superficial lymphatic vessels

The **great saphenous vein** on the medial thigh runs superiorly to join the femoral vein.

Femoral triangle

The **superficial inguinal nodes** are inferior to the inguinal ligament and drain to the deep inguinal nodes.

The **deep inguinal nodes** lie alongside the femoral artery within the femoral triangle.

Deep lymph vessels

The **femoral artery** and **vein** run together with the femoral nerve deep to the inguinal ligament and through the femoral triangle.

Femoral artery and vein and deep lymph vessels

Great saphenous vein

The **popliteal nodes** are embedded in the popliteal fossa of the posterior knee.

The **anterior tibial artery** serves the lower leg.

FIGURE 5-17 · Femoral triangle

Implications of Shortened and/or Lengthened/Weak Muscle

Shortened: Inability to fully abduct the thigh is noted. When the hip adductor muscles are shortened, they are more susceptible to tearing, which is a common occurrence when the muscle is overstretched quickly. Such a tear is called a groin pull. Chronic groin pulls, or recent groin pulls that have healed to the extent that inflammation is no longer present, can be addressed. Friction to the area of the tear can assist healing, limit scar tissue formation, and reduce the likelihood of repeat injury.

Lengthened: Limited ability to adduct the thigh is noted.

Palpation and Massage

The adductors of the thigh are easy to palpate as a group. They comprise the bulk of the medial thigh. Effleurage and pétrissage are appropriate strokes to apply to the hip adductor muscles. In addition, friction can be applied with care, as the medial thigh can be a tender, vulnerable area. Teaching your client to provide self-massage to the hip adductor muscles can be a useful way to address the more proximal aspect of these muscles.

How to Stretch This Muscle

Abduct the thigh.

Synergists

Adductor magnus, pectineus, and gracilis

Antagonists

Gluteus medius, gluteus minimus, tensor fascia latae, and sartorius

Innervation and Arterial Supply

Innervation: sciatic nerve
Arterial supply: femoral and obturator arteries

PECTINEUS (pek-tin-e-us)

Meaning of Name

Comb

Location

Pectineus is located in the femoral triangle.

Origin and Insertion

Origin: superior pubic ramus
Insertion: pectineal line on the proximal, posterior femur

Actions

Flexes and adducts the thigh

Explanation of Actions

Because the origin on the superior pubis is anterior and superior to the insertion on the femur, the femur is pulled anteriorly, causing flexion of the hip. In addition, the origin is medial to the insertion on the pectineal line of the femur. By pulling the femur medially, the muscle adducts the thigh.

Notable Muscle Facts

This muscle is designed to accomplish its actions of adduction and flexion with power, rather than speed.

Implications of Shortened and/or Lengthened/ Weak Muscle

Shortened: A shortened pectineus can cause an anterior pelvic tilt. In addition, when pectineus is shortened, one has limited ability to abduct the thigh and assumes a posture in which the feet are close together. When any of the hip adductor muscles are shortened, they are more susceptible to tearing, which is a common occurrence when a muscle is overstretched quickly. Such a tear is called a groin pull. Chronic groin pulls, or recent groin pulls that have healed to the extent that inflammation is no longer present, can be addressed. Friction to the area of the tear can assist healing, limit scar tissue formation, and reduce the likelihood of repeat injury. It may be best to teach your client to apply friction to this muscle on his or her own, rather than for you to touch this sensitive area so close to the genital area.
Lengthened: Reduced ability to flex and adduct the thigh is noted.

Palpation and Massage

This muscle lies right in the femoral triangle and thus is difficult to palpate or massage due to the femoral artery, vein, and nerve in this area (see Fig. 5-17). Find the inguinal ligament just lateral to the pubic symphysis, and palpate just inferior to the inguinal ligament. Gentle pressure to pectineus

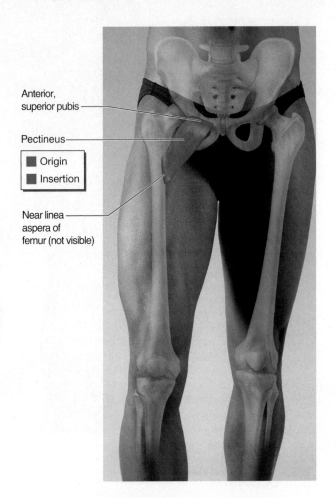

Anterior, superior pubis

Pectineus

■ Origin
■ Insertion

Near linea aspera of femur (not visible)

FIGURE 5-18 · Pectineus

is possible in this area, when done with care. Many times, it is more appropriate to teach self-massage to a client rather than massage in this delicate area.

How to Stretch This Muscle

Abduct the thigh with the knee flexed. Additional stretch can be achieved by extending the hip.

Synergists

Adductor magnus, adductor longus, adductor brevis, and gracilis

Antagonists

Gluteus medius, gluteus minimus, tensor fascia latae, and sartorius

Innervation and Arterial Supply

Innervation: femoral nerve
Arterial supply: femoral and obturator arteries

GRACILIS (gras-i-lis)

Meaning of Name
Slender

Location
Gracilis is the most superficial, medial thigh muscle.

Origin and Insertion
Origin: body and inferior ramus of the pubis
Insertion: pes anserinus

Actions
Adducts the hip and flexes and medially rotates the knee

Explanation of Actions
Gracilis is a hip adductor because the origin is medial to the insertion; thus, contraction pulls the femur medially, causing hip adduction. Gracilis crosses the posterior aspect of the knee, and its origin is above the insertion. Thus, this muscle flexes the knee. Finally, the proximal, medial, anterior tibia is pulled posteriorly, thus causing the tibia to rotate medially.

Notable Muscle Facts
Gracilis is the second longest muscle in the body, next to sartorius. Gracilis has a role in stabilizing the medial aspect of the knee, due to the placement of its tendon of insertion.

Implications of Shortened and/or Lengthened/ Weak Muscle
Shortened: Limited ability to abduct the thigh is noted.
Lengthened: Due to the relative weakness of this muscle, lengthening of gracilis results in no substantial loss of function. In fact, gracilis is a common muscle for surgeons to use in muscle replacement surgery, especially to replace a muscle in the hand.

Palpation and Massage
This muscle can be palpated along the most medial superficial aspect of the thigh. It runs as a pant seam does, along the inner thigh and leg.

How to Stretch This Muscle
Abduct the thigh.

Synergists
Adductor magnus, adductor longus, adductor brevis, and pectineus (abduct the hip); hamstrings, gastrocnemius, sartorius, popliteus, and plantaris (flex the knee); semitendinosus and semimembranosus (medially rotate the knee)

Antagonists
Gluteus medius, gluteus minimus, tensor fascia latae, and sartorius (abduct the hip); quadriceps femoris group (extend the knee); biceps femoris (laterally rotates the knee)

Innervation and Arterial Supply
Innervation: obturator nerve
Arterial supply: deep femoral and obturator arteries

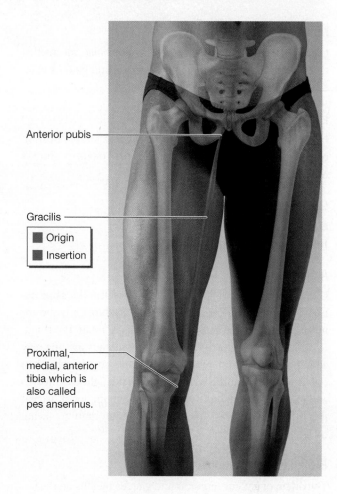

Anterior pubis

Gracilis
■ Origin
■ Insertion

Proximal, medial, anterior tibia which is also called pes anserinus.

FIGURE 5-19 · Gracilis

GLUTEUS MINIMUS (glut-e-us min-i-mis)

Meaning of Name

Gluteus refers to the buttock region, and *minimus* means that this muscle is smaller than gluteus medius and gluteus maximus.

Location

In the lateral hip, gluteus minimus covers a sizable portion of the external surface of the ilium. It is deep to gluteus medius.

Origin and Insertion

Origin: external surface of the lateral ilium
Insertion: greater trochanter

Actions

Gluteus minimus and gluteus medius perform the same actions: abduction and medial rotation of the hip. Only the anterior fibers of these muscles can medially rotate the thigh. In addition, both gluteus minimus and gluteus medius play an important role in stabilization of the hip, particularly when one is walking. On the weight-bearing side, gluteus medius and gluteus minimus contract to pull the ilium down, so that the other ilium rises, allowing the other limb to swing through when walking.

Explanation of Actions

The origin of gluteus minimus and gluteus medius on the lateral ilium is superior to the greater trochanter of the femur. In addition, these muscles cross the lateral side of the hip joint. Thus, the greater trochanter is pulled out to the side, resulting in hip abduction. It is the same line of pull that allows gluteus medius and gluteus medius to pull the ilium down when weight is on the limb and thus the femur cannot move. The anterior portions of gluteus medius and gluteus minimus perform medial rotation of the hip because the anterior aspect of the origin attachments of these muscles are more anterior than the greater trochanter. Thus, the muscles pull the greater trochanter forward, causing the femur to rotate medially.

Notable Muscle Facts

The anterior section of gluteus minimus is thicker and stronger than the posterior portion.

Implications of Shortened and/or Lengthened/ Weak Muscle

Shortened: When gluteus minimus and gluteus medius are shortened, a wider stance and medial rotation of hip, as shown by toes that point inwardly, may be noted. There is

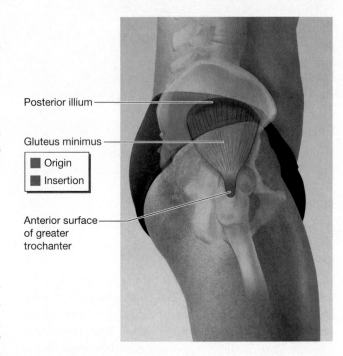

Posterior illium
Gluteus minimus
■ Origin
■ Insertion
Anterior surface of greater trochanter

FIGURE 5-20 · Gluteus minimus

limited ability to adduct and laterally rotate the hip, and low back pain may be present.
Lengthened: Limited ability to abduct the thigh is noted.

Palpation and Massage

Gluteus minimis and medius can be palpated by pressing into the lateral ilium. Direct pressure and friction are easily applied to these muscles.

How to Stretch This Muscle

Adduct the hip.

Synergists

Gluteus medius, tensor fascia latae (medially rotate the hip), and sartorius (abducts the hip)

Antagonists

Piriformis, gemellus superior, gemellus inferior, obturator internus, obturator externus, quadratus femoris, iliopsoas, sartorius, and gluteus maximus (laterally rotate the hip); adductor magnus, adductor longus, adductor brevis, pectineus, and gracilis (adduct the hip)

Innervation and Arterial Supply

Innervation: superior gluteal nerve
Arterial supply: superior gluteal artery

GLUTEUS MEDIUS (glut-e-us me-de-us)

Meaning of Name

Gluteus refers to the buttock region, and *medius* refers to the fact that this muscle is the medium-sized gluteus muscle. It is smaller than gluteus maximus and larger than gluteus minimus.

Location

Gluteus medius is located on the lateral hip, on the external surface of the ilium. Gluteus medius is larger than and superficial to gluteus minimus.

Origin and Insertion

Origin: external surface of the lateral ilium
Insertion: greater trochanter

Actions

Gluteus minimus and gluteus medius perform the same actions: abduction and medial rotation of the hip. Only the anterior fibers of these muscles can medially rotate the thigh. In addition, both gluteus minimus and gluteus medius play an important role in stabilization of the hip, particularly when one is walking. On the weight-bearing side, gluteus medius and gluteus minimus contract to pull the ilium down, so that the other ilium rises, allowing the other limb to swing through when walking.

Explanation of Actions

The origin of gluteus minimus and gluteus medius on the lateral ilium is superior to the greater trochanter of the femur. In addition, these muscles cross the lateral side of the hip joint. Thus, the greater trochanter is pulled out to the side, resulting in hip abduction. It is the same line of pull that allows gluteus minimus and gluteus medius to pull the ilium down when the weight is on the limb, and thus the femur cannot move. The anterior portion of gluteus medius and gluteus minimus perform medial rotation of the hip because the anterior aspect of the origin attachments of these muscles is more anterior than the greater trochanter. Thus, the muscles pull the greater trochanter forward, causing the femur to rotate medially.

Notable Muscle Facts

Because gluteus medius pulls the ilium down, tension in the muscle can affect the SI joint and contribute to low back pain.

Implications of Shortened and/or Lengthened/Weak Muscle

Shortened: A shortened gluteus medius results in a wider stance, medial rotation of the hip, as shown by toes that point inwardly, and low back pain.
Lengthened: Limited ability to abduct the thigh is noted.

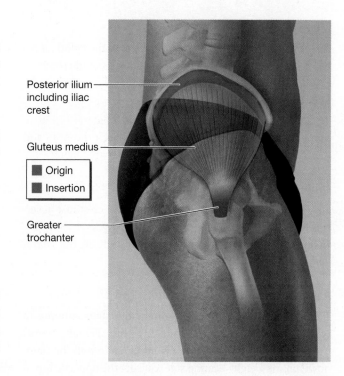

Posterior ilium including iliac crest
Gluteus medius
■ Origin
■ Insertion
Greater trochanter

FIGURE 5-21 · Gluteus medius

Palpation and Massage

Gluteus minimis and medius can be palpated by pressing into the lateral ilium. Direct pressure and friction are easily applied to these muscles.

How to Stretch This Muscle

Adduct the hip.

Synergists

Gluteus minimus, tensor fascia latae (medially rotate the hip), and sartorius (abducts the hip)

Antagonists

Piriformis, gemellus superior, gemellus inferior, obturator internus, obturator externus, quadratus femoris, iliopsoas, sartorius, and gluteus maximus (laterally rotate the hip); adductor magnus, adductor longus, adductor brevis, pectineus, and gracilis (adduct the hip)

Innervation and Arterial Supply

Innervation: superior gluteal nerve
Arterial supply: superior gluteal artery

TENSOR FASCIA LATAE (ten-sor fash-e la-te)

Meaning of Name

Tensor means to tighten. *Fascia latae* refers to the broad (latae) band of fascia that surrounds all the muscles of the thigh.

Location

Tensor fascia latae is located in the anterolateral hip area. More specifically, it lies superficially between the ASIS and the IT band, and is superficial to the greater trochanter.

Origin and Insertion

Origin: ASIS and a small portion of the iliac crest just posterior to the ASIS

Insertion: IT band, which attaches distally to the lateral condyle of the tibia

Actions

The TFL works with gluteus medius and gluteus minimus to medially rotate the hip and abduct the hip. TFL also works with gluteus medius and gluteus minimus to pull the ilium down on the weight-bearing side, causing the opposite hip to rise, so that the leg can swing through without hitting the ground when walking. In addition, TFL is located anterior enough to flex the hip. And, TFL helps to keep the IT band tight enough to help stabilize the lateral aspect of the knee joint.

Explanation of Actions

Because the origin of TFL is both more medial and anterior to the final bony attachment on the lateral tibia, TFL pulls the lateral tibia anteriorly, thus causing medial rotation of the hip joint. TFL abducts the hip because the origin is superior or proximal to the insertion and crosses the lateral aspect of the joint. Thus, the lateral proximal tibia is pulled laterally, causing abduction of the hip. TFL is a hip flexor because the origin is superior to the insertion, and the muscle crosses the anterior (as well as lateral) aspect of the joint. Pulling the tibia anteriorly causes hip flexion. Even though the bone moved by the shortening of TFL is the tibia, the femur must move as well. TFL keeps tension in the IT band, which crosses the lateral aspect of the knee joint. This helps maintain the stability of the knee joint.

Notable Muscle Facts

The TFL's ability to tighten the fascia latae, particularly to the IT band, helps to keep the major thigh muscles, which are surrounded by the fascia latae, close to the femur, thus increasing their efficiency.

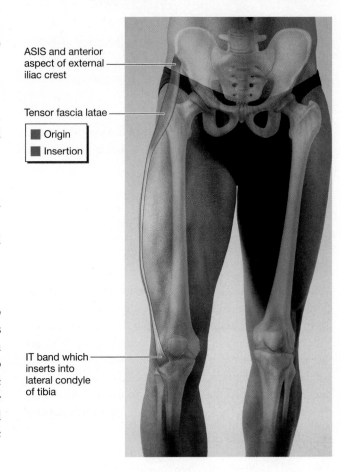

ASIS and anterior aspect of external iliac crest

Tensor fascia latae

■ Origin
■ Insertion

IT band which inserts into lateral condyle of tibia

FIGURE 5-22 · Tensor fascia latae

Implications of Shortened and/or Lengthened/ Weak Muscle

Shortened: A shortened TFL can cause an anterior pelvic tilt. It can also cause the hip to be medially rotated, as indicated by toes pointing inward. In addition, a wide stance is a possible manifestation of a short TFL, as the muscle is a hip abductor.

Lengthened: A lengthened TFL is not typically observed posturally or by a deficiency in the ability to perform the muscle's actions, but may contribute to instability in the lateral knee.

Palpation and Massage

The TFL can be palpated and massaged by finding the ASIS and pressing into the iliac crest just posterior to the ASIS, and by tracing the muscle toward the greater trochanter. Friction is an appropriate stroke to use for this muscle. It may be possible to note the fusiform nature of the muscle fibers.

How to Stretch This Muscle

Extend, laterally rotate, and adduct the thigh.

Synergists

Iliopsoas, rectus femoris, sartorius, and pectineus (flex the hip); gluteus medius and minimus (medially rotate the hip); and sartorius and gluteus medius and minimus (abduct the hip)

Antagonists

Gluteus maximus, semimembranosus, semitendinosus, and biceps femoris (extend the hip); gluteus maximus, piriformis, obturator internus, obturator externus, gemellus superior, gemellus inferior, quadrates femoris, iliopsoas, and sartorius (laterally rotate the hip); and adductor magnus, adductor longus, adductor brevis, pectineus, and gracilis (adduct the hip)

Innervation and Arterial Supply

Innervation: superior gluteal nerve
Arterial supply: superior gluteal artery

GLUTEUS MAXIMUS (glut-e-us maks-i-mus)

Meaning of Name

Gluteus means buttock region, and *maximus* indicates that this muscle is the largest muscle of the gluteal region.

Location

Gluteus maximus is located in the superficial buttock region.

Origin and Insertion

Origin: posterior ilium and posterior iliac crest, posterior sacrum, and posterior coccyx

Insertion: gluteal tuberosity and IT band

Actions

Laterally rotates and forcefully extends the hip

Explanation of Actions

Because the origin is superior to the insertion, and the muscle crosses the back of the hip joint, the gluteal tuberosity is pulled posteriorly, causing hip extension.

Because the origin is medial to the insertion, and the muscle crosses the posterior aspect of the hip joint, a shortening of gluteus maximus pulls the gluteal tuberosity on the posterior femur posteriorly or back, thus causing lateral rotation of the hip.

Notable Muscle Facts

Gluteus maximus allows forceful extension of the hip, as needed for running, climbing stairs, and rising up from a sitting position. Gluteus maximus is also important in walking, as it contracts each time the heel strikes the ground, to halt the forward moving momentum of the trunk and upper body, thus allowing us to remain upright. This muscle contains primarily slow-twitch muscle fibers, allowing for great endurance. Outside of the quadricep group—which some consider a single muscle, gluteus maximus is the largest muscle of the body.

Implications of Shortened and/or Lengthened/ Weak Muscle

Shortened: Posterior tilt of the pelvis and a posture of hip lateral rotation, with toes pointed out to the side is noted.

Lengthened: Potential anterior tilt of the pelvis and inability to forcefully extend and laterally rotate the hip is noted.

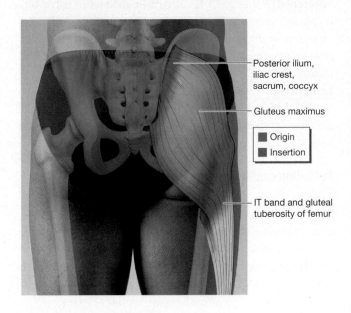

Posterior ilium, iliac crest, sacrum, coccyx

Gluteus maximus

■ Origin
■ Insertion

IT band and gluteal tuberosity of femur

FIGURE 5-23 · Gluteus maximus

Palpation and Massage

Gluteus maximus is easy to palpate and massage, as it is large and superficial in the buttock region. Find the PSIS and sacrum and work laterally and inferiorly toward the proximal posterior femur. Effleurage, pétrissage, friction, and tapotement are all appropriate strokes to be used for this muscle. Of course, good communication is essential when working in this potentially emotionally sensitive area.

How to Stretch This Muscle

Medially rotate and flex the hip.

Synergists

Semimembranosus, semitendinosus, and biceps femoris (extend the hip); and piriformis, obturator internus, obturator externus, gemellus superior, gemellus inferior, quadratus femoris, iliopsoas, and sartorius (laterally rotate the hip)

Antagonists

Iliopsoas, rectus femoris, sartorius, and TFL (flex the hip); and gluteus medius and minimus (medially rotate the hip)

Innervation and Arterial Supply

Innervation: inferior gluteal nerve
Arterial supply: superior gluteal artery

HAMSTRINGS: SEMIMEMBRANOSUS (ham-strings: sem-e-mem-bra-no-sus)

Meaning of Name

The term "hamstrings" is due to the fact these three thick muscles, known as the *ham*, have long tendons of insertion. In abattoir and butcher shops, the muscles of hogs were hung by their tendons (strings). *Semi* refers to half and *membranosis* refers to the fact that the tendon of origin of the muscle is thick and wide and expands into a membrane-like aponeurosis that surrounds the proximal part of the muscle. This muscle is almost half membrane.

Location

The hamstrings are located in the posterior thigh. Semimembranosus is the deeper of the two medial hamstrings.

Origin and Insertion

Origin: ischial tuberosity
Insertion: proximal, medial, posterior tibia

Actions

All three hamstrings extend the hip and flex the knee. Depending on which opposing muscles are contracting simultaneously, hamstrings can perform hip extension only, knee flexion only, or both actions at once. To be more specific, if the quadriceps are contracting, the action of knee flexion will be held in check, and the hamstrings will extend the hip. If the hip flexors are contracting, the action of hip extension will be held in check, and the hamstrings will only be able to flex the knee. When no opposing muscles contract, the hamstrings can cause both knee flexion and hip extension simultaneously.

Explanation of Actions

Because the hamstrings cross the posterior aspect of the hip joint, they are hip extensors, and because they cross the posterior aspect of the knee, they flex the knee.

Notable Muscle Facts

Semimembranosus is the largest of the three hamstrings. Semimembranosus works with semitendinosus, popliteus, and gracilis to medially rotate the knee (see popliteus). All three hamstrings are active at heel strike, pulling the pelvis posteriorly and helping to keep the body upright.

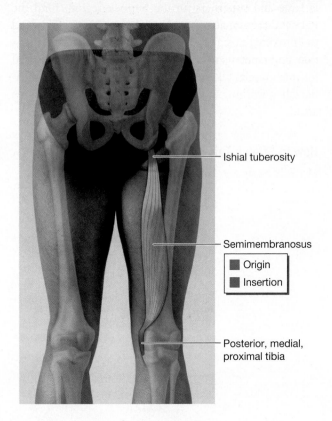

Ishial tuberosity

Semimembranosus

■ Origin
■ Insertion

Posterior, medial, proximal tibia

FIGURE 5-24 · Hamstrings: semimembranosus

Implications of Shortened and/or Lengthened/ Weak Muscle

Shortened: A posterior pelvic tilt is noted. Shortened hamstrings can also cause difficulty flexing the hip when the knee is extended. This is frequently demonstrated as difficulty touching one's toes with knees extended.

Lengthened: Limited ability to flex the knee and/or extend the hip is noted.

Palpation and Massage

The hamstrings are easy to access in the posterior thigh. Find the ischial tuberosity. Friction is a good stroke to apply to the hamstring's thick tendons of origin. Effleurage, pétrissage, friction, and tapotement are all appropriate strokes to apply to the bellies of the muscles. The tendon of insertion can be palpated at the medial, posterior knee. The tendon is deep to the tendon of semitendinosus. It is recommended to apply pressure gently in this potentially sensitive area.

How to Stretch This Muscle

Flex the hip with the knee extended.

Synergists

The other hamstrings (semitendinosus and biceps femoris), gastrocnemius, plantaris, gracilis, sartorius, and popliteus (flex the knee); the other hamstrings (semitendinosus and biceps femoris) and gluteus maximus (extend the hip)

Antagonists

The quadriceps group: vastus intermedius, vastus medialis, vastus lateralis, and rectus femoris (extend the knee); and iliopsoas, rectus femoris, TFL, pectineus, and sartorius (flex the hip)

Innervation and Arterial Supply

Innervation: sciatic nerve
Arterial supply: inferior gluteal artery

HAMSTRINGS: SEMITENDINOSUS (ham-strings: sem-e-ten-di-no-sus)

Meaning of Name

Semi means one half, and *tendinosis* refers to the fact that this muscle has a long tendon of origin. Thus, the muscle is almost half tendon.

Location

Semitendinosus is located in the superficial, medial thigh, directly superficial to semimembranosus.

Origin and Insertion

Origin: ischial tuberosity
Insertion: pes anserinus, a flat area on the proximal, medial, anterior tibia

Actions

All three hamstrings extend the hip and flex the knee. Depending on which opposing muscles are contracting simultaneously, hamstrings can perform hip extension only, knee flexion only, or both actions at once. To be more specific, if the quadriceps are contracting, the action of knee flexion will be held in check, and the hamstrings will extend the hip. If the hip flexors are contracting, the action of hip extension will be held in check, and the hamstrings will only be able to flex the knee. When no opposing muscles contract, the hamstrings can cause both knee flexion and hip extension simultaneously.

Explanation of Actions

Because the hamstrings cross the posterior aspect of the hip joint, they are hip extensors, and because they cross the posterior aspect of the knee, they flex the knee.

Notable Muscle Facts

Semitendinosus works with semimembranosus, popliteus, and gracilis in medially rotating the tibia (see popliteus). All three hamstrings are active at heel strike, pulling the pelvis posteriorly and helping to keep the body upright.

Implications of Shortened and/or Lengthened/ Weak Muscle

Shortened: Posterior pelvic tilt is noted. Shortened hamstrings can also cause difficulty flexing the hip when the knee is extended. This is frequently demonstrated as difficulty touching one's toes with knees extended.
Lengthened: Limited ability to flex the knee and/or extend the hip is noted.

Palpation and Massage

The hamstrings are easy to access in the posterior thigh. Find the ischial tuberosity. Friction is a good stroke to apply to the hamstring's thick tendons of origin. Effleurage, pétrissage,

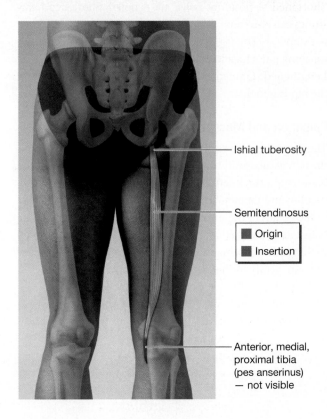

Ishial tuberosity

Semitendinosus

■ Origin
■ Insertion

Anterior, medial, proximal tibia (pes anserinus) — not visible

FIGURE 5-25 · Hamstrings: semitendinosus

friction, and tapotement are all appropriate strokes to apply to the bellies of the muscles. The tendon of insertion can be palpated at the medial, proximal, anterior tibia. The tendon is superficial to the tendon of semimembranosus.

How to Stretch This Muscle

Flex the hip with the knee extended.

Synergists

The other hamstrings (semimembranosus and biceps femoris), gastrocnemius, plantaris, gracilis, sartorius, and popliteus (flex the knee); and the other hamstrings (semimembranosus and biceps femoris) and gluteus maximus (extend the hip)

Antagonists

The quadriceps group: vastus intermedius, vastus medialis, vastus lateralis, and rectus femoris (extend the knee); and iliopsoas, rectus femoris, TFL, pectineus, and sartorius (flex the hip)

Innervation and Arterial Supply

Innervation: sciatic nerve
Arterial supply: inferior gluteal artery

HAMSTRINGS: BICEPS FEMORIS (ham-strings: bi-sepz fem-o-ris)

Meaning of Name

Biceps means two heads, and femoris referring to the femur.

Location

Biceps femoris is located in the lateral aspect of the posterior thigh.

Origin and Insertion

Origin: ischial tuberosity and distal half of the linea aspera
Insertion: head of the fibula

Actions

All three hamstrings extend the hip and flex the knee. Depending on which opposing muscles are contracting simultaneously, hamstrings can perform hip extension only, knee flexion only, or both actions at once. To be more specific, if the quadriceps are contracting, the action of knee flexion will be held in check, and the hamstrings will extend the hip. If the hip flexors are contracting, the action of hip extension will be held in check, and the hamstrings will only be able to flex the knee. When no opposing muscles contract, the hamstrings can cause both knee flexion and hip extension simultaneously.

Explanation of Actions

Because the hamstrings cross the posterior aspect of the hip joint, they are hip extensors, and because they cross the posterior aspect of the knee, they flex the knee.

Notable Muscle Facts

Biceps femoris performs lateral rotation of the knee. All three hamstrings are active at heel strike, pulling the pelvis posteriorly and helping to keep the body upright.

Implications of Shortened and/or Lengthened/ Weak Muscle

Shortened: Posterior pelvic tilt is noted. Shortened hamstrings can also cause difficulty flexing the hip when the knee is extended. This is frequently demonstrated as difficulty touching one's toes with knees extended.
Lengthened: Limited ability to flex the knee and/or extend the hip is noted.

Palpation and Massage

The hamstrings are easy to access in the posterior thigh. Find the ischial tuberosity. Friction is a good stroke to apply to the hamstring's thick tendons of origin. Effleurage, pétrissage, friction, and tapotement are all appropriate strokes to apply to the bellies of the muscles. The tendon of insertion can be

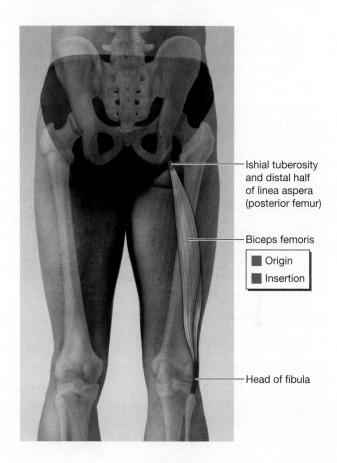

Ishial tuberosity and distal half of linea aspera (posterior femur)

Biceps femoris
■ Origin
■ Insertion

Head of fibula

FIGURE 5-26 · Hamstrings: biceps femoris

palpated at the lateral, posterior knee. The tendon is easily palpable just proximal to the head of the fibula

How to Stretch This Muscle

Flex the hip with the knee extended.

Synergists

The other hamstrings (semimembranosus and semitendinosus), gastrocnemius, plantaris, gracilis, sartorius, and popliteus (flex the knee); and the other hamstrings (semimembranosus and semitendinosus) and gluteus maximus (extend the hip)

Antagonists

The quadriceps group: vastus intermedius, vastus medialis, vastus lateralis, and rectus femoris (extend the knee); and iliopsoas, rectus femoris, TFL, pectineus, and sartorius (flex the hip)

Innervation and Arterial Supply

Innervation: sciatic nerve
Arterial supply: inferior gluteal artery

ILIOPSOAS (PSOAS MAJOR AND ILIACUS) (il-e-o-so-as)

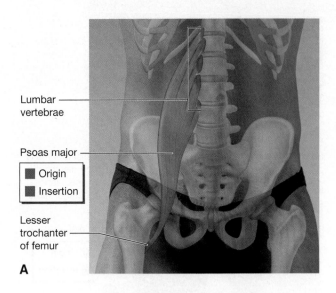

Lumbar vertebrae

Psoas major

☐ Origin
☐ Insertion

Lesser trochanter of femur

A

Iliac fossa (not visible)

Iliacus

Origin (not visible)
☐ Insertion

Lesser trochanter of femur

B

FIGURE 5-27 · **Iliopsoas. A:** psoas major **B:** iliacus

Meaning of Name

Ilio refers to the iliacus muscle and tells us that this muscle attaches to much of the ilium, namely the iliac fossa. *Psoas* means loins or the area of the lower trunk or low back between rib 12 and the ilium.

Location

Iliopsoas is located deep in the abdominal area. Noting a line between the navel and the ASIS and working deep to abdominal organs in this area will allow one to access the iliopsoas muscle.

Origin and Insertion

Origin of the iliacus portion: iliac fossa
Origin of the psoas major portion: bodies and transverse processes of T12–L5
Insertion: lesser trochanter

Actions

The actions of iliopsoas include hip flexion and lateral rotation of the hip. Iliopsoas is our strongest hip flexor.

Explanation of Actions

Because origin is superior to insertion, and because this muscle crosses the anterior aspect of the hip, shortening of iliopsoas pulls the femur forward, resulting in hip flexion. Because

the insertion attachment is on the lesser trochanter of the femur, and this bone marking is medial and a bit posterior on the femur, a forward pull to the insertion on the lesser trochanter will cause the femur to rotate laterally.

Notable Muscle Facts

There are differing opinions about how psoas major affects the position of the pelvis. When the lower limb is fixed, the shortening of psoas major shortens and pulls the lower lumbar vertebrae anteriorly, causing flexion. In some people with a significant lumbar curve, psoas major pulls on the upper lumbar vertebrae and T12 posteriorly, causing extension. Both psoas major and iliacus can cause an anterior pelvic curve by pulling the pelvis forward, iliacus directly and psoas major indirectly. Iliacus pulls the ilium forward, and psoas major pulls the lower lumbar spine forward, which is joined to the sacrum and additionally to the pelvis.

Implications of Shortened and/or Lengthened/ Weak Muscle

Shortened: Anterior pelvic tilt and inability to fully extend the thigh is noted.
Lengthened: Limited hip flexion is noted.

Palpation and Massage

Iliopsoas can be a difficult muscle to palpate and massage. Good communication with your client is essential! Find the navel and ASIS. With client supine, press gently into the linear space between the ASIS and navel as he or she exhales. Work around the intestinal organs to allow you to reach the dense fibers of the psoas major muscle. Asking the client to flex his or her hip can confirm that you have found the muscle.

How to Stretch This Muscle
Extend the hip.

Synergists
Rectus femoris, sartorius, pectineus, and TFL (flex the hip); and gluteus maximus, piriformis, obturator internus, obtura-tor externus, gemellus superior, gemellus inferior, quadrates femoris, and sartorius (laterally rotate the hip)

Antagonists
Gluteus maximus and the three hamstrings (extend the hip); and gluteus medius, gluteus minimus, and TFL (medially rotate the hip)

Innervation and Arterial Supply
Innervation: lumbar plexus
Arterial supply: lumbar arteries

QUADRICEPS GROUP: VASTUS INTERMEDIUS (kwad-dri-cep grup: vas-tus in-ter-me-de-us)

Meaning of Name

Quad means four. The quadriceps group, commonly called *the quads*, is considered by some to be four muscles, and by others to be a single, large, four-headed muscle. *Vastus* means very large, and *intermedius* refers to the fact that the vastus intermedius muscle is located between vastus lateralis and vastus medialis.

Location

The quadriceps group is located in the anterior thigh. More specifically, vastus intermedius is the deepest quad, located centrally in the anterior thigh. Vastus intermedius is completely covered by the other three quadriceps muscles.

Origin and Insertion

Origin: anterior shaft of the femur
Insertion: tibial tuberosity via the patellar ligament

Actions

Extends the knee

Explanation of Actions

Because vastus intermedius crosses the anterior aspect of the knee joint, and because the origin is proximal to the insertion, this muscle pulls the anterior leg toward the anterior thigh, thus causing knee extension.

Notable Muscle Facts

Vastus intermedius contains a small amount of muscle and a long and wide tendon of insertion. As a group, the quadriceps muscles are strong knee extensors. Knee extension requires much strength when the knees are flexed and the lower limbs are fixed. In this instance, the quadriceps muscles lift the weight of the whole body. The quadriceps group is important in gait, as these muscles pull the knee into full extension (locked position) at heel strike, in order for the lower limb to support full weight. In addition, the quadriceps group determines the position of the patella. The position of the patella contributes to the efficiency of the pull of the quadriceps tendon of insertion. And the patella is designed to slide in the groove of the proximal femur. A quadriceps muscle can pull the patella out of its track, causing friction and pain.

Implications of Shortened and/or Lengthened/ Weak Muscle

Shortened: When the quadriceps group is shortened, limited knee flexion is noted. In addition, shortened quadriceps muscles can pull the patella out of line, causing anterior knee pain.
Lengthened: Limited ability to extend the knee is noted.

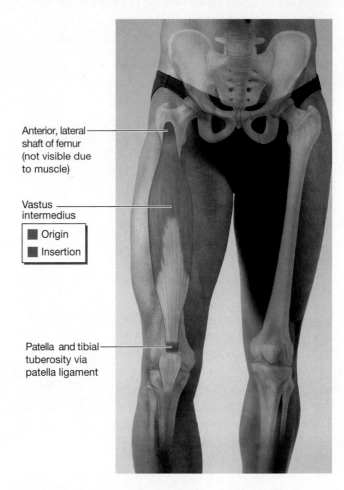

Anterior, lateral shaft of femur (not visible due to muscle)

Vastus intermedius

■ Origin
■ Insertion

Patella and tibial tuberosity via patella ligament

FIGURE 5-28 · Quadriceps group: vastus intermedius

Palpation and Massage

As a group, the quads are easy to palpate and massage in the anterior thigh. Effleurage, pétrissage, friction, and tapotement are all appropriate strokes for these muscles.

How to Stretch This Muscle

Flex the knee.

Synergists

The other quadriceps group muscles: vastus medialis, vastus lateralis, and rectus femoris

Antagonists

Semimembranosus, semitendinosus, biceps femoris, gastrocnemius, plantaris, gracilis, sartorius, and popliteus (flex the knee)

Innervation and Arterial Supply

Innervation: femoral nerve
Arterial supply: femoral and deep femoral arteries

QUADRICEPS GROUP: VASTUS MEDIALIS (kwad-dri-cep grup: vas-tus me-de-a-lis)

Meaning of Name

Vastus means very large, and *medialis* refers to the fact that this muscle is the most medial quadriceps muscle.

Location

The quadriceps group is located in the anterior thigh. More specifically, vastus medialis is in the anteromedial thigh, as it wraps around the medial aspect of the thigh from posterior to anterior.

Origin and Insertion

Origin: linea aspera
Insertion: tibial tuberosity via the patellar ligament

Actions

Extends the knee

Explanation of Actions

Because vastus medialis crosses the anterior aspect of the knee joint, and because the origin is proximal to the insertion, this muscle pulls the anterior leg toward the anterior thigh, thus causing knee extension.

Notable Muscle Facts

As a group, the quadriceps muscles are strong knee extensors. Knee extension requires much strength when the knees are flexed and the lower limbs are fixed. In this instance, the quadriceps muscles lift the weight of the whole body. The quadriceps group is important in gait, as these muscles pull the knee into full extension (locked position) at heel strike, in order for the lower limb to support full weight. In addition, the quadriceps group determines the position of the patella. The position of the patella contributes to the efficiency of the pull of the quadriceps tendon of insertion. And, the patella is designed to slide in the groove of the proximal femur. A quadriceps muscle can pull the patella out of its track, causing friction and pain.

Implications of Shortened and/or Lengthened/ Weak Muscle

Shortened: When the quadriceps group is shortened, limited knee flexion is noted. In addition, shortened quadriceps muscles can pull the patella out of line, causing anterior knee pain.
Lengthened: Limited ability to extend the knee is noted.

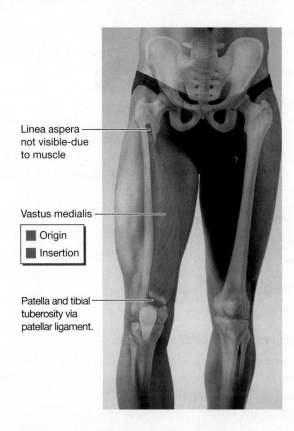

Linea aspera not visible-due to muscle

Vastus medialis

■ Origin
■ Insertion

Patella and tibial tuberosity via patellar ligament.

FIGURE 5-29 · Quadriceps group: vastus medialis

Palpation and Massage

As a group, the quads are easy to palpate and massage in the anterior thigh. Effleurage, pétrissage, friction, and tapotement are all appropriate strokes for these muscles.

How to Stretch This Muscle

Flex the knee.

Synergists

The other quadriceps group muscles: vastus intermedius, vastus lateralis, and rectus femoris

Antagonists

Semimembranosus, semitendinosus, biceps femoris, gastrocnemius, plantaris, gracilis, sartorius, and popliteus (flex the knee)

Innervation and Arterial Supply

Innervation: femoral nerve
Arterial supply: femoral and deep femoral arteries

QUADRICEPS GROUP: VASTUS LATERALIS (kwad-dri-cep grup: vas-tus lat-ar-a-lis)

Meaning of Name

Vastus means very large, and *lateralis* refers to the fact that this muscle is the most lateral quadriceps muscle.

Location

The quadriceps group is located in the anterior thigh. More specifically, vastus lateralis is in the anterolateral thigh, as it wraps around the lateral aspect of the thigh from posterior to anterior. Vastus lateralis is the only muscle in the lateral thigh.

Origin and Insertion

Origin: linea aspera
Insertion: tibial tuberosity via the patellar ligament

Actions

Extends the knee

Explanation of Actions

Because vastus lateralis crosses the anterior aspect of the knee joint, and because the origin is proximal to the insertion, this muscle pulls the anterior leg toward the anterior thigh, thus causing knee extension.

Notable Muscle Facts

Vastus lateralis can adhere to the more superficial IT band. Thus, friction in this area can be helpful. As a group, the quadriceps muscles are strong knee extensors. Knee extension requires much strength when the knees are flexed and the lower limbs are fixed. In this instance, the quadriceps muscles lift the weight of the whole body. The quadriceps group is important in gait, as these muscles pull the knee into full extension (locked position) at heel strike, in order for the lower limb to support full weight. In addition, the quadriceps group determines the position of the patella. The position of the patella contributes to the efficiency of the pull of the quadriceps tendon of insertion. And, the patella is designed to slide in the groove of the proximal femur. A quadriceps muscle can pull the patella out of its track, causing friction and pain.

Implications of Shortened and/or Lengthened/Weak Muscle

Shortened: When the quadriceps group is shortened, limited knee flexion is noted. In addition, shortened quadriceps muscles can pull the patella out of line, causing anterior knee pain.
Lengthened: Limited ability to extend the knee is noted.

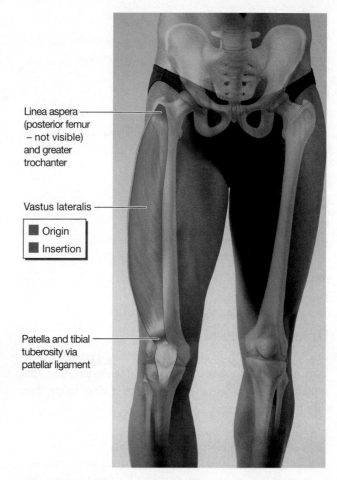

Linea aspera (posterior femur – not visible) and greater trochanter

Vastus lateralis

■ Origin
■ Insertion

Patella and tibial tuberosity via patellar ligament

FIGURE 5-30 · Quadriceps group: vastus lateralis

Palpation and Massage

As a group, the quads are easy to palpate and massage in the anterior thigh. Effleurage, pétrissage, friction, and tapotement are all appropriate strokes for these muscles.

How to Stretch This Muscle

Flex the knee.

Synergists

The other quadriceps group muscles: vastus intermedius, vastus medialis, and rectus femoris

Antagonists

Semimembranosus, semitendinosus, biceps femoris, gastrocnemius, plantaris, gracilis, sartorius, and popliteus (flex the knee)

Innervation and Arterial Supply

Innervation: femoral nerve
Arterial supply: femoral and deep femoral arteries

QUADRICEPS GROUP: RECTUS FEMORIS (kwad-dri-cep grup: rek-tus fem-o-ris)

Meaning of Name

Rectus means straight and usually refers to the vertical or straight up and down orientation of a muscle. Femoris refers to the fact that this muscle is located in the area of the femur.

Location

Superficial anterior thigh

Origin and Insertion

Origin: AIIS and a small area close to the acetabulum
Insertion: tibial tuberosity via the patellar ligament

Actions

Extends the knee and flexes the hip

Explanation of Actions

Rectus femoris crosses the anterior aspect of the hip joint, with origin superior to insertion. Thus, it pulls the thigh anteriorly, resulting in hip flexion. In addition, rectus femoris crosses the anterior aspect of the knee joint, and because the origin is proximal to the insertion, this muscle pulls the anterior leg toward the anterior thigh, thus causing knee extension.

Notable Muscle Facts

Rectus femoris is the only quadriceps group member that crosses two joints. Thus, it has two actions. The quadriceps muscles are strong knee extensors. Knee extension requires much strength when the knees are flexed and the lower limbs are fixed. In this instance, the quadriceps muscles lift the weight of the whole body. The quadriceps group is important in gait, as these muscles pull the knee into full extension (locked position) at heel strike, in order for the lower limb to support full weight. In addition, the quadriceps group determines the position of the patella. The position of the patella contributes to the efficiency of the pull of the quadriceps tendon of insertion. And, the patella is designed to slide in the groove of the proximal femur. A quadriceps muscle can pull the patella out of its track, causing friction and pain.

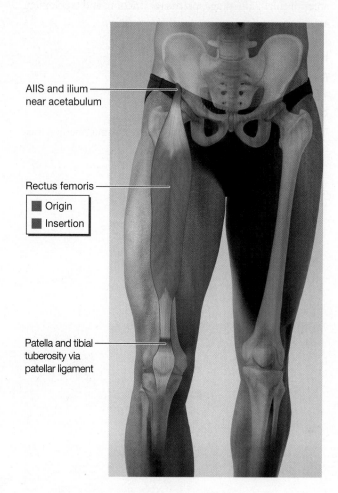

AIIS and ilium near acetabulum

Rectus femoris

■ Origin
■ Insertion

Patella and tibial tuberosity via patellar ligament

FIGURE 5-31 · Quadriceps group: rectus femoris

Implications of Shortened and/or Lengthened/ Weak Muscle

Shortened: When the quadriceps group is shortened, limited knee flexion is noted. In addition, shortened quadriceps muscles can pull the patella out of line, causing anterior knee pain. A shortened rectus femoris can also cause an anterior pelvic tilt.

Lengthened: Limited ability to extend the knee is noted.

Palpation and Massage

To find the origin of rectus femoris, find the AIIS. Because the AIIS is difficult to palpate, find the ASIS first, and move about 2 inches inferiorly and about a 1/2–inch medially. You can feel the tendon of origin of rectus femoris, a bit deeper than the tendon of origin of sartorius. Effleurage, pétrissage, friction, and tapotement are all appropriate strokes for the belly of rectus femoris, located in the superficial anterior thigh.

How to Stretch This Muscle

Flex the knee while extending the hip.

Synergists

The other quadriceps group muscles: vastus intermedius, vastus medialis, and vastus lateralis; and the hip flexors: iliopsoas, sartorius, TFL, and pectineus

Antagonists

Semimembranosus, semitendinosus, biceps femoris, gastrocnemius, plantaris, gracilis, sartorius, and popliteus (flex the knee); and gluteus maximus, semimembranosus, semitendinosus, and biceps femoris (extend the hip)

Innervation and Arterial Supply

Innervation: femoral nerve
Arterial supply: femoral and deep femoral arteries

SARTORIUS (sar-to-re-us)

Meaning of Name

Sartor refers to a tailor. The muscle has this name because the combined movements of sartorius results in a sitting position with crossed knees that was commonly used by tailors as they sewed.

Location

Sartorius is a thin strip of muscle that runs from lateral to medial as it runs distally across the superficial, anterior thigh. As the muscle reaches the medial side of the distal thigh, its tendon of insertion passes behind the knee before emerging again anteriorly and inserting into pes anserinus. Sartorius forms the lateral border of the femoral triangle (see Fig. 5-17).

Origin and Insertion

Origin: ASIS
Insertion: pes anserinus, the flat area on the proximal, medial, anterior tibia

Actions

Sartorius performs hip flexion, lateral rotation of the hip, abduction of the hip, and flexion of the knee. These actions combine to create the movement of crossing one's legs, as was done by tailors when sewing.

Explanation of Actions

Because origin is superior to insertion, and sartorius crosses the anterior aspect of the hip joint, it flexes the hip. Because origin is more lateral than insertion, as well as superior to insertion, it performs abduction. Because origin is more lateral than insertion, and this muscles crosses the anterior thigh, and because the insertion is on the medial tibia, sartorius pulls the medial tibia anteriorly. This causes the hip joint to rotate laterally. Finally, because sartorius crosses the posterior aspect of the knee joint, this muscle flexes the knee.

Notable Muscle Facts

Sartorius is the longest muscle in the body.

Implications of Shortened and/or Lengthened/ Weak Muscle

Shortened: Anterior pelvic tilt is noted.
Lengthened: A weak, lengthened sartorius will not typically cause functional deficits.

Palpation and Massage

Find the ASIS, and feel distally for the tendon of origin. It can be hard to distinguish the muscle belly of sartorius from

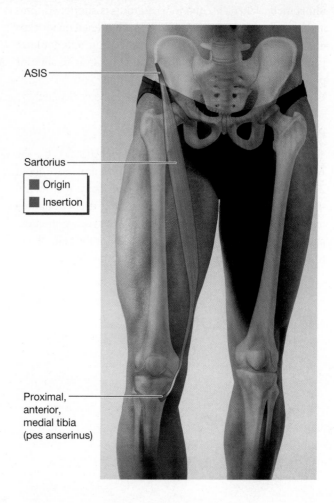

ASIS

Sartorius

■ Origin
■ Insertion

Proximal, anterior, medial tibia (pes anserinus)

FIGURE 5-32 · Sartorius

the quadriceps muscles. However, providing effleurage, pétrissage, and friction to the entire anterior thigh will ensure that sartorius is addressed.

How to Stretch This Muscle

Sartorius can be difficult to stretch, as it performs so many actions. Extend the thigh, then adduct the thigh behind the opposite lower limb, while medially rotating it. Keep the knee extended.

Synergists

Lateral rotators of the hip: gluteus maximus, piriformis, obturator internus, obturator externus, gemellus superior, gemellus inferior, quadratus femoris, and iliopsoas; hip abductors: gluteus medius, gluteus minimus, and TFL; hip

flexors: iliopsoas, pectineus, rectus femoris, and TFL; knee flexors: semimembranosus, semitendinosus, biceps femoris, gastrocnemius, plantaris, gracilis, and popliteus

Antagonists

Medial rotators of the hip: gluteus medius, gluteus minimus, and TFL; hip adductors: adductor magnus, adductor longus, adductor brevis, pectineus, and gracilis; hip extensors: semimembranosus, semitendinosus, biceps femoris, and gluteus maximus; knee extensors: rectus femoris, vastus intermedius, vastus medialis, and vastus lateralis

Innervation and Arterial Supply

Innervation: femoral nerve
Arterial supply: femoral artery

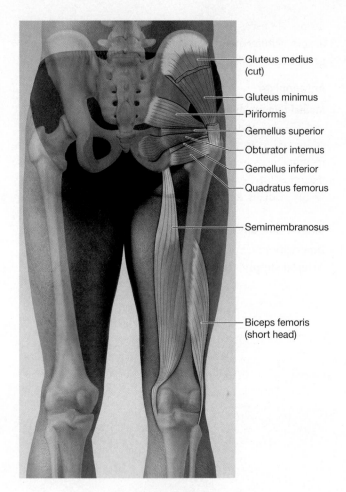

Gluteus medius (cut)
Gluteus minimus
Piriformis
Gemellus superior
Obturator internus
Gemellus inferior
Quadratus femorus
Semimembranosus
Biceps femoris (short head)

FIGURE 5-33 · Deep posterior thigh muscles

Regional Illustrations of Muscles
Figure 5-33 shows the deep posterior thigh muscles.
Figure 5-34 shows the superficial posterior thigh muscles.
Figure 5-35 shows the deep anterior thigh muscles.
Figure 5-36 shows the superficial anterior thigh muscles.
Figure 5-37 shows the lateral thigh muscles.

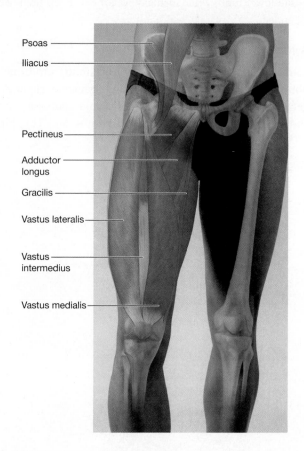

Psoas
Iliacus
Pectineus
Adductor longus
Gracilis
Vastus lateralis
Vastus intermedius
Vastus medialis

FIGURE 5-35 · Deep anterior thigh muscles

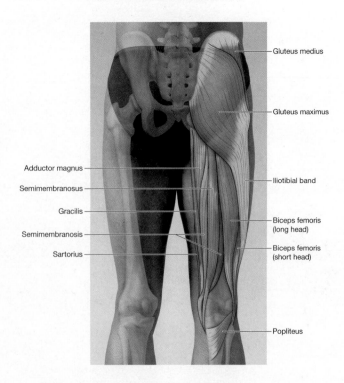

Gluteus medius
Gluteus maximus
Adductor magnus
Semimembranosus
Gracilis
Semimembranosis
Sartorius
Iliotibial band
Biceps femoris (long head)
Biceps femoris (short head)
Popliteus

FIGURE 5-34 · Superficial posterior thigh muscles

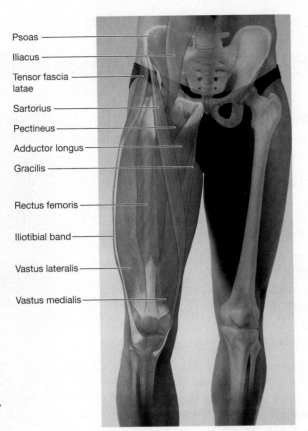

Psoas

Iliacus

Tensor fascia latae

Sartorius

Pectineus

Adductor longus

Gracilis

Rectus femoris

Iliotibial band

Vastus lateralis

Vastus medialis

FIGURE 5-36 · Superficial anterior thigh muscles

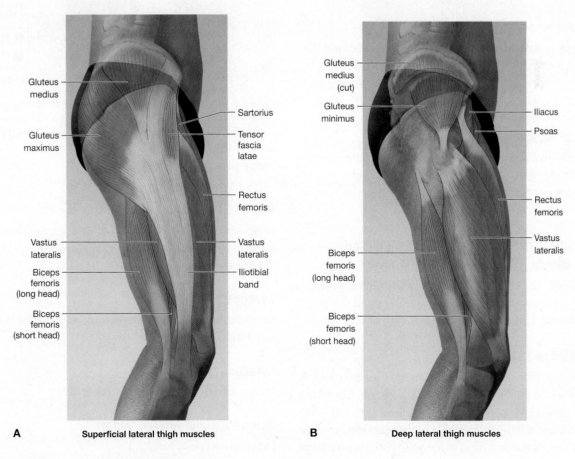

Gluteus medius

Gluteus maximus

Vastus lateralis

Biceps femoris (long head)

Biceps femoris (short head)

Sartorius

Tensor fascia latae

Rectus femoris

Vastus lateralis

Iliotibial band

Gluteus medius (cut)

Gluteus minimus

Iliacus

Psoas

Rectus femoris

Vastus lateralis

Biceps femoris (long head)

Biceps femoris (short head)

A Superficial lateral thigh muscles

B Deep lateral thigh muscles

FIGURE 5-37 · Lateral thigh muscles

Posterior Knee and Superficial Posterior Leg Muscles

POPLITEUS (pop-lit-e-us)

Meaning of Name

Popliteus refers to the "ham" of the knee, which is another way of naming the posterior knee.

Location

Popliteus is a flat, triangular muscle, deep in the popliteal fossa, which is located in the posterior knee area.

Origin and Insertion

Origin: lateral epicondyle of the humerus
Insertion: proximal, medial, posterior tibia and lateral meniscus of the knee

Actions

This muscle medially rotates the knee, which is equivalent to lateral rotation of the femur when the tibia is fixed. This movement is necessary to "unlock" the knee from a fully extended position. In addition, popliteus is a weak flexor of the knee.

Explanation of Actions

Popliteus pulls the medial aspect of the tibia posteriorly, thus causing it to turn medially. Popliteus also flexes the knee because it crosses the knee joint posteriorly, and its insertion is inferior to origin.

Notable Muscle Facts

Popliteus has a role in stabilizing the knee joint. It reinforces the job of the posterior cruciate ligament in preventing the femur from moving too far anterior in relation to the tibia.

Implications of Shortened and/or Lengthened/ Weak Muscle

Shortened: Limited lateral rotation of the tibia is noted. A short popliteus inhibits our ability to fully extend the knee.
Lengthened: Limited medial rotation of the tibia is noted.

Palpation and Massage

Popliteus is difficult to massage and/or palpate because it is located in the popliteal fossa, an endangerment site due to the presence of the popliteal artery, popliteal vein, and many lymph nodes in the area. In addition, the tibial and common fibular nerves and the small saphenous vein are present in this area.

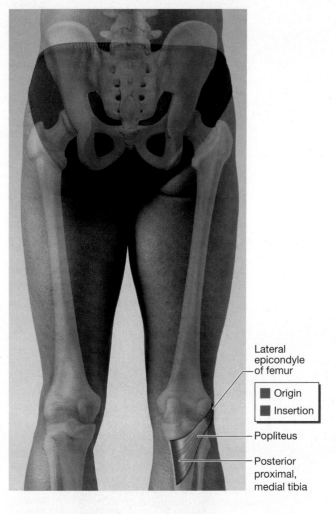

FIGURE 5-38 · Popliteus

Lateral epicondyle of femur
■ Origin
■ Insertion
Popliteus
Posterior proximal, medial tibia

How to Stretch This Muscle

A pin-and-stretch technique is possible for popliteus, which requires pressure to the muscle with knee flexed and then extending the knee.

Synergists

Semimembranosus, semitendinosus, and gracilis (medially rotate and flex the knee)

Antagonists

Biceps femoris (laterally rotates the knee)

Innervation and Arterial Supply

Innervation: tibial nerve
Arterial supply: branches of the popliteal artery

PLANTARIS (plan-tar-is)

Meaning of Name

Plantaris refers the plantar surface of the foot and the action of plantarflexion.

Location

Plantaris is located superficially in the posterior knee area. This muscle has a small, fleshy muscle belly and a long tendon of insertion that lies between gastrocnemius and soleus in the superficial posterior leg compartment. At its distal aspect, plantaris' tendon of insertion becomes part of the Achilles tendon. The muscle belly of plantaris is located superficial to popliteus.

Origin and Insertion

Origin: lateral epicondyle of the femur
Insertion: posterior calcaneus via the Achilles tendon

Actions

The actions of plantaris include knee flexion and plantarflexion of the ankle.

Explanation of Actions

Because plantaris crosses the posterior aspect of the knee, and the origin is superior to the insertion, plantaris pulls the posterior leg toward the posterior thigh, resulting in knee flexion. Plantaris crosses the posterior aspect of the ankle joint, with its origin proximal to insertion. Thus, plantaris pulls the calcaneus posteriorly, resulting in plantarflexion.

Notable Muscle Facts

Plantaris is variably present, and occasionally can be doubly present. Its long tendon of insertion can be surgically transplanted to replace other damaged tissue.

Implications of Shortened and/or Lengthened/ Weak Muscle

Shortened: Possible pain or tension in the superficial posterior knee is noted.
Lengthened: No consequences, as this muscle has very limited functional purpose.

Palpation and Massage

Palpate and/or massage this muscle carefully, as it is located in the popliteal fossa. Recall that this area in the posterior knee is an endangerment site, as the popliteal artery and vein are superficial.

How to Stretch This Muscle

Dorsiflex the ankle with the knee extended.

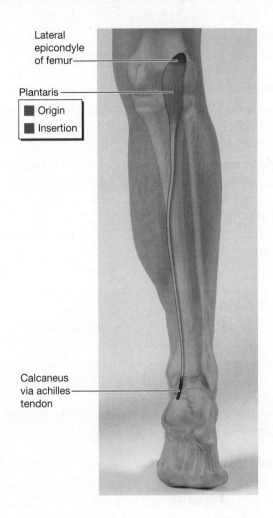

Lateral epicondyle of femur

Plantaris

■ Origin
■ Insertion

Calcaneus via achilles tendon

FIGURE 5-39 · Plantaris

Synergists

Knee flexors: semimembranosus, semitendinosus, biceps femoris, gastrocnemius, popliteus, gracilis, sartorius, and sartorius; plantarflexors: gastrocnemius, soleus, tibialis posterior, flexor hallucis longus, flexor digitorum longus, peroneus longus, and peroneus brevis

Antagonists

Knee extensors: rectus femoris, vastus intermedius, vastus medialis, and vastus lateralis; dorsiflexors: tibialis anterior, extensor digitorum longus, extensor hallucis longus, and peroneus tertius

Innervation and Arterial Supply

Innervation: tibial nerve
Arterial supply: branches of the popliteal artery

GASTROCNEMIUS (gas-trok-ne-me-us)

Meaning of Name

Gastro means belly, and *cnemius* refers to the leg.

Location

Gastrocnemius is located superficially in the posterior knee.

Origin and Insertion

Origin of medial head: medial epicondyle of the femur
Origin of lateral head: lateral epicondyle of the femur
Insertion: posterior aspect of the calcaneus via the Achilles tendon

Actions

Flexes the knee and plantarflexes the ankle

Explanation of Actions

Because gastrocnemius crosses the posterior aspect of the knee, and the origin is superior to the insertion, this muscle pulls the posterior leg toward the posterior thigh, resulting in knee flexion. Gastrocnemius crosses the posterior aspect of the ankle joint, with its origin proximal to insertion. Thus, gastrocnemius pulls the calcaneus posteriorly, resulting in plantarflexion.

Notable Muscle Facts

This muscle is a very strong plantarflexor and is engaged when forceful plantarflexion is needed. When minimal strength of plantarflexion is required, gastrocnemius may not be involved, especially if the knee is flexed. Gastrocnemius plays an important role in stabilization of the ankle joint. It stabilizes the ankle joint from a posterior perspective, preventing the tibia from sliding forward over the talus. In addition, the gastrocnemius muscle is a frequent site of muscle cramps, particularly at night. Such cramps may be relieved by stretching the muscle and by engaging the opposing muscles. Finally, gastrocnemius is notable as it forms the contour of the posterior leg.

Implications of Shortened and/or Lengthened/ Weak Muscle

Shortened: Limited dorsiflexion is noted when the knee is extended.
Lengthened: Limited ability to perform forceful plantarflexion is noted.

Palpation and Massage

Gastrocnemius is a fleshy muscle that is easy to palpate and massage. The two proximal parts of the muscle emerge be-

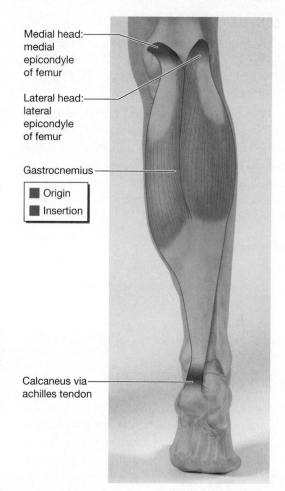

Medial head:
medial
epicondyle
of femur

Lateral head:
lateral
epicondyle
of femur

Gastrocnemius

■ Origin
■ Insertion

Calcaneus via
achilles tendon

FIGURE 5-40 · Gastrocnemius

tween the distal aspects of the hamstrings. Gastrocnemius is the most superficial muscle in the posterior leg. Effleurage, pétrissage, and friction are all appropriate strokes to apply to this muscle. Friction to a taut Achilles tendon can be helpful to relieve adhesions and relax the muscle.

How to Stretch This Muscle
Dorsiflex the ankle while the knee is extended.

Synergists
Knee flexors: semimembranosus, semitendinosus, biceps femoris, plantaris, popliteus, gracilis, and sartorius; plan-tarflexors: soleus, plantaris, tibialis posterior, flexor hallucis longus, flexor digitorum longus, peroneus longus, and peroneus brevis

Antagonists
Knee extensors: rectus femoris, vastus intermedius, vastus medialis, and vastus lateralis; dorsiflexors: tibialis anterior, extensor digitorum longus, extensor hallucis longus, and peroneus tertius

Innervation and Arterial Supply
Innervation: tibial nerve
Arterial supply: branches of the popliteal artery

SOLEUS (so-le-us)

Meaning of Name

Soleus refers to the fish named sole, which is flat like the soleus muscle.

Location

Most of soleus is directly deep to gastrocnemius and is thus the deepest muscle in the superficial posterior leg compartment. However, the distal portion of soleus is wider than gastrocnemius, and thus is superficial and easier to palpate.

Origin and Insertion

Origin: soleal line of the tibia and the head and posterior proximal shaft of the fibula

Insertion: posterior calcaneus, via the Achilles tendon

Actions

Plantarflexes the ankle

Explanation of Actions

Soleus crosses the posterior ankle joint, with its origin superior to the insertion on the calcaneus. Thus, soleus pulls the calcaneus posteriorly, causing plantarflexion.

Notable Muscle Facts

Soleus has been dubbed "the second heart," as this muscle is well positioned to assist venous return from the posterior leg. Contraction of the soleus helps push blood from the posterior legs back toward the heart. In addition, soleus assists gastrocnemius in stabilizing the ankle joint from a posterior perspective. Soleus, in combination with gastrocnemius, results in a "three-headed" muscular structure called *triceps surae*. Because soleus crosses the ankle joint, and no other joint, it is able to plantarflex the ankle regardless of the position of the knee or any other joint. Finally, soleus and the other plantarflexors work with the dorsiflexors to help us maintain balance as we shift our weight on our feet.

Implications of Shortened and/or Lengthened/ Weak Muscle

Shortened: Inability to dorsiflex the ankle, both while the knee is flexed and while the knee is extended.

Lengthened: A lengthened soleus can limit ability to plantarflex the ankle.

Palpation and Massage

Soleus can be palpated and massaged through the gastrocnemius in the posterior leg. As already mentioned, the distal edges of soleus are palpable, as they are wider than gastrocnemius.

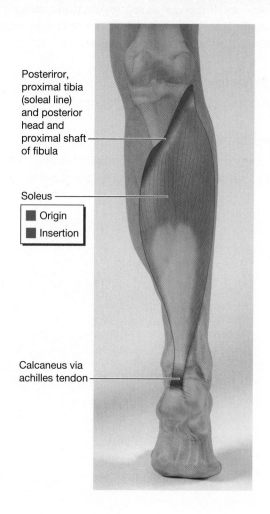

Posteriror, proximal tibia (soleal line) and posterior head and proximal shaft of fibula

Soleus

■ Origin
■ Insertion

Calcaneus via achilles tendon

FIGURE 5-41 · **Soleus**

When a client contracts his or her plantarflexors isometrically, the border between gastrocnemius and soleus is more palpable. Massage to the posterior leg with the intention to address the deeper muscles can affect the soleus muscle. Effleurage, pétrissage, and friction are all appropriate strokes to apply to this area.

How to Stretch This Muscle

Dorsiflex the ankle with the knee flexed. Flexion of the knee gives slack to gastrocnemius, so that the stretch is focused on soleus.

Synergists

Plantarflexors: gastrocnemius, plantaris, tibialis posterior, flexor hallucis longus, flexor digitorum longus, peroneus longus, and peroneus brevis

Antagonists

Dorsiflexors: tibialis anterior, extensor digitorum longus, extensor hallucis longus, and peroneus tertius

Innervation and Arterial Supply

Innervation: tibial nerve
Arterial supply: branches of the popliteal artery

Muscles of the Leg That Move the Foot and Toes

Muscles of the leg that move the foot and toes are covered in this section. These include the tibialis posterior, flexor digitorum longus, flexor hallucis longus, peroneus longus, peroneus brevis, peroneus tertius, extensor digitorum longus, extensor hallucis longus, and tibialis anterior.

TIBIALIS POSTERIOR (tib-e-a-lis po-ster-e-or)

Meaning of Name

Tibialis refers to the tibia, and *posterior* reflects the fact that this muscle is located in the posterior leg, covering much of the tibia.

Location

Tibialis posterior is the deepest muscle in the deep posterior leg compartment. Its tendon of insertion passes posterior and inferior to the medial malleolus as it continues toward the plantar surface of the foot.

Origin and Insertion

Origin: posterior tibia, fibula, and interosseus membrane
Insertion: plantar surface of the navicular, all three cuneiforms, and the cuboid, and the bases of the second, third, and fourth metatarsals.

Actions

Inverts the foot and plantarflexes the ankle

Explanation of Actions

Tibialis posterior crosses the posterior ankle joint with its origin proximal to insertion. Thus, the muscle pulls the plantar surface of the foot toward the posterior leg, which results in plantarflexion of the ankle. In addition, the tendon of insertion of tibialis posterior crosses the medial side of the foot. Thus, the muscle pulls the plantar surface of the foot medially, which results in inversion of the foot.

Notable Muscle Facts

Tibialis posterior has a very unique tendon of insertion, which attaches to 8 bones. The placement of this tendon serves to support the medial longitudinal arch.

Implications of Shortened and/or Lengthened/ Weak Muscle

Shortened: A shortened tibialis posterior can cause a higher medial longitudinal arch. Difficulty dorsiflexing and inverting can also result.
Lengthened: A lengthened tibialis posterior can cause difficulty inverting the foot and could cause a weakened medial longitudinal arch.

Palpation and Massage

Because tibialis posterior is located deep in the posterior leg, the muscle can be addressed by massaging the posterior leg with the intention to address the deeper muscles. Effleurage, pétrissage, and friction are all appropriate strokes to apply to this muscle.

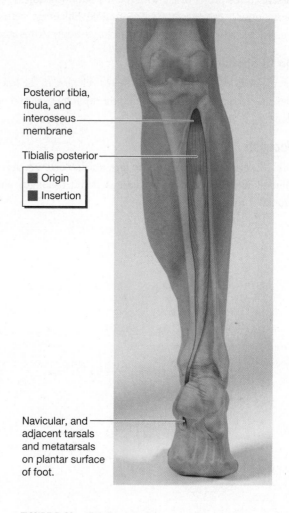

Posterior tibia, fibula, and interosseus membrane

Tibialis posterior

- ■ Origin
- ■ Insertion

Navicular, and adjacent tarsals and metatarsals on plantar surface of foot.

FIGURE 5-42 · Tibialis posterior

How to Stretch This Muscle

Dorsiflex the ankle while everting the foot.

Synergists

Plantarflexors: gastrocnemius, soleus, plantaris, flexor hallucis longus, flexor digitorum longus, peroneus longus, and peroneus brevis

Antagonists

Dorsiflexors: tibialis anterior, extensor digitorum longus, extensor hallucis longus, and peroneus tertius

Innervation and Arterial Supply

Innervation: tibial nerve
Arterial supply: posterior tibial artery

FLEXOR DIGITORUM LONGUS (flex-or dij-i-to-rum long-gus)

Meaning of Name

Flexor indicates the action of flexion. *Digitorum* indicates that the muscle moves four digits, in this case the four lateral toes. *Longus* refers to the fact that the muscle is longer than flexor digitorum brevis.

Location

This muscle is located in the deep posterior leg compartment. The tendon of insertion passes posterior and inferior to the medial malleolus as it continues toward the plantar surface of the foot.

Origin and Insertion

Origin: midsection of the posterior tibia
Insertion: plantar surface of the distal phalanges of the four lateral toes

Actions

Flexes the four lateral toes and plantarflexes the ankle

Explanation of Actions

The muscle originates on the posterior leg, crosses the posterior side of the ankle joint, and inserts onto the plantar side of the foot. Thus, contraction pulls the plantar surface of the foot toward the origin on the posterior leg, resulting in plantarflexion. In addition, the muscle crosses the plantar surface of all joints within the toes. Thus, muscle contraction causes flexion of the toes.

Notable Muscle Facts

The curling or flexing action of flexor digitorum longus helps us maintain balance when standing and helps us to push off when walking. This muscle flexes the distal phalanges of the four lateral toes with much more force than the proximal or middle phalanges.

Implications of Shortened and/or Lengthened/Weak Muscle

Shortened: Limited ability to dorsiflex the ankle and/or extend the four lateral toes is noted. A shortened flexor digitorum longus can increase susceptibility to toe cramps.
Lengthened: A lengthened flexor digitorum longus can weaken the action of push-off when walking.

Palpation and Massage

Because flexor digitorum longus is located deep in the posterior leg, the muscle can be addressed by massaging the posterior leg with the intention of addressing the deeper muscles. Effleurage, pétrissage, and friction are all appropriate strokes to apply to this muscle.

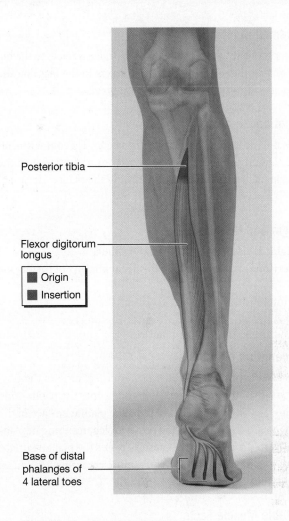

Posterior tibia

Flexor digitorum longus

■ Origin
■ Insertion

Base of distal phalanges of 4 lateral toes

FIGURE 5-43 · Flexor digitorum longus

How to Stretch This Muscle

Dorsiflex the ankle and extend the toes.

Synergists

Plantarflexors: gastrocnemius, soleus, plantaris, tibialis posterior, flexor hallucis longus, peroneus longus, and peroneus brevis; toe flexor: flexor digitorum brevis

Antagonists

Dorsiflexors: tibialis anterior, extensor digitorum longus, extensor hallucis longus, and peroneus tertius; toe extensors: extensor digitorum longus and extensor digitorum brevis

Innervation and Arterial Supply

Innervation: tibial nerve
Arterial supply: posterior tibial artery

FLEXOR HALLUCIS LONGUS (fleks-or hal-u-sis long-gus)

Meaning of Name

Flexor indicates the action of flexion. *Hallucis* refers to the big toe or first digit of the foot. *Longus* refers to the fact that the muscle is longer than flexor hallucis brevis.

Location

This muscle is located in the deep posterior leg compartment. The tendon of insertion passes posterior and inferior to the medial malleolus as it continues toward the plantar surface of the foot.

Origin and Insertion

Origin: midsection of the posterior fibula
Insertion: plantar surface of the distal phalanx of the big toe

Actions

Flexes the big toe and plantarflexes the ankle

Explanation of Actions

The muscle originates on the posterior leg, crosses the posterior side of the ankle joint, and inserts onto the plantar side of the foot. Thus, contraction pulls the plantar surface of the foot toward the origin on the posterior leg, resulting in plantarflexion. In addition, the muscle crosses the plantar surface of all joints of the big toe. Thus, muscle contraction causes flexion of the big toe.

Notable Muscle Facts

The curling or flexing action of flexor hallucis longus helps us maintain balance when standing and helps us to push off when walking. This muscle flexes the distal phalanges of the great toe with greater strength than the proximal or middle phalanx of the great toe.

Implications of Shortened and/or Lengthened/ Weak Muscle

Shortened: Limited ability to dorsiflex the ankle and/or extend the great toe is noted. A shortened flexor hallucis longus can increase susceptibility to cramps in the big toe.

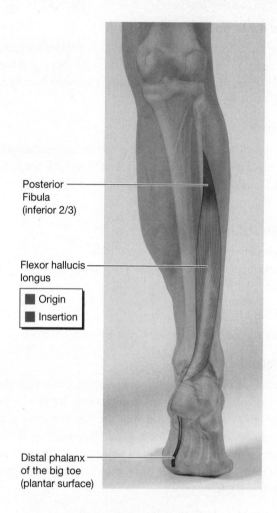

Posterior Fibula (inferior 2/3)

Flexor hallucis longus

■ Origin
■ Insertion

Distal phalanx of the big toe (plantar surface)

FIGURE 5-44 · Flexor hallucis longus

Lengthened: A lengthened flexor hallucis longus can weaken the action of push-off when walking.

Palpation and Massage

Because flexor hallucis longus is located deep in the posterior leg, the muscle can be addressed by massaging the posterior leg, with the intention of addressing the deeper muscles. Effleurage, pétrissage, and friction are all appropriate strokes to apply to this muscle.

How to Stretch This Muscle

Dorsiflex the ankle and extend the big toe.

Synergists

Plantarflexors: gastrocnemius, soleus, plantaris, tibialis posterior, flexor hallucis longus, peroneus longus, and peroneus brevis; flexor of the big toe: flexor hallucis brevis

Antagonists

Dorsiflexors: tibialis anterior, extensor digitorum longus, extensor hallucis longus, and peroneus tertius; extensors of the first digit of the foot: extensor hallucis longus and extensor hallucis brevis

Innervation and Arterial Supply

Innervation: tibial nerve
Arterial supply: posterior tibial artery

PERONEUS LONGUS (per-o-ne-us long-gus)

Meaning of Name

Peroneus refers to the fibula, and *longus* indicates that this muscle is longer than peroneus brevis. Peroneus longus is also called Fibularis longus.

Location

Both peroneus longus and peroneus brevis are located in the lateral leg compartment, along the lateral fibula. Peroneus longus covers the proximal portion of the lateral fibula and is superficial to peroneus brevis. The tendon of insertion of peroneus longus runs distally along the fibula, posterior to the lateral malleolus, and all the way across the plantar surface of the foot to the medial cuneiform and first metatarsal. This muscle is sometimes called the *stirrup muscle* due to the fact that the long tendon of insertion can be compared to a stirrup that runs along the bottom of the foot.

Origin and Insertion

Origin: head of the fibula and the lateral, proximal fibula
Insertion: base of the first metatarsal and the medial cuneiform

Actions

Everts the foot and plantarflexes the ankle

Explanation of Actions

Because peroneus longus is located along the lateral leg and its tendon of insertion crosses the lateral aspect of the ankle and inserts on the plantar surface of the foot, the muscle pulls the plantar surface of the foot toward the lateral leg. This causes eversion of the foot. In addition, because the tendon of insertion passes posterior to the lateral malleolus, the plantar surface of the foot is pulled posteriorly, resulting in plantarflexion.

Notable Muscle Facts

The long tendon of insertion of peroneus longus provides support to the transverse arch. Both peroneus longus and brevis play a role in allowing the feet to be placed flat upon the floor. Because the hips are often wider than the feet, the angle of the lower limbs, when walking or standing, is such that the feet will not land or rest flat upon the floor unless eversion of the foot occurs. Peroneus longus and brevis cause this eversion. Finally, peroneus longus and brevis support the lateral aspect of the ankle joint.

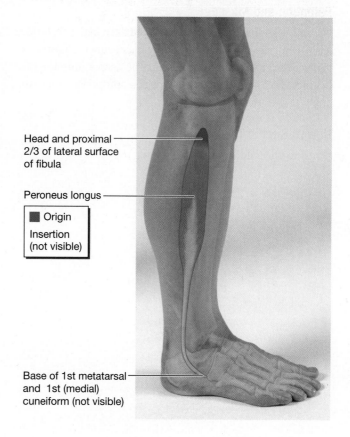

Head and proximal 2/3 of lateral surface of fibula

Peroneus longus

■ Origin
Insertion (not visible)

Base of 1st metatarsal and 1st (medial) cuneiform (not visible)

FIGURE 5-45 · Peroneus longus

Implications of Shortened and/or Lengthened/ Weak Muscle

Shortened: Lower medial longitudinal arch is noted. One's shoes can become more worn on the insides with shortened foot evertors.

Lengthened: Limited ability to evert the foot is noted.

Palpation and Massage

Peroneus longus can be palpated along the proximal, lateral fibula. Friction to this area and gentle cross-fiber friction just distal to the head of the fibula are effective ways to address the muscle.

How to Stretch This Muscle

Inverting the foot while the ankle is dorsiflexed can stretch peroneus longus and peroneus brevis.

Synergists

Evertors of the foot: peroneus brevis and peroneus tertius; plantarflexors: gastrocnemius, soleus, plantaris, tibialis posterior, flexor digitorum longus, flexor hallucis longus, and peroneus brevis

Antagonists

Dorsiflexors: tibialis anterior, extensor digitorum longus, extensor hallucis longus, and peroneus tertius; invertors of the foot: tibialis anterior and tibialis posterior

Innervation and Arterial Supply

Innervation: superficial fibular (peroneal) nerve
Arterial supply: fibular artery

PERONEUS BREVIS (per-o-ne-us bre-vis)

Meaning of Name

Peroneus refers to the fibula, and *brevis* indicates that this muscle is shorter than peroneus longus. Peroneus brevis is also called Fibularis brevis.

Location

Both peroneus longus and peroneus brevis are located in the lateral leg compartment, along the lateral fibula. Peroneus brevis covers the distal portion of the lateral fibula and is deep to peroneus longus. The tendon of insertion runs distally along the fibula, posterior to the lateral malleolus, to the lateral base of the fifth metatarsal.

Origin and Insertion

Origin: distal lateral aspect of the fibula
Insertion: lateral side of the base of the fifth metatarsal

Actions

Everts the foot and plantarflexes the ankle

Explanation of Actions

Because peroneus brevis is located along the lateral leg, and its tendon of insertion crosses the lateral aspect of the ankle and inserts on the lateral side of the fifth metatarsal, the muscle pulls the fifth metatarsal toward the lateral leg. This causes eversion of the foot. In addition, because the tendon of insertion passes posterior to the lateral malleolus, the foot is pulled posteriorly, resulting in plantarflexion.

Notable Muscle Facts

Both peroneus longus and brevis play a role in allowing the feet to be placed flat upon the floor. Because the hips are often wider than the feet, the angle of the lower limbs, when walking or standing, is such that the feet will not land or rest flat upon the floor unless eversion of the foot occurs. Peroneus longus and brevis cause this eversion. Finally, peroneus longus and brevis support the lateral aspect of the ankle joint.

Implications of Shortened and/or Lengthened/Weak Muscle

Shortened: When peroneus longus and brevis are shortened, the medial longitudinal arch can be higher.
Lengthened: Limited ability to evert the foot and possible ankle instability when lengthened, one can experience lateral ankle instability and difficulty everting the foot.

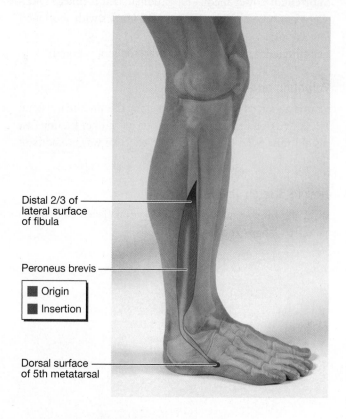

Distal 2/3 of lateral surface of fibula

Peroneus brevis

■ Origin
■ Insertion

Dorsal surface of 5th metatarsal

FIGURE 5-46 · Peroneus brevis

Palpation and Massage

Peroneus brevis can be palpated along the distal, lateral fibula. Friction to this area is an effective way to address the muscle.

How to Stretch This Muscle

Invert the foot while the ankle is dorsiflexed.

Synergists

Evertors of the foot: peroneus brevis and peroneus tertius; plantarflexors: gastrocnemius, soleus, plantaris, tibialis posterior, flexor digitorum longus, flexor hallucis longus, and peroneus longus

Antagonists

Dorsiflexors: tibialis anterior, extensor digitorum longus, extensor hallucis longus, and peroneus tertius; invertors of the foot: tibialis anterior and tibialis posterior

Innervation and Arterial Supply

Innervation: superficial fibular (peroneal) nerve
Arterial supply: fibular artery

PERONEUS TERTIUS (per-o-ne-us ter-shus)

Meaning of Name

Peroneus refers to the fibula, and *tertius* means third. Peroneus tertius is also called Fibularis tertius.

Location

Peroneus tertius is located along the distal aspect of the anterior fibula. The tendon of insertion runs anterior to the lateral malleolus. This muscle often blends in with the distal end of the extensor hallucis muscle. Peroneus tertius is located within the anterior leg compartment.

Origin and Insertion

Origin: distal anterior fibula
Insertion: anterior aspect of the base of the fifth metatarsal

Actions

Everts the foot and dorsiflexes the ankle

Explanation of Actions

Because peroneus tertius crosses the lateral aspect of the ankle and its origin is proximal to insertion, this muscle causes foot eversion. Because the tendon of insertion of peroneus tertius crosses the anterior aspect of the ankle joint, it causes dorsiflexion of the ankle.

Notable Muscle Facts

Peroneus tertius blends with the extensor digitorum longus muscle.

Implications of Shortened and/or Lengthened/ Weak Muscle

Shortened: Lower medial longitudinal arch is noted.
Lengthened: No notable movement limitations is noted.

Palpation and Massage

Peroneus tertius can be palpated along the distal anterior fibula. It is nearly impossible to distinguish from the distal portion of extensor digitorum longus. Direct pressure to the anterior distal fibula is one way to address this muscle.

How to Stretch This Muscle

Invert the foot while plantarflexing the ankle.

Synergists

Evertors of the foot: peroneus longus and peroneus brevis; dorsiflexors: tibialis anterior, extensor digitorum longus and extensor hallucis longus

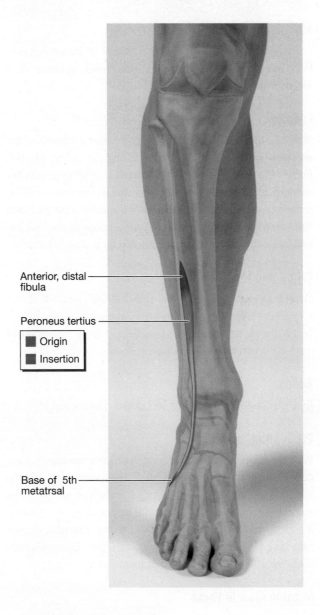

Anterior, distal fibula

Peroneus tertius

■ Origin
■ Insertion

Base of 5th metatrsal

FIGURE 5-47 · **Peroneus tertius**

Antagonists

Plantarflexors: gastrocnemius, soleus, plantaris, tibialis posterior, flexor digitorum longus, flexor hallucis longus, peroneus longus, and peroneus brevis; invertors of the foot: tibialis anterior and tibialis posterior

Innervation and Arterial Supply

Innervation: deep fibular (peroneal) nerve
Arterial supply: anterior tibial artery

EXTENSOR DIGITORUM LONGUS (eks-ten-sor dij-i-to-rum long-gus)

Meaning of Name

Extensor indicates the action of extension. *Digitorum* refers to four digits, and *longus* means that this muscle is longer than extensor digitorum brevis.

Location

Extensor digitorum longus is the most lateral muscle of the anterior leg compartment. It lies along the entire anterior fibula. The proximal part of the muscle is deep to tibialis anterior, but the distal portion is superficial. The tendon of insertion crosses the anterior aspect of the ankle joint and then splits into four distinct tendons, one per digit of the four lateral toes. The tendons are surrounded by a synovial sheath.

Origin and Insertion

Origin: lateral condyle of the tibia and the proximal three-fourths of the anterior fibula
Insertion: dorsal side of the middle and distal phalanges of the four lateral toes

Actions

Extends the four lateral toes and dorsiflexes the ankle

Explanation of Actions

Because extensor digitorum longus crosses the anterior aspect of the ankle, with the origin on the anterior leg and the insertion more distal on the dorsal surface of the toes, the muscle pulls the dorsal side of the foot toward the anterior leg, thus causing dorsiflexion. In addition, extensor digitorum longus pulls the dorsal aspect of the four lateral toes toward the anterior leg, thus extending the toes.

Notable Muscle Facts

Extensor digitorum longus is important during the swing phase of walking, as it helps to keep the foot lifted off of the floor. Likewise, this muscle helps to control the rate of descent of the foot as it comes to the floor just after heel strike.

Implications of Shortened and/or Lengthened/ Weak Muscle

Shortened: Limited ability to flex the toes is noted
Lengthened: Weakness in extension of the metatarsophalangeal joints of the four lateral toes.

Palpation and Massage

Extensor digitorum longus can be palpated easily along the anterior fibula. Friction and direct pressure are reasonable strokes to apply to this muscle.

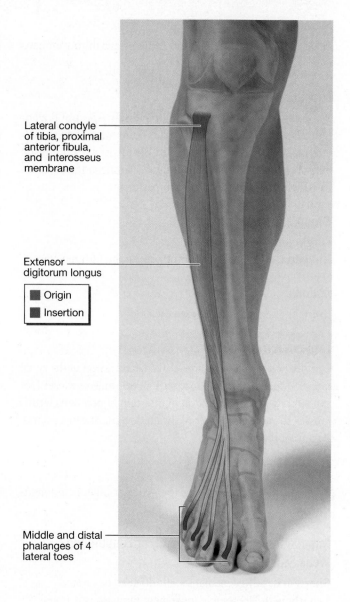

Lateral condyle of tibia, proximal anterior fibula, and interosseus membrane

Extensor digitorum longus

■ Origin
■ Insertion

Middle and distal phalanges of 4 lateral toes

FIGURE 5-48 · Extensor digitorum longus

How to Stretch This Muscle

Plantarflex the ankle while flexing the toes.

Synergists

Extensor of the four lateral toes: extensor digitorum brevis, which acts on the metacarpophalangeal (MP) joints of the foot; dorsiflexors of the ankle: tibialis anterior, extensor hallucis longus, and peroneus tertius

Antagonists

Toe flexors: flexor digitorum longus and flexor digitorum brevis; plantarflexors: gastrocnemius, soleus, plantaris, tibialis posterior, flexor hallucis longus, flexor digitorum longus, peroneus longus, and peroneus brevis

Innervation and Arterial Supply

Innervation: deep peroneal nerve
Arterial supply: anterior tibial artery

EXTENSOR HALLUCIS LONGUS (eks-ten-sor hal-u-sis long-gus)

Meaning of Name

Extensor indicates the action of extension. *Hallucis* refers to the big toe or the first digit of the foot. And longus means that this muscle is longer than extensor hallucis brevis.

Location

Extensor hallucis longus is located in the anterior leg compartment, deep to extensor digitorum longus and tibialis anterior. The tendon of insertion of extensor hallucis longus crosses the anterior aspect of the ankle joint and runs along the dorsal surface of the big toe to the distal phalanx.

Origin and Insertion

Origin: middle of the shaft of the anterior fibula and the interosseus membrane
Insertion: dorsal aspect of the distal phalanx of the big toe

Actions

Extends the great (big) toe and dorsiflexes the ankle

Explanation of Actions

Because extensor hallucis longus crosses the anterior aspect of the ankle, with the origin on the anterior leg and the insertion more distal on the dorsal surface of big toe, the muscle pulls the dorsal side of the foot toward the anterior leg, thus causing dorsiflexion. In addition, extensor digitorum longus pulls the dorsal aspect of the big toe toward the anterior leg, thus extending the first digit.

Notable Muscle Facts

Extensor hallucis longus is important during the swing phase of walking, as it helps to keep the foot lifted off of the floor. Likewise, this muscle helps to control the rate of descent of the foot as it comes to the floor just after heel stake.

Implications of Shortened and/or Lengthened/ Weak Muscle

Shortened: Limited ability to flex the great/big toe is noted.
Lengthened: Limited ability to extend the big/great toe is noted.

Palpation and Massage

Extensor hallucis longus may be palpated and massaged deep in the anterior leg compartment. Friction and direct pressure are reasonable strokes to apply to this muscle.

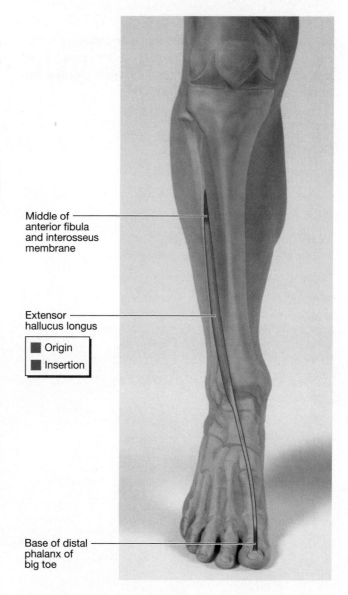

Middle of anterior fibula and interosseus membrane

Extensor hallucus longus

■ Origin
■ Insertion

Base of distal phalanx of big toe

FIGURE 5-49 · Extensor hallucis longus

How to Stretch This Muscle

Plantarflex the ankle while flexing the great toe.

Synergists

Extensor of the first digit: extensor hallucis brevis, which acts on the MP joint of the big toe; dorsiflexors of the ankle: tibialis anterior, extensor digitorum longus, and peroneus tertius

Antagonists

Toe flexors: flexor hallucis longus and flexor hallucis brevis; plantarflexors: gastrocnemius, soleus, plantaris, tibialis posterior, flexor hallucis longus, flexor digitorum longus, peroneus longus, and peroneus brevis

Innervation and Arterial Supply

Innervation: deep peroneal nerve
Arterial supply: anterior tibial artery

TIBIALIS ANTERIOR (tib-e-a-lis an-ter-e-or)

Meaning of Name

Tibialis anterior attaches to a significant portion of the front of the tibia.

Location

Tibialis anterior is the largest and most superficial muscle in the anterior leg compartment. It is one of the strongest muscles per volume unit in the body. The tendon of insertion of tibialis anterior crosses the anterior aspect of the ankle joint on its way to the medial side of the foot.

Origin and Insertion

Origin: lateral condyle and lateral shaft of the tibia and interosseus membrane
Insertion: base of the first metatarsal and medial cuneiform

Actions

Dorsiflexes the ankle and inverts the foot

Explanation of Actions

Because tibialis anterior crosses the anterior aspect of the ankle, it is a dorsiflexor. Because it inserts on the medial aspect of the foot, it pulls the medial aspect of the foot superiorly, causing inversion. As the strongest dorsiflexor, tibialis anterior is important in walking. It is used concentrically when we pull the dorsal side of the foot closer to the anterior leg as we swing our leg with each step. Also, we use tibialis anterior eccentrically right after our heel strikes the ground, to control the rate of descent of the foot to the ground. We use tibialis anterior even more when going uphill and more eccentric contraction is required when going downhill.

Notable Muscle Facts

Tibialis anterior is one of the strongest muscles in the body (per unit of volume). Along with the plantarflexors, tibialis anterior helps us maintain balance as we shift our weight on our feet.

Implications of Shortened and/or Lengthened/ Weak Muscle

Shortened: A shortened tibialis anterior can cause a high medial longitudinal arch, as well as difficulty everting the foot and plantarflexing the ankle.

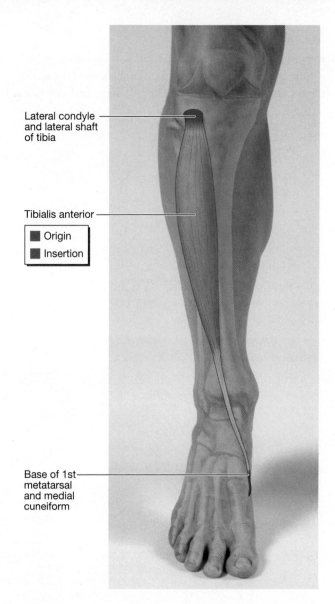

Lateral condyle and lateral shaft of tibia

Tibialis anterior

■ Origin
■ Insertion

Base of 1st metatarsal and medial cuneiform

FIGURE 5-50 · Tibialis anterior

Lengthened: Inability to fully dorsiflex the foot; this limitation can be noticed during gait. A lengthened or weakened tibialis anterior causes the foot to slap or drop to the ground, just after heel strike when walking.

Palpation and Massage

Tibialis anterior is easy to palpate and massage in the anterior leg, between the tibia and fibula. Effleurage, friction, and direct pressure are all effective strokes to apply to this muscle.

How to Stretch This Muscle

Plantarflex the ankle while everting the foot.

Synergists

Dorsiflexors: extensor digitorum longus, extensor hallucis longus, and peroneus tertius; inverter: tibialis posterior

Antagonists

Plantarflexors: gastrocnemius, soleus, plantaris, tibialis posterior, flexor hallucis longus, flexor digitorum longus, peroneus longus, and peroneus brevis; evertors of the foot: peroneus longus, peroneus brevis, and peroneus tertius

Innervation and Arterial Supply

Innervation: deep peroneal nerve
Arterial supply: anterior tibial nerve

Regional Illustrations of Muscles

Figure 5-51 shows a deep view of the posterior leg.
Figure 5-52 shows a superficial view of the posterior leg.
Figure 5-53 shows a superficial view of the lateral leg.

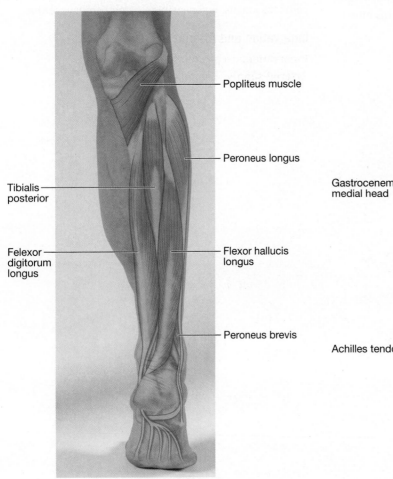

Popliteus muscle

Peroneus longus

Tibialis posterior

Felexor digitorum longus

Flexor hallucis longus

Peroneus brevis

FIGURE 5-51 · A deep view of the posterior leg

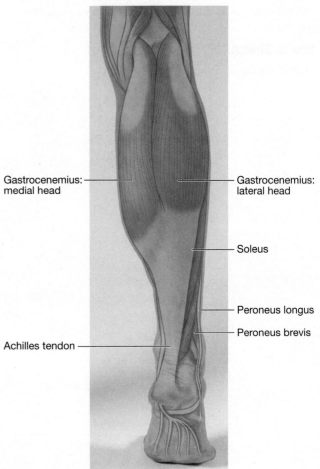

Gastrocenemius: medial head

Gastrocenemius: lateral head

Soleus

Peroneus longus

Peroneus brevis

Achilles tendon

FIGURE 5-52 · A superficial view of the posterior leg

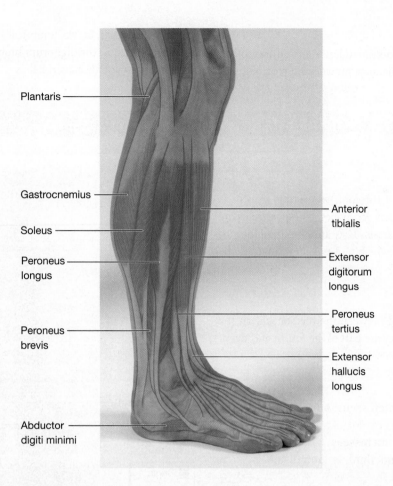

Plantaris

Gastrocnemius

Soleus

Peroneus
longus

Peroneus
brevis

Abductor
digiti minimi

Anterior
tibialis

Extensor
digitorum
longus

Peroneus
tertius

Extensor
hallucis
longus

FIGURE 5-53 · A superficial view of the lateral leg

Intrinsic Foot Muscles

Intrinsic muscles of the foot include the dorsal interossei, plantar interossei, flexor hallucis brevis, adductor hallucis, flexor digiti minimi brevis, lumbricals, quadratus plantae, abductor hallucis, flexor digitorum brevis, and abductor digiti minimi. These are discussed below.

DORSAL INTEROSSEI (dor-sal in-ter-ahs-e-i)

Meaning of Name

Dorsal refers to the top of the foot, where this muscle is located. *Interossei* means between bones. These muscles are located between the metatarsals. They are a group of four interosseus muscles, each of which moves a single digit in one direction.

Location

These muscles are located between the metatarsals on the dorsal side of the foot. They are part of the fourth and deepest layer of intrinsic foot muscles.

Origin and Insertion

Origin of each dorsal interosseus: adjacent sides of the metatarsals it lies between

Insertion of each dorsal interosseus: base of the proximal phalanx of either the second, third, or forth digit

Actions

The sum of the actions of dorsal interossei is said to be abduction of the toes, which is the movements of the digits away from the midline of the foot, defined as the second digit. In reality, each interosseus muscle moves a single digit either medially or laterally. One muscle moves the fourth digit laterally, one moves the third digit laterally, one moves the second digit medially, and one moves the second digit laterally.

Explanation of Actions

Each interosseus muscle is located on one particular side (either the medial or lateral side) of the proximal phalanx it moves, and it inserts into that same side of the proximal phalanx. The three interossei located on the lateral side of digits 2, 3, and 4 pull the proximal phalanges of those digits laterally, and the interosseus muscle that is located on the medial side of the proximal phalanx of digit 2 pulls the proximal phalanx of digit 2 medially.

Notable Muscle Facts

"DAB" is a useful acronym for remembering that the Dorsal interossei ABduct the toes.

Implications of Shortened and/or Lengthened/ Weak Muscle

Shortened: Limited ability to adduct the toes is noted.
Lengthened: Limited ability to abduct the toes is noted.

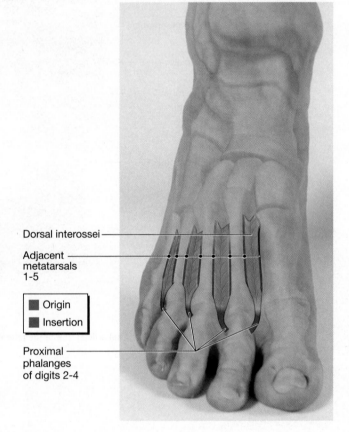

Dorsal interossei

Adjacent metatarsals 1-5

■ Origin
■ Insertion

Proximal phalanges of digits 2-4

FIGURE 5-54 · Dorsal interossei

Palpation and Massage

Palpating and frictioning deep between the metatarsals on the dorsal side of the foot will find and address dorsal interossei.

How to Stretch This Muscle

Adduct the toes.

Synergists

There are no other abductors of digits 2, 3, and 4 of the foot.

Antagonists

Plantar interossei (adducts the toes)

Innervation and Arterial Supply

Innervation: lateral plantar nerve
Arterial supply: branches of the plantar arch

PLANTAR INTEROSSEI (plan-tar in-ter-ahs-e-i)

Meaning of Name

Plantar refers to the plantar side of the foot, and *interossei* means between bones. In this case, the bones of reference are the metatarsals.

Location

The plantar interossei are located on the plantar side of the foot, deep between the metatarsals. They are part of the fourth and deepest layer of intrinsic foot muscles.

Origin and Insertion

Origin: metatarsals 3, 4, and 5
Insertion: plantar sides of the proximal phalanges of digits 3, 4, and 5

Actions

As a group, the plantar interossei adduct the toes. Individually, each plantar interosseus moves either the third, fourth, or fifth digit toward the second digit, which is the midline of the foot.

Explanation of Actions

One plantar interosseus muscle originates on the medial side of the third metatarsal. This interosseus muscle inserts on the medial side of the proximal phalanx of the third digit. When the muscle shortens, it pulls the proximal phalanx of the second digit medially. The plantar interosseus muscle that originates on the medial side of the fourth metatarsal inserts on the medial side of the proximal phalanx of the fourth digit. Thus, when it shortens, it pulls the proximal phalanx of the fourth digit medially. The plantar interosseus muscle that originates on the medial side of the fifth metacarpal inserts on the medial side of the proximal phalanx of the fifth digit, and thus pulls the fifth digit medially when it shortens. The combined movements of the three interossei muscles is to bring digits 3, 4, and 5 closer to digit 2, which is the same as adducting the toes.

Notable Muscle Facts

"PAD" is a useful acronym to remember: the Plantar interossei ADduct the toes.

Implications of Shortened and/or Lengthened/ Weak Muscle

Shortened: Limited ability to abduct the toes is noted.
Lengthened: Limited ability to adduct the toes is noted.

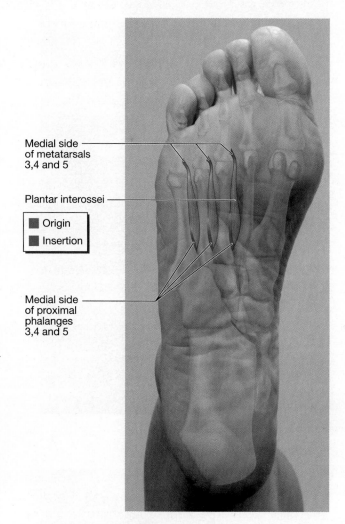

Medial side of metatarsals 3, 4 and 5

Plantar interossei

☐ Origin
☐ Insertion

Medial side of proximal phalanges 3, 4 and 5

FIGURE 5-55 · Plantar interossei

Palpation and Massage

Palpating and providing friction to the plantar side of the foot, deep between the metatarsals, allows us to access and massage the plantar interossei.

How to Stretch This Muscle

Abduct the toes.

Synergists

There are no other adductors of digits 3, 4, and 5 of the foot.

Antagonists

Dorsal interossei (abducts the toes)

Innervation and Arterial Supply

Innervation: lateral plantar nerve
Arterial supply: branches of the plantar arch

LAYER 3 INTRINSIC FOOT MUSCLES

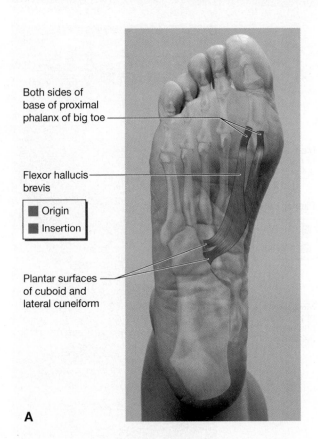

Both sides of
base of proximal
phalanx of big toe

Flexor hallucis
brevis

■ Origin
■ Insertion

Plantar surfaces
of cuboid and
lateral cuneiform

A

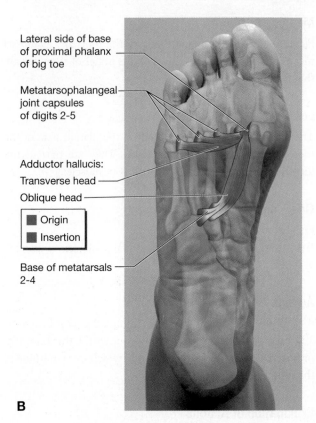

Lateral side of base
of proximal phalanx
of big toe

Metatarsophalangeal
joint capsules
of digits 2-5

Adductor hallucis:

Transverse head

Oblique head

■ Origin
■ Insertion

Base of metatarsals
2-4

B

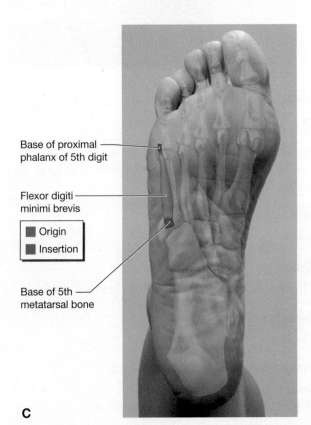

Base of proximal
phalanx of 5th digit

Flexor digiti
minimi brevis

■ Origin
■ Insertion

Base of 5th
metatarsal bone

C

FIGURE 5-56 · **Layer 3 intrinsic foot muscles A:** Flexor hallucis brevis;
B: Adductor hallucis; **C:** Flexor digiti minimi brevis.

FLEXOR HALLUCIS BREVIS (fleks-or hal-u-sis bre-vis)

Meaning of Name

Flexor refers to the action of flexion. *Hallucis* refers to the big toe. The word *brevis* informs us that this muscle is shorter than flexor hallucis longus.

Location

Flexor hallucis brevis is a third-layer intrinsic foot muscle, located on the plantar surface of the foot and covering the first metatarsal.

Origin and Insertion

Origin: plantar surfaces of the cuboid and the lateral cuneiform
Insertion: both sides of the base of the proximal phalanx of the big toe

Actions

Flexes the MP joint of the big toe at the MP joint

Explanation of Actions

Because the muscle crosses the plantar side of the MP joint, and because the insertion on the plantar surface of the proximal phalanx of the big toe is pulled toward the origin on the plantar surface of the cuboid and lateral cuneiform, flexion of the big toe results.

Notable Muscle Facts

There are two tendons of insertion of flexor hallucis brevis, each of which contains a sesamoid bone.

Implications of Shortened and/or Lengthened/ Weak Muscle

Shortened: Limited ability to extend the MP joint of the great toe is noted.
Lengthened: Limited ability to flex the MP joint of the great toe is noted.

Palpation and Massage

This muscle can be palpated on the plantar side of the first metatarsal. Direct pressure and friction are appropriate strokes to apply to this muscle.

How to Stretch This Muscle

Extend the MP joint of the big toe.

Synergists

Flexor hallucis longus (flexes the big toe)

Antagonists

Extensor hallucis longus and brevis (extend the big toe)

Innervation and Arterial Supply

Innervation: medial plantar nerve
Arterial supply: medial plantar artery

ADDUCTOR HALLUCIS (a-duk-tor hal-u-sis)

Meaning of Name

Adductor refers to the action of adduction, and *hallucis* refers to the big toe.

Location

Adductor hallucis is a third-layer intrinsic foot muscle, located on the plantar surface of the foot. It covers the MP joint capsules and much of the second and third metatarsals of the foot (see Fig. 5-57).

Origin and Insertion

Origin of the oblique head: base of metatarsals 2–4
Origin of the transverse head: joint capsules of the MP joints
Insertion: lateral side of the base of the proximal phalanx of the big toe

Actions

Adducts and flexes the big toe at the MP joint

Explanation of Actions

Because the origin is medial to the insertion, and because adductor hallucis crosses the MP joints on the plantar surface of the foot, this muscle adducts the big toe. Because the origin is proximal to the insertion, and the muscle crosses the plantar surface of the big toe, adductor hallucis also flexes the big toe.

Notable Muscle Facts

Adductor hallucis helps to support the transverse arch of the foot. Adductor hallucis is similar to adductor pollicis in that both muscles have a transverse head and an oblique head.

Implications of Shortened and/or Lengthened/Weak Muscle

Shortened: Inability to abduct the great toe is noted.
Lengthened: Limited ability to adduct the bit toe.

Palpation and Massage

Adductor hallucis may be palpated on the plantar surface of the foot, focusing on the areas of the MP joint capsules and metatarsals 2 and 3. Friction and direct pressure are appropriate strokes for this muscle.

How to Stretch This Muscle

Abduct the big toe.

Synergists

There are no other major adductors of the big toe.

Antagonists

Abductor hallucis (abducts the big toe)

Innervation and Arterial Supply

Innervation: lateral plantar nerve
Arterial supply: branches of the planter arch

FLEXOR DIGITI MINIMI BREVIS (flexs-or dij-i-ti min-i-mi bre-vis)

Meaning of Name

Flexor refers to the action of flexion. *Digiti minimi* refers to the smallest digit, the fifth digit. *Brevis* indicates that the digiti minimi of the foot is smaller than that of the hand. Not all sources include the word brevis in this muscle's name.

Location

Flexor digiti minimi brevis is a third-layer intrinsic foot muscle, located on the plantar surface of the foot. It covers the fifth metatarsal of the foot (see Fig. 5-57).

Origin and Insertion

Origin: base of the fifth metatarsal
Insertion: base of the proximal phalanx of the fifth digit

Actions

Flexes the fifth digit of the foot at the MP joint

Explanation of Actions

Flexor digiti minimi brevis crosses the plantar surface of the MP joint of the fifth digit, with its origin more proximal than insertion. Thus, the plantar surface of the proximal phalanx is pulled toward the fifth metatarsal. The result is flexion of the fifth digit.

Notable Muscle Facts

It is unusual that this muscle name includes the word "brevis," as muscles with "brevis" are typically paired with muscles with the word "longus," and there is no flexor digiti minimi longus in the foot.

Implications of Shortened and/or Lengthened/ Weak Muscle

Shortened: Limited ability to extend the MP joint of the fifth digit is noted.
Lengthened: Limited ability to flex the MP joint of the fifth digit is noted.

Palpation and Massage

Flexor digiti minimi brevis can be palpated and massaged by applying direct pressure or friction to the muscle on the plantar surface of the fifth digit.

How to Stretch This Muscle

Extend the fifth digit of the foot.

Synergists

Flexor digitorum longus and flexor digitorum brevis (flex the MP joint of the fifth digit)

Antagonists

Extensor digitorum longus and extensor digitorum brevis (extend the fifth digit of the foot at the MP joint)

Innervation and Arterial Supply

Innervation: lateral plantar nerve
Arterial supply: lateral plantar artery

LUMBRICALS (lum-bri-kals)

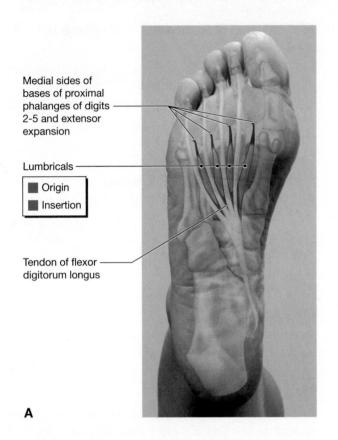

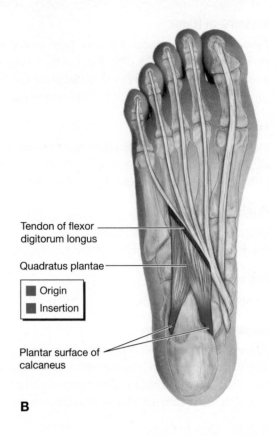

FIGURE 5-57 · Layer 2 intrinsic foot muscles. A: Lumbricals **B:** Quadratus plantae

Meaning of Name

Earthworms

Location

Lumbricals are located quite centrally on the plantar surface of the foot. They are part of the second layer of intrinsic foot muscles.

Origin and Insertion

Origin: tendon of origin of flexor digitorum longus
Insertion: plantar aspect of the proximal phalanges of digits 2–5 and the extensor expansion, which covers the dorsal surface of the toes

Actions

Flex the MP joints of digits 2–5 and extend the proximal interphalangeal (PIP) and distal interphalangeal (DIP) joints of digits 2–5

Explanation of Actions

Lumbricals flex the MP joints of the four lateral toes because the tendons of origin cross the plantar aspect of these joints, with origin more proximal to insertion. Lumbricals extend the DIP and PIP joints of digits 2–5 because they pull on the extensor expansion, which pulls the dorsal sides of the toes toward the dorsal side of the foot.

Notable Muscle Facts

Lumbrical muscles in the hand have the same actions as the lumbricals of the foot. However, the lumbricals of the hand typically have greater mobility. Lumbricals in the foot add stability to the distal joints of the foot.

Implications of Shortened and/or Lengthened/ Weak Muscle

There are no common or obvious implications of shortened or lengthened lumbrical muscles.

Palpation and Massage

Lumbricals can be palpated and massaged by providing direct pressure or friction to the central area on the plantar side of the foot.

How to Stretch This Muscle

Extend the MP joints of digits 2–5 of the foot while flexing the DIP joints and PIP joints of the same digits.

Synergists

Flexor digitorum longus and flexor digitorum brevis (flex the MP joints of the four lateral toes) and extensor digitorum (extends the PIP and DIP joints of these digits)

Antagonists

Extensor digitorum longus and extensor digitorum brevis (extend the MP joints of the four lateral toes) and flexor digitorum longus (flexes the PIP and DIP joints of these digits)

Innervation and Arterial Supply

Innervation: medial and lateral plantar nerves
Arterial supply: medial and lateral plantar arteries

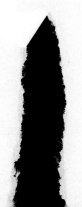

QUADRATUS PLANTAE (kwah-drat-us plan-te)

Meaning of Name

Quadratus refers to square, which is the shape of this muscle. *Plantae* refers to the fact that this muscle is located on the plantar surface of the foot (see Fig. 5-58).

Location

Quadratus plantae is located on the proximal or posterior third of the plantar surface of the foot. This muscle is part of the second layer of intrinsic foot muscles.

Origin and Insertion

Origin: calcaneus
Insertion: tendon of insertion of flexor digitorum longus

Actions

Quadratus plantae assists flexor digitorum longus in flexing the four lateral toes by providing additional pull on the flexor digitorum longus' tendon of insertion and by adjusting the angle of pull on this tendon to make it more efficient.

Explanation of Actions

By anchoring on the calcaneus and by pulling the tendon of flexor digitorum longus directly toward the calcaneus, quadratus plantae helps to flex the toes.

Notable Muscle Facts

Quadratus plantae's ability to flex the four lateral toes is especially important when the ankle is dorsiflexed, as such an ankle position decreases the strength of flexor digitorum longus.

Implications of Shortened and/or Lengthened/ Weak Muscle

Shortened: Tension is felt in the heel area.
Lengthened: Reduced ability to flex the four lateral toes is noted, particularly when the ankle is dorsiflexed.

Palpation and Massage

Quadratus plantae can be palpated and massaged by applying friction and direct pressure to the plantar surface of the calcaneus.

How to Stretch This Muscle

Extend the four lateral toes.

Synergists

Toe flexors: flexor digitorum longus and flexor digitorum brevis

Antagonists

Toe extensors: extensor digitorum longus and extensor digitorum brevis

Innervation and Arterial Supply

Innervation: lateral plantar nerve
Arterial supply: medial and lateral plantar arteries

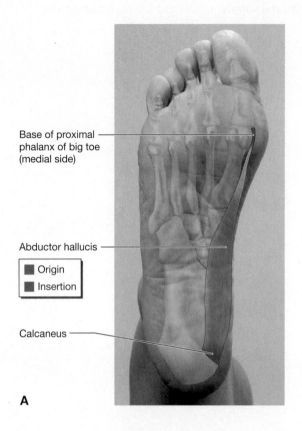

Base of proximal phalanx of big toe (medial side)

Abductor hallucis

■ Origin
■ Insertion

Calcaneus

A

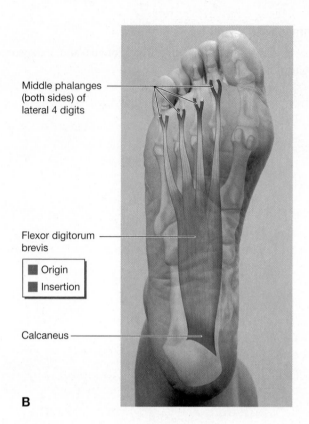

Middle phalanges (both sides) of lateral 4 digits

Flexor digitorum brevis

■ Origin
■ Insertion

Calcaneus

B

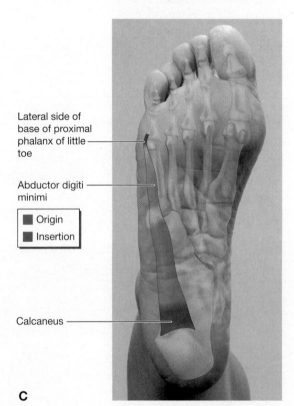

Lateral side of base of proximal phalanx of little toe

Abductor digiti minimi

■ Origin
■ Insertion

Calcaneus

C

FIGURE 5-58 · **Layer 1 intrinsic foot muscles. A:** Abductor hallucis; **B:** Flexor digitorum brevis; **C:** Abductor digiti minimi

ABDUCTOR HALLUCIS (ab-duk-ter hal-u-sis)

Meaning of Name

Abduction refers to the action of abduction, and *hallucis* refers to the big toe.

Location

Abductor hallucis is located on the medial side of the plantar surface of the foot. It is a first-layer intrinsic foot muscle. The muscular portion lies between the calcaneus and the medial cuneiform.

Origin and Insertion

Origin: tuberosity of the calcaneus
Insertion: medial side of the base of the proximal phalanx of the big toe

Actions

Abducts and flexes the big toe

Explanation of Actions

Because abductor hallucis attaches to the medial side of the proximal phalanx of the big toe and because the origin is proximal to the insertion, the muscle has the leverage to pull the proximal phalanx of the big toe medially, thus causing abduction. Because the origin is proximal to the insertion, abductor hallucis flexes the MP joint of the big toe.

Notable Muscle Facts

Abductor hallucis supports the medial longitudinal arch. This muscle is a stronger flexor than abductor of the MP joint of the big toe.

Implications of Shortened and/or Lengthened/ Weak Muscle

Shortened: Limited ability to adduct and/or extend the big toe is noted.
Lengthened: When abductor hallucis is weak or overlengthened, one can experience difficulty abducting the big toe fully.

Palpation and Massage

Abductor hallucis can be palpated and massaged by applying friction and direct pressure to the medial side of the calcaneus.

How to Stretch This Muscle

Adduct and extend digit one of the foot.

Synergists

There is no other major abductor of the great toe.

Antagonists

Adductor hallucis (adducts the big toe)

Innervation and Arterial Supply

Innervation: medial plantar nerve
Arterial supply: medial and plantar artery

FLEXOR DIGITORUM BREVIS (fleks-or dij-i-to-rum bre-vis)

Meaning of Name

Flexor refers to the action of flexion. *Digitorum* tells us that this muscle acts upon the four digits, in this case the four lateral toes. Also, *brevis* tells us that the flexor digitorum brevis is shorter than the flexor digitorum longus.

Location

Flexor digitorum brevis is located on the plantar surface of the foot, from the calcaneus to the PIP joints of the four lateral toes (see Fig. 5-59). It is a first-layer intrinsic foot muscle.

Origin and Insertion

Origin: tuberosity of the calcaneus
Insertion: medial and lateral sides of the proximal phalanges of digits 2–5

Actions

Flexes digits 2–5 of the foot at the PIP joints

Explanation of Actions

Because flexor digitorum brevis crosses the plantar side of the PIP joints of the four lateral toes, and because its origin is proximal to the insertion, the plantar sides of the middle phalanges are pulled toward the plantar side of the foot. The result is toe flexion at the PIP joints.

Notable Muscle Facts

Flexor digitorum brevis helps to stabilize the longitudinal arch. The tendons of insertion of flexor digitorum brevis can be compared to the tendons of insertion of flexor digitorum superficialis (located in the hand), as both split to create a tunnel for a deeper tendon to pass beneath.

Implications of Shortened and/or Lengthened/ Weak Muscle

Shortened: Limited ability to extend the PIP joints of the four lateral toes is noted.
Lengthened: A weak or overlengthened flexor digitorum brevis will weaken the action of toe flexion at the PIP joints.

Palpation and Massage

Flexor digitorum brevis can be palpated and massaged by applying direct pressure and friction to the plantar surface of the foot from the calcaneus to the MP joints.

How to Stretch This Muscle

Extend the four lateral toes.

Synergists

Flexor digitorum longus (flexes four lateral toes)

Antagonists

Extensor digitorum longus (extends PIP joints of the four lateral toes)

Innervation and Arterial Supply

Innervation: medial plantar nerve
Arterial supply: medial and lateral plantar arteries

ABDUCTOR DIGITI MINIMI (ab-duk-ter dij-i-ti min-i-mi)

Meaning of Name

Abduction refers to the action of abduction, and *digiti minimi* refers to the smallest digit, in this case the fifth digit of the foot.

Location

Abductor digiti minimi is located on the lateral side of the plantar surface of the foot, from the calcaneus to the MP joint of the fifth digit (see Fig. 5-59). It is a first-layer intrinsic foot muscle.

Origin and Insertion

Origin: tuberosity of the calcaneus
Insertion: lateral side of the base of the proximal phalanx of the fifth digit of the foot

Actions

Abducts the fifth digit of the foot

Explanation of Actions

Because abductor digiti minimi inserts on the lateral aspect of the proximal phalanx of the fifth digit, and because the origin is proximal to this insertion, the muscle pulls the proximal phalanx of the fifth digit laterally, thus causing abduction of the smallest toe.

Notable Muscle Facts

Abductor digiti minimi helps stabilize the lateral portion of the longitudinal arch.

Implications of Shortened and/or Lengthened/ Weak Muscle

Shortened: Limited ability to adduct the fifth digit is noted.
Lengthened: Limited ability to abduct the fifth digit is noted.

Palpation and Massage

Abductor digiti minimi can be palpated and massaged by applying direct pressure and friction to the lateral plantar aspect of the foot.

How to Stretch This Muscle

Adduct the fifth digit of the foot.

Synergists

There is no other muscle that abducts the fifth digit of the foot.

Antagonists

Plantar interossei

Innervation and Arterial Supply

Innervation: lateral plantar nerve
Arterial supply: lateral plantar artery

Regional Illustrations of Muscles

Figure 5-59 shows the muscle attachment sites on bones of the pelvis, thigh & knee.

Figure 5-60 shows the muscle attachment sites on anterior pelvis, thigh, leg and dorsal side of foot.

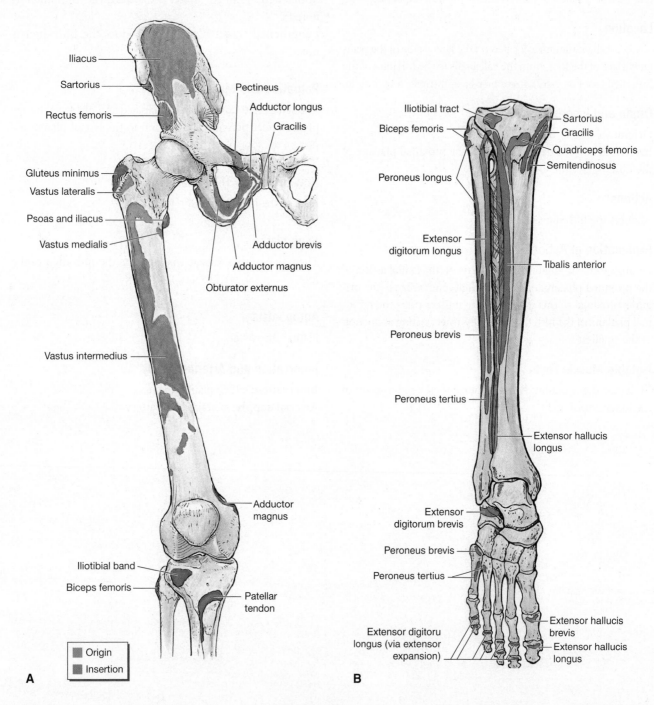

FIGURE 5-59 · **Muscle attachment sites on bones of the pelvis, thigh, and knee. A:** Anterior view of thigh; **B:** Anterior view of leg and dorsal side of foot.

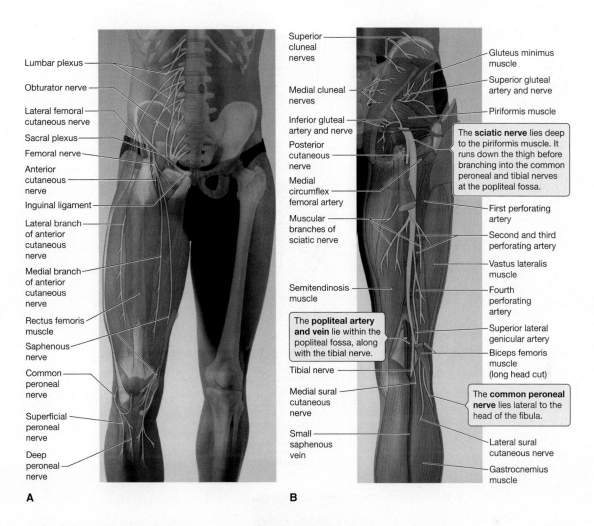

FIGURE 5-60 · **Nerves that serve the lower extremity A:** Anterior thigh; **B:** Posterior thigh (*continued*)

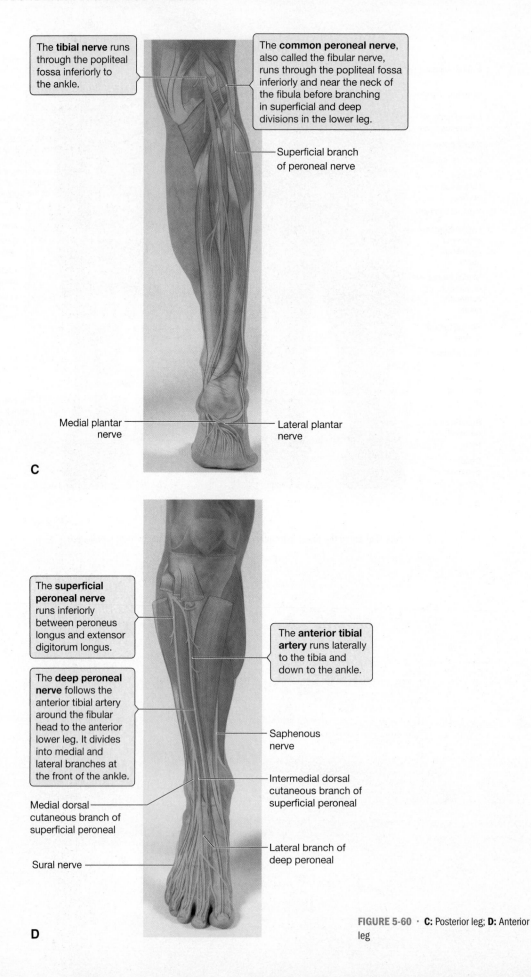

The **tibial nerve** runs through the popliteal fossa inferiorly to the ankle.

The **common peroneal nerve**, also called the fibular nerve, runs through the popliteal fossa inferiorly and near the neck of the fibula before branching in superficial and deep divisions in the lower leg.

Superficial branch of peroneal nerve

Medial plantar nerve

Lateral plantar nerve

C

The **superficial peroneal nerve** runs inferiorly between peroneus longus and extensor digitorum longus.

The **deep peroneal nerve** follows the anterior tibial artery around the fibular head to the anterior lower leg. It divides into medial and lateral branches at the front of the ankle.

Medial dorsal cutaneous branch of superficial peroneal

Sural nerve

The **anterior tibial artery** runs laterally to the tibia and down to the ankle.

Saphenous nerve

Intermedial dorsal cutaneous branch of superficial peroneal

Lateral branch of deep peroneal

D

FIGURE 5-60 · C: Posterior leg; **D:** Anterior leg

ILLUSTRATIONS OF NERVE SUPPLY AND ARTERIAL SUPPLY TO LOWER LIMB

Figure 5-61 shows both arterial supply and veins of the lower limb

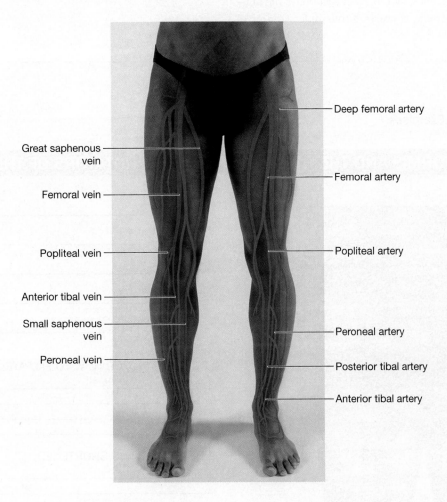

FIGURE 5-61 · Vessels of the lower limb.

■ CHAPTER SUMMARY

This chapter has provided you with much information about the bones and joints of the lower extremity and the muscles that move the hip, knee, ankle, foot, and toes.

Memorizing the names, locations, and actions of the muscles covered is important. However, a true understanding of how these muscles affect our posture and our ability to move is essential to use this information to guide our massage therapy treatments to best assist our clients.

■ WORKBOOK

Muscle Drawing Exercises

PIRIFORMIS AND THE OTHER DEEP LATERAL ROTATORS OF THE HIP

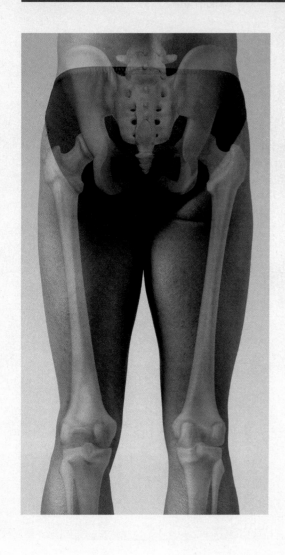

ORIGIN: _____

INSERTION: _____

ACTION(S): _____

NERVE: _____

ARTERIAL SUPPLY: _____

LOCATION AND/OR HOW TO PALPATE:
_____
_____
_____
_____

WHEN MUSCLE IS SHORTENED:
_____
_____
_____

WHEN MUSCLE IS LENGTHENED:
_____
_____
_____

HOW TO STRETCH THIS MUSCLE:
_____
_____

SYNERGIST(S):
_____
_____

ANTAGONIST(S):
_____
_____
_____

NOTES: _____
_____
_____

ADDUCTOR MAGNUS

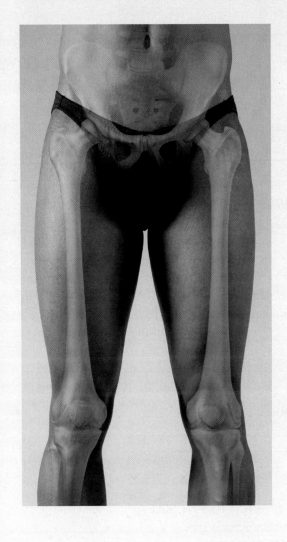

ORIGIN: _____

INSERTION: _____

ACTION(S): _____

NERVE: _____

ARTERIAL SUPPLY: _____

LOCATION AND/OR HOW TO PALPATE:
_____
_____
_____
_____
_____

WHEN MUSCLE IS SHORTENED:
_____
_____
_____
_____

WHEN MUSCLE IS LENGTHENED:
_____
_____
_____
_____

HOW TO STRETCH THIS MUSCLE:
_____
_____

SYNERGIST(S):
_____
_____

ANTAGONIST(S):
_____
_____
_____
_____

NOTES: _____
_____
_____
_____
_____
_____
_____

ADDUCTOR LONGUS AND BREVIS

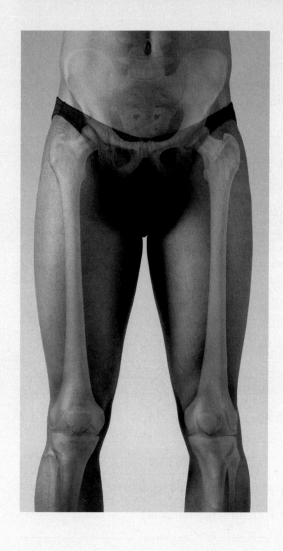

ORIGIN: _____

INSERTION: _____

ACTION(S): _____

NERVE: _____

ARTERIAL SUPPLY: _____

LOCATION AND/OR HOW TO PALPATE:
_____
_____
_____
_____
_____

WHEN MUSCLE IS SHORTENED:
_____
_____
_____
_____

WHEN MUSCLE IS LENGTHENED:
_____
_____
_____
_____

HOW TO STRETCH THIS MUSCLE:
_____
_____

SYNERGIST(S):
_____
_____

ANTAGONIST(S):
_____
_____
_____
_____

NOTES: _____
_____
_____
_____
_____
_____

PECTINEUS

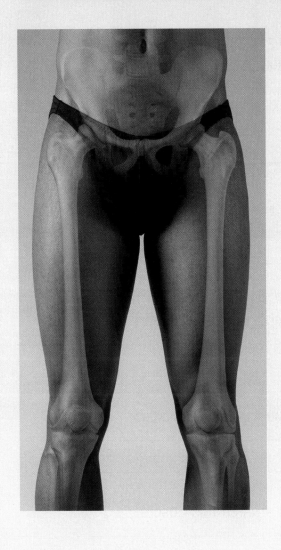

ORIGIN: _____

INSERTION: _____

ACTION(S): _____

NERVE: _____

ARTERIAL SUPPLY: _____

LOCATION AND/OR HOW TO PALPATE:
_____
_____
_____
_____
_____

WHEN MUSCLE IS SHORTENED:
_____
_____
_____
_____

WHEN MUSCLE IS LENGTHENED:
_____
_____
_____
_____

HOW TO STRETCH THIS MUSCLE:
_____
_____

SYNERGIST(S):
_____
_____

ANTAGONIST(S):
_____
_____
_____
_____

NOTES: _____
_____
_____
_____
_____
_____
_____

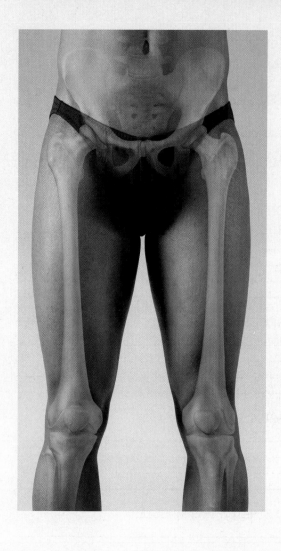

ORIGIN: _____

INSERTION: _____

ACTION(S): _____

NERVE: _____

ARTERIAL SUPPLY: _____

LOCATION AND/OR HOW TO PALPATE:
_____
_____
_____
_____

WHEN MUSCLE IS SHORTENED:
_____
_____
_____
_____

WHEN MUSCLE IS LENGTHENED:
_____
_____
_____
_____

HOW TO STRETCH THIS MUSCLE:
_____
_____

SYNERGIST(S):
_____
_____

ANTAGONIST(S):
_____
_____
_____

NOTES: _____
_____
_____
_____
_____
_____

GLUTEUS MINIMUS

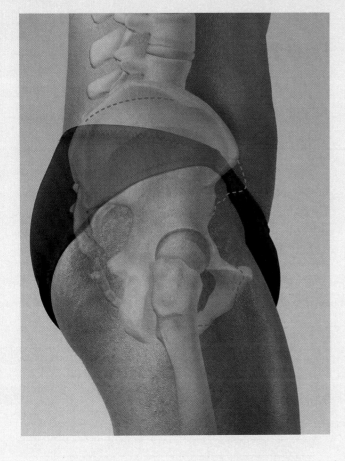

ORIGIN: _____

INSERTION: _____

ACTION(S): _____

NERVE: _____

ARTERIAL SUPPLY: _____

LOCATION AND/OR HOW TO PALPATE:
_____
_____
_____
_____
_____

WHEN MUSCLE IS SHORTENED:
_____
_____
_____
_____

WHEN MUSCLE IS LENGTHENED:
_____
_____
_____
_____

HOW TO STRETCH THIS MUSCLE:
_____
_____

SYNERGIST(S):
_____
_____

ANTAGONIST(S):
_____
_____
_____
_____

NOTES: _____
_____
_____
_____
_____
_____

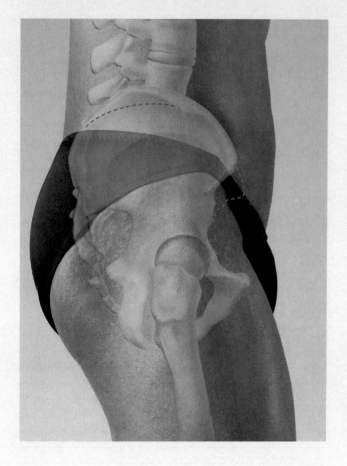

ORIGIN: _____

INSERTION: _____

ACTION(S): _____

NERVE: _____

ARTERIAL SUPPLY: _____

LOCATION AND/OR HOW TO PALPATE:
_____
_____
_____
_____
_____

WHEN MUSCLE IS SHORTENED:
_____
_____
_____
_____

WHEN MUSCLE IS LENGTHENED:
_____
_____
_____
_____

HOW TO STRETCH THIS MUSCLE:
_____
_____

SYNERGIST(S):
_____
_____

ANTAGONIST(S):
_____
_____
_____
_____

NOTES: _____
_____
_____
_____
_____
_____
_____

TENSOR FASCIA LATAE

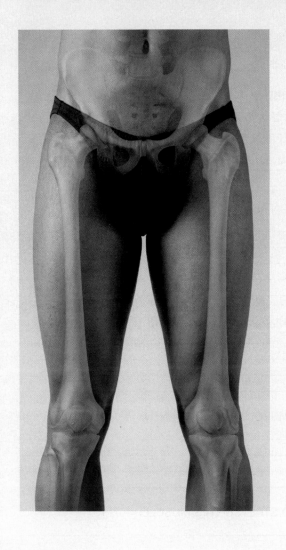

ORIGIN: _____

INSERTION: _____

ACTION(S): _____

NERVE: _____

ARTERIAL SUPPLY: _____

LOCATION AND/OR HOW TO PALPATE:
_____
_____
_____
_____
_____

WHEN MUSCLE IS SHORTENED:
_____
_____
_____
_____

WHEN MUSCLE IS LENGTHENED:
_____
_____
_____
_____

HOW TO STRETCH THIS MUSCLE:
_____
_____

SYNERGIST(S):
_____
_____

ANTAGONIST(S):
_____
_____
_____
_____

NOTES: _____
_____
_____
_____
_____
_____
_____

GLUTEUS MAXIMUS

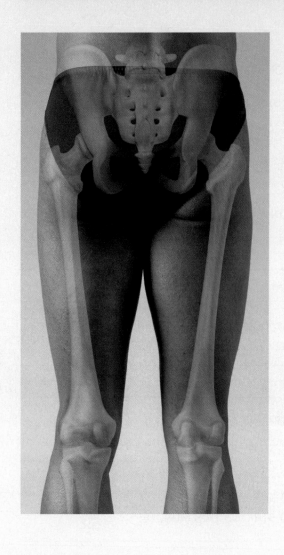

ORIGIN: _____

INSERTION: _____

ACTION(S): _____

NERVE: _____

ARTERIAL SUPPLY: _____

LOCATION AND/OR HOW TO PALPATE:
_____
_____
_____
_____
_____

WHEN MUSCLE IS SHORTENED:
_____
_____
_____
_____

WHEN MUSCLE IS LENGTHENED:
_____
_____
_____
_____

HOW TO STRETCH THIS MUSCLE:
_____
_____

SYNERGIST(S):
_____
_____

ANTAGONIST(S):
_____
_____
_____
_____

NOTES: _____
_____
_____
_____
_____
_____

HAMSTRINGS: SEMIMEMBRANOSUS

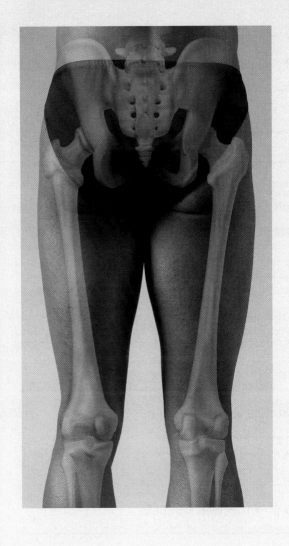

ORIGIN: _____

INSERTION: _____

ACTION(S): _____

NERVE: _____

ARTERIAL SUPPLY: _____

LOCATION AND/OR HOW TO PALPATE:
_____
_____
_____
_____
_____

WHEN MUSCLE IS SHORTENED:
_____
_____
_____
_____

WHEN MUSCLE IS LENGTHENED:
_____
_____
_____
_____

HOW TO STRETCH THIS MUSCLE:
_____
_____

SYNERGIST(S):
_____
_____

ANTAGONIST(S):
_____
_____
_____
_____

NOTES: _____
_____
_____
_____
_____
_____

HAMSTRINGS: SEMITENDINOSUS

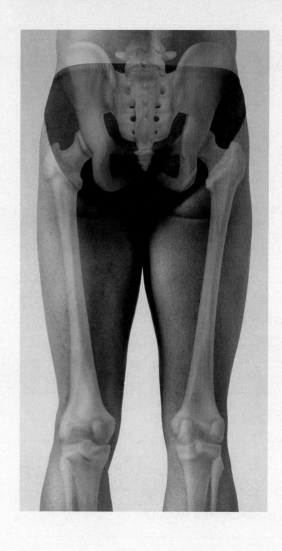

ORIGIN: _____

INSERTION: _____

ACTION(S): _____

NERVE: _____

ARTERIAL SUPPLY: _____

LOCATION AND/OR HOW TO PALPATE:
_____
_____
_____
_____

WHEN MUSCLE IS SHORTENED:
_____
_____
_____
_____

WHEN MUSCLE IS LENGTHENED:
_____
_____
_____
_____

HOW TO STRETCH THIS MUSCLE:
_____
_____

SYNERGIST(S):
_____
_____

ANTAGONIST(S):
_____
_____
_____
_____

NOTES: _____
_____
_____
_____
_____
_____

HAMSTRINGS: BICEPS FEMORIS

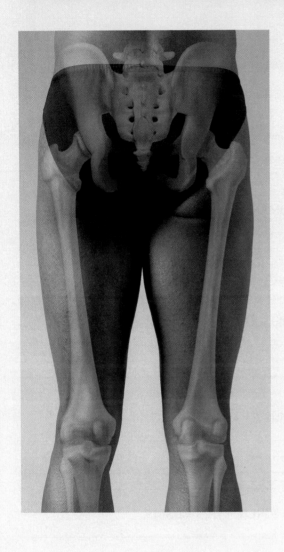

ORIGIN: _____

INSERTION: _____

ACTION(S): _____

NERVE: _____

ARTERIAL SUPPLY: _____

LOCATION AND/OR HOW TO PALPATE:
_____
_____
_____
_____
_____

WHEN MUSCLE IS SHORTENED:
_____
_____
_____
_____

WHEN MUSCLE IS LENGTHENED:
_____
_____
_____
_____

HOW TO STRETCH THIS MUSCLE:
_____
_____

SYNERGIST(S):
_____
_____

ANTAGONIST(S):
_____
_____
_____
_____

NOTES: _____
_____
_____
_____
_____
_____

ILIOPSOAS

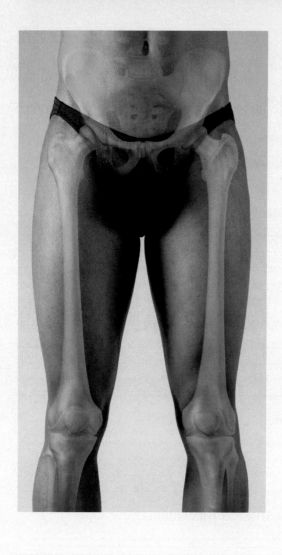

ORIGIN: _____

INSERTION: _____

ACTION(S): _____

NERVE: _____

ARTERIAL SUPPLY: _____

LOCATION AND/OR HOW TO PALPATE:

_____
_____
_____
_____
_____

WHEN MUSCLE IS SHORTENED:

_____
_____
_____
_____

WHEN MUSCLE IS LENGTHENED:

_____
_____
_____
_____

HOW TO STRETCH THIS MUSCLE:

_____
_____

SYNERGIST(S):

_____
_____

ANTAGONIST(S):

_____
_____
_____
_____

NOTES: _____
_____
_____
_____
_____
_____

QUADRICEPS GROUP: VASTUS INTERMEDIUS

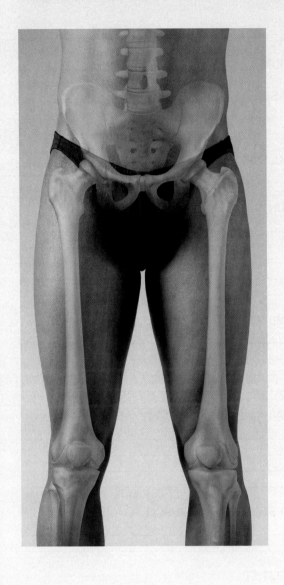

ORIGIN: _____

INSERTION: _____

ACTION(S): _____

NERVE: _____

ARTERIAL SUPPLY: _____

LOCATION AND/OR HOW TO PALPATE:

_____
_____
_____
_____
_____

WHEN MUSCLE IS SHORTENED:

_____
_____
_____
_____

WHEN MUSCLE IS LENGTHENED:

_____
_____
_____
_____

HOW TO STRETCH THIS MUSCLE:

_____
_____

SYNERGIST(S):

_____
_____

ANTAGONIST(S):

_____
_____
_____
_____

NOTES: _____

_____
_____
_____
_____
_____
_____

QUADRICEPS GROUP: VASTUS MEDIALIS

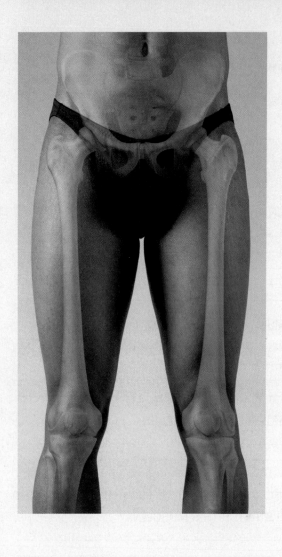

ORIGIN: _____

INSERTION: _____

ACTION(S): _____

NERVE: _____

ARTERIAL SUPPLY: _____

LOCATION AND/OR HOW TO PALPATE:
_____
_____
_____
_____
_____

WHEN MUSCLE IS SHORTENED:
_____
_____
_____
_____

WHEN MUSCLE IS LENGTHENED:
_____
_____
_____
_____

HOW TO STRETCH THIS MUSCLE:
_____
_____

SYNERGIST(S):
_____
_____

ANTAGONIST(S):
_____
_____
_____
_____

NOTES: _____
_____
_____
_____
_____
_____
_____

QUADRICEPS GROUP: VASTUS LATERALIS

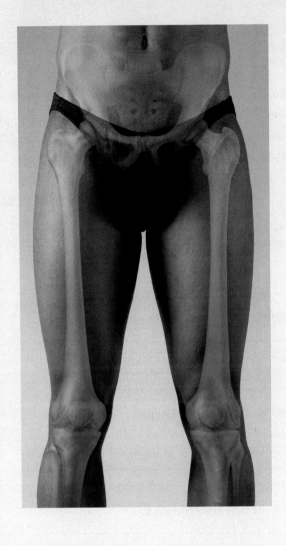

ORIGIN: _____

INSERTION: _____

ACTION(S): _____

NERVE: _____

ARTERIAL SUPPLY: _____

LOCATION AND/OR HOW TO PALPATE:

_____
_____
_____
_____
_____

WHEN MUSCLE IS SHORTENED:

_____
_____
_____
_____

WHEN MUSCLE IS LENGTHENED:

_____
_____
_____
_____

HOW TO STRETCH THIS MUSCLE:

_____
_____

SYNERGIST(S):

_____
_____

ANTAGONIST(S):

_____
_____
_____
_____

NOTES: _____

_____
_____
_____
_____
_____
_____
_____

QUADRICEPS GROUP: RECTUS FEMORIS

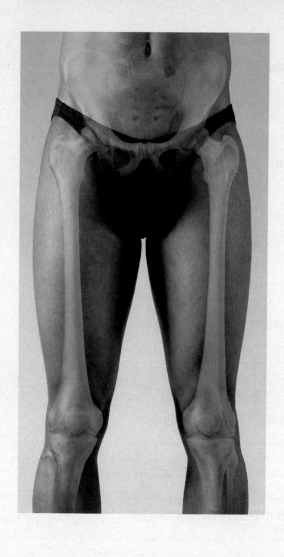

ORIGIN: _____

INSERTION: _____

ACTION(S): _____

NERVE: _____

ARTERIAL SUPPLY: _____

LOCATION AND/OR HOW TO PALPATE:

_____
_____
_____
_____
_____

WHEN MUSCLE IS SHORTENED:

_____
_____
_____
_____

WHEN MUSCLE IS LENGTHENED:

_____
_____
_____
_____

HOW TO STRETCH THIS MUSCLE:

_____
_____

SYNERGIST(S):

_____
_____

ANTAGONIST(S):

_____
_____
_____
_____

NOTES: _____
_____
_____
_____
_____
_____

SARTORIUS

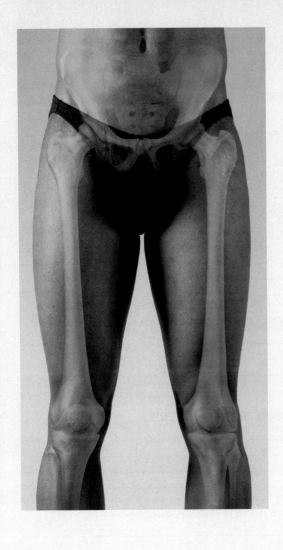

ORIGIN: _____

INSERTION: _____

ACTION(S): _____

NERVE: _____

ARTERIAL SUPPLY: _____

LOCATION AND/OR HOW TO PALPATE:
_____
_____
_____
_____
_____

WHEN MUSCLE IS SHORTENED:
_____
_____
_____
_____

WHEN MUSCLE IS LENGTHENED:
_____
_____
_____
_____

HOW TO STRETCH THIS MUSCLE:
_____
_____

SYNERGIST(S):
_____
_____

ANTAGONIST(S):
_____
_____
_____
_____

NOTES: _____
_____
_____
_____
_____
_____
_____

POPLITEUS

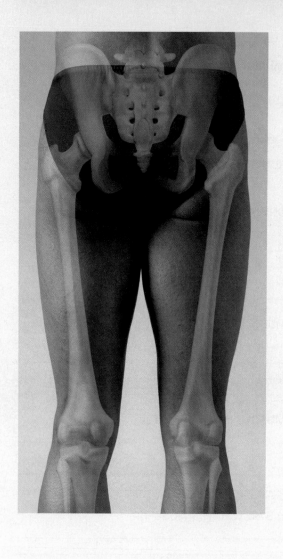

ORIGIN: _____

INSERTION: _____

ACTION(S): _____

NERVE: _____

ARTERIAL SUPPLY: _____

LOCATION AND/OR HOW TO PALPATE:

_____
_____
_____
_____
_____

WHEN MUSCLE IS SHORTENED:

_____
_____
_____
_____

WHEN MUSCLE IS LENGTHENED:

_____
_____
_____
_____

HOW TO STRETCH THIS MUSCLE:

_____
_____

SYNERGIST(S):

_____
_____

ANTAGONIST(S):

_____
_____
_____
_____

NOTES: _____
_____
_____
_____
_____
_____

PLANTARIS

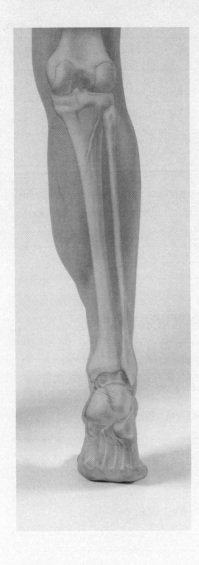

ORIGIN: _____

INSERTION: _____

ACTION(S): _____

NERVE: _____

ARTERIAL SUPPLY: _____

LOCATION AND/OR HOW TO PALPATE:
_____
_____
_____
_____
_____

WHEN MUSCLE IS SHORTENED:
_____
_____
_____
_____

WHEN MUSCLE IS LENGTHENED:
_____
_____
_____
_____

HOW TO STRETCH THIS MUSCLE:
_____
_____

SYNERGIST(S):
_____
_____

ANTAGONIST(S):
_____
_____
_____
_____

NOTES: _____
_____
_____
_____
_____
_____

GASTROCNEMIUS

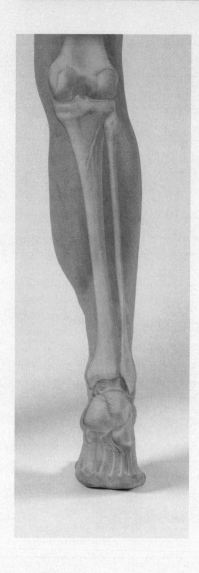

ORIGIN: _____

INSERTION: _____

ACTION(S): _____

NERVE: _____

ARTERIAL SUPPLY: _____

LOCATION AND/OR HOW TO PALPATE:
_____
_____
_____
_____

WHEN MUSCLE IS SHORTENED:
_____
_____
_____
_____

WHEN MUSCLE IS LENGTHENED:
_____
_____
_____
_____

HOW TO STRETCH THIS MUSCLE:
_____
_____

SYNERGIST(S):
_____
_____

ANTAGONIST(S):
_____
_____
_____
_____

NOTES: _____
_____
_____
_____
_____
_____

SOLEUS

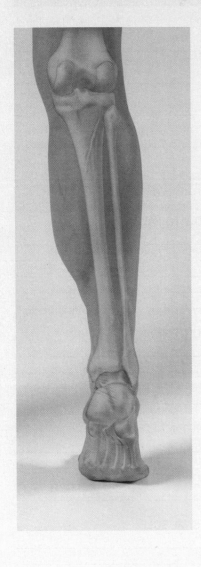

ORIGIN: _____

INSERTION: _____

ACTION(S): _____

NERVE: _____

ARTERIAL SUPPLY: _____

LOCATION AND/OR HOW TO PALPATE:
_____
_____
_____
_____
_____

WHEN MUSCLE IS SHORTENED:
_____
_____
_____
_____

WHEN MUSCLE IS LENGTHENED:
_____
_____
_____
_____

HOW TO STRETCH THIS MUSCLE:
_____
_____

SYNERGIST(S):
_____
_____

ANTAGONIST(S):
_____
_____
_____
_____

NOTES: _____
_____
_____
_____
_____
_____

TIBIALIS POSTERIOR

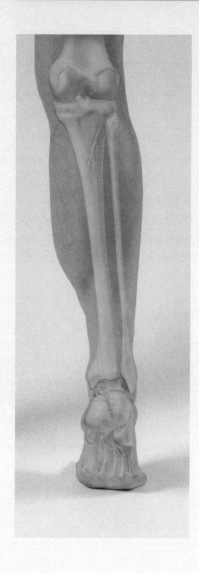

ORIGIN: _____

INSERTION: _____

ACTION(S): _____

NERVE: _____

ARTERIAL SUPPLY: _____

LOCATION AND/OR HOW TO PALPATE:

_____
_____
_____
_____

WHEN MUSCLE IS SHORTENED:

_____
_____
_____
_____

WHEN MUSCLE IS LENGTHENED:

_____
_____
_____
_____

HOW TO STRETCH THIS MUSCLE:

_____
_____

SYNERGIST(S):

_____
_____

ANTAGONIST(S):

_____
_____
_____
_____

NOTES: _____
_____
_____
_____
_____
_____

FLEXOR DIGITORUM LONGUS

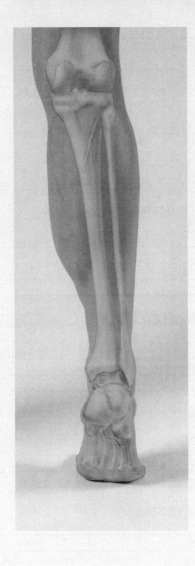

ORIGIN: _____

INSERTION: _____

ACTION(S): _____

NERVE: _____

ARTERIAL SUPPLY: _____

LOCATION AND/OR HOW TO PALPATE:
_____
_____
_____
_____
_____

WHEN MUSCLE IS SHORTENED:
_____
_____
_____
_____

WHEN MUSCLE IS LENGTHENED:
_____
_____
_____
_____

HOW TO STRETCH THIS MUSCLE:
_____
_____

SYNERGIST(S):
_____
_____

ANTAGONIST(S):
_____
_____
_____
_____

NOTES: _____
_____
_____
_____
_____
_____

FLEXOR HALLUCIS LONGUS

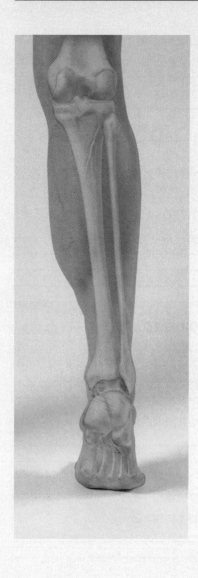

ORIGIN: _____

INSERTION: _____

ACTION(S): _____

NERVE: _____

ARTERIAL SUPPLY: _____

LOCATION AND/OR HOW TO PALPATE:
_____
_____
_____
_____
_____

WHEN MUSCLE IS SHORTENED:
_____
_____
_____
_____

WHEN MUSCLE IS LENGTHENED:
_____
_____
_____
_____

HOW TO STRETCH THIS MUSCLE:
_____
_____

SYNERGIST(S):
_____
_____

ANTAGONIST(S):
_____
_____
_____
_____

NOTES: _____
_____
_____
_____
_____
_____
_____

PERONEUS LONGUS

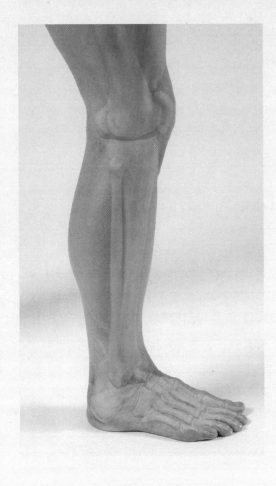

ORIGIN: _____

INSERTION: _____

ACTION(S): _____

NERVE: _____

ARTERIAL SUPPLY: _____

LOCATION AND/OR HOW TO PALPATE:
_____
_____
_____
_____
_____

WHEN MUSCLE IS SHORTENED:
_____
_____
_____
_____

WHEN MUSCLE IS LENGTHENED:
_____
_____
_____
_____

HOW TO STRETCH THIS MUSCLE:
_____
_____

SYNERGIST(S):
_____
_____

ANTAGONIST(S):
_____
_____
_____
_____

NOTES: _____
_____
_____
_____
_____
_____

PERONEUS BREVIS

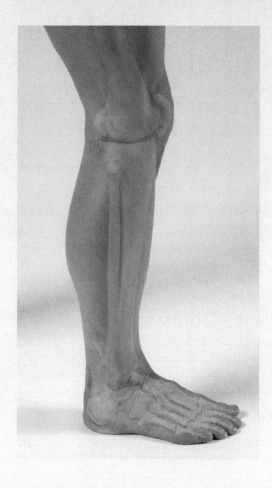

ORIGIN: _____

INSERTION: _____

ACTION(S): _____

NERVE: _____

ARTERIAL SUPPLY: _____

LOCATION AND/OR HOW TO PALPATE:
_____
_____
_____
_____
_____

WHEN MUSCLE IS SHORTENED:
_____
_____
_____
_____

WHEN MUSCLE IS LENGTHENED:
_____
_____
_____
_____

HOW TO STRETCH THIS MUSCLE:
_____
_____

SYNERGIST(S):
_____
_____

ANTAGONIST(S):
_____
_____
_____
_____

NOTES: _____
_____
_____
_____
_____
_____

PERONEUS TERTIUS

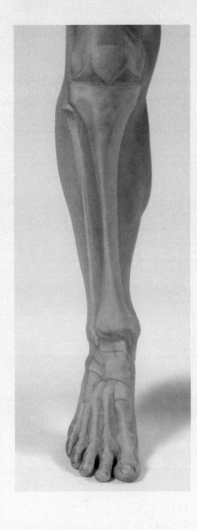

ORIGIN: _____

INSERTION: _____

ACTION(S): _____

NERVE: _____

ARTERIAL SUPPLY: _____

LOCATION AND/OR HOW TO PALPATE:
_____
_____
_____
_____
_____

WHEN MUSCLE IS SHORTENED:
_____
_____
_____
_____

WHEN MUSCLE IS LENGTHENED:
_____
_____
_____
_____

HOW TO STRETCH THIS MUSCLE:
_____
_____

SYNERGIST(S):
_____
_____

ANTAGONIST(S):
_____
_____
_____
_____

NOTES: _____
_____
_____
_____
_____
_____
_____

EXTENSOR DIGITORUM LONGUS

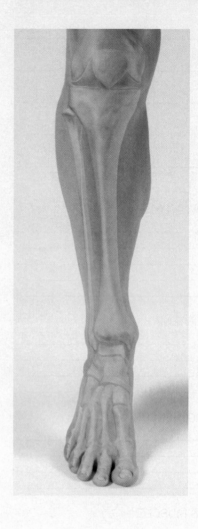

ORIGIN: _____

INSERTION: _____

ACTION(S): _____

NERVE: _____

ARTERIAL SUPPLY: _____

LOCATION AND/OR HOW TO PALPATE:
_____
_____
_____
_____
_____

WHEN MUSCLE IS SHORTENED:
_____
_____
_____
_____

WHEN MUSCLE IS LENGTHENED:
_____
_____
_____
_____

HOW TO STRETCH THIS MUSCLE:
_____
_____

SYNERGIST(S):
_____
_____

ANTAGONIST(S):
_____
_____
_____
_____

NOTES: _____
_____
_____
_____
_____
_____
_____

EXTENSOR HALLUCIS LONGUS

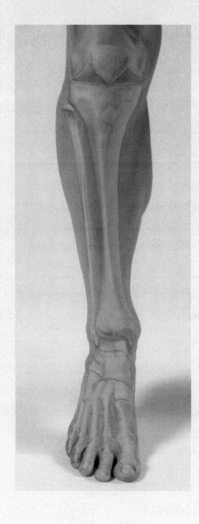

ORIGIN: _____

INSERTION: _____

ACTION(S): _____

NERVE: _____

ARTERIAL SUPPLY: _____

LOCATION AND/OR HOW TO PALPATE:

_____
_____
_____
_____
_____

WHEN MUSCLE IS SHORTENED:

_____
_____
_____
_____

WHEN MUSCLE IS LENGTHENED:

_____
_____
_____
_____

HOW TO STRETCH THIS MUSCLE:

_____
_____
_____

SYNERGIST(S):

_____
_____

ANTAGONIST(S):

_____
_____
_____
_____

NOTES: _____

_____
_____
_____
_____
_____
_____

TIBIALIS ANTERIOR

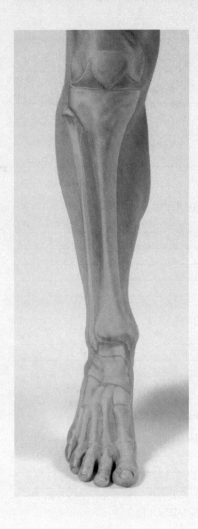

ORIGIN: _____

INSERTION: _____

ACTION(S): _____

NERVE: _____

ARTERIAL SUPPLY: _____

LOCATION AND/OR HOW TO PALPATE:
_____
_____
_____
_____
_____

WHEN MUSCLE IS SHORTENED:
_____
_____
_____
_____

WHEN MUSCLE IS LENGTHENED:
_____
_____
_____
_____

HOW TO STRETCH THIS MUSCLE:
_____
_____

SYNERGIST(S):
_____
_____

ANTAGONIST(S):
_____
_____
_____
_____

NOTES: _____
_____
_____
_____
_____
_____
_____

DORSAL INTEROSSEI

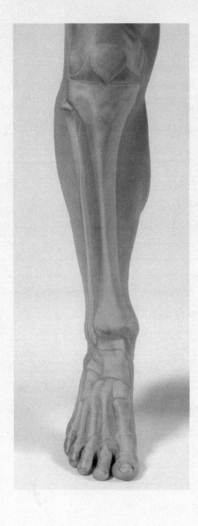

ORIGIN: _____

INSERTION: _____

ACTION(S): _____

NERVE: _____

ARTERIAL SUPPLY: _____

LOCATION AND/OR HOW TO PALPATE:
_____
_____
_____
_____
_____

WHEN MUSCLE IS SHORTENED:
_____
_____
_____
_____

WHEN MUSCLE IS LENGTHENED:
_____
_____
_____
_____

HOW TO STRETCH THIS MUSCLE:
_____
_____

SYNERGIST(S):
_____
_____

ANTAGONIST(S):
_____
_____
_____
_____

NOTES: _____
_____
_____
_____
_____
_____
_____

PLANTAR INTEROSSEI

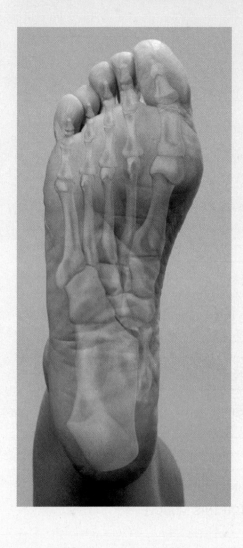

ORIGIN: _____

INSERTION: _____

ACTION(S): _____

NERVE: _____

ARTERIAL SUPPLY: _____

LOCATION AND/OR HOW TO PALPATE:
_____
_____
_____
_____
_____

WHEN MUSCLE IS SHORTENED:
_____
_____
_____
_____

WHEN MUSCLE IS LENGTHENED:
_____
_____
_____
_____

HOW TO STRETCH THIS MUSCLE:
_____
_____

SYNERGIST(S):
_____
_____

ANTAGONIST(S):
_____
_____
_____
_____

NOTES: _____
_____
_____
_____
_____
_____

FLEXOR HALLUCIS BREVIS

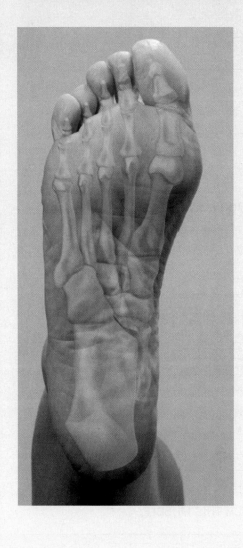

ORIGIN: _____

INSERTION: _____

ACTION(S): _____

NERVE: _____

ARTERIAL SUPPLY: _____

LOCATION AND/OR HOW TO PALPATE:
_____
_____
_____
_____
_____

WHEN MUSCLE IS SHORTENED:
_____
_____
_____
_____

WHEN MUSCLE IS LENGTHENED:
_____
_____
_____
_____

HOW TO STRETCH THIS MUSCLE:
_____
_____

SYNERGIST(S):
_____
_____

ANTAGONIST(S):
_____
_____
_____
_____

NOTES: _____
_____
_____
_____
_____
_____

ADDUCTOR HALLUCIS

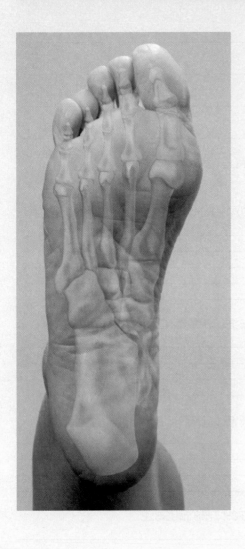

ORIGIN: _____

INSERTION: _____

ACTION(S): _____

NERVE: _____

ARTERIAL SUPPLY: _____

LOCATION AND/OR HOW TO PALPATE:
_____
_____
_____
_____
_____

WHEN MUSCLE IS SHORTENED:
_____
_____
_____
_____

WHEN MUSCLE IS LENGTHENED:
_____
_____
_____
_____

HOW TO STRETCH THIS MUSCLE:
_____
_____
_____

SYNERGIST(S):
_____
_____

ANTAGONIST(S):
_____
_____
_____
_____

NOTES: _____
_____
_____
_____
_____
_____

FLEXOR DIGITI MINIMI BREVIS

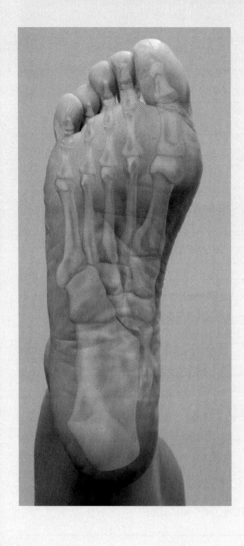

ORIGIN: _____

INSERTION: _____

ACTION(S): _____

NERVE: _____

ARTERIAL SUPPLY: _____

LOCATION AND/OR HOW TO PALPATE:
_____
_____
_____
_____

WHEN MUSCLE IS SHORTENED:
_____
_____
_____
_____

WHEN MUSCLE IS LENGTHENED:
_____
_____
_____
_____

HOW TO STRETCH THIS MUSCLE:
_____
_____

SYNERGIST(S):
_____
_____

ANTAGONIST(S):
_____
_____
_____

NOTES: _____
_____
_____
_____
_____
_____

LUMBRICALS

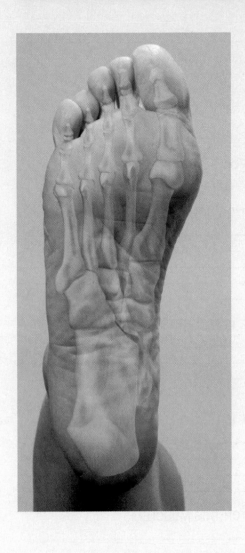

ORIGIN: _____

INSERTION: _____

ACTION(S): _____

NERVE: _____

ARTERIAL SUPPLY: _____

LOCATION AND/OR HOW TO PALPATE:
_____
_____
_____
_____
_____

WHEN MUSCLE IS SHORTENED:
_____
_____
_____
_____

WHEN MUSCLE IS LENGTHENED:
_____
_____
_____
_____

HOW TO STRETCH THIS MUSCLE:
_____
_____

SYNERGIST(S):
_____
_____

ANTAGONIST(S):
_____
_____
_____
_____

NOTES: _____
_____
_____
_____
_____
_____

QUADRATUS PLANTAE

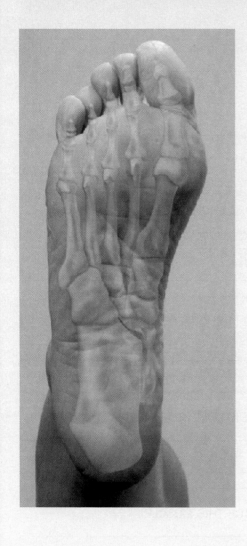

ORIGIN: _____

INSERTION: _____

ACTION(S): _____

NERVE: _____

ARTERIAL SUPPLY: _____

LOCATION AND/OR HOW TO PALPATE:
_____
_____
_____
_____
_____

WHEN MUSCLE IS SHORTENED:
_____
_____
_____
_____

WHEN MUSCLE IS LENGTHENED:
_____
_____
_____
_____

HOW TO STRETCH THIS MUSCLE:
_____
_____

SYNERGIST(S):
_____
_____

ANTAGONIST(S):
_____
_____
_____

NOTES: _____
_____
_____
_____
_____
_____

ABDUCTOR HALLUCIS

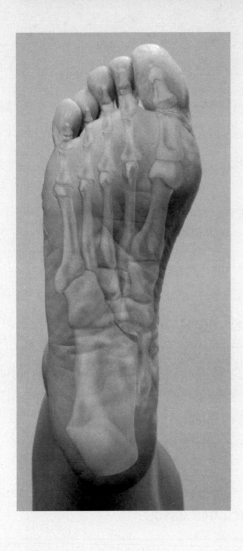

ORIGIN: _____

INSERTION: _____

ACTION(S): _____

NERVE: _____

ARTERIAL SUPPLY: _____

LOCATION AND/OR HOW TO PALPATE:
_____
_____
_____
_____
_____

WHEN MUSCLE IS SHORTENED:
_____
_____
_____
_____

WHEN MUSCLE IS LENGTHENED:
_____
_____
_____
_____

HOW TO STRETCH THIS MUSCLE:
_____
_____

SYNERGIST(S):
_____
_____

ANTAGONIST(S):
_____
_____
_____
_____

NOTES: _____
_____
_____
_____
_____
_____

FLEXOR DIGITORUM BREVIS

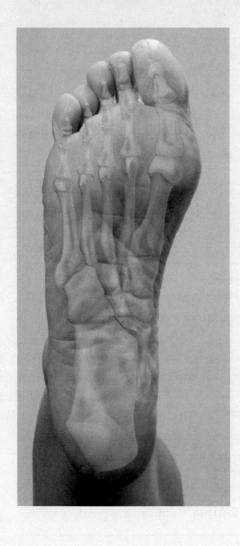

ORIGIN: _____

INSERTION: _____

ACTION(S): _____

NERVE: _____

ARTERIAL SUPPLY: _____

LOCATION AND/OR HOW TO PALPATE:

_____
_____
_____
_____

WHEN MUSCLE IS SHORTENED:

_____
_____
_____
_____

WHEN MUSCLE IS LENGTHENED:

_____
_____
_____
_____

HOW TO STRETCH THIS MUSCLE:

_____
_____

SYNERGIST(S):

_____
_____

ANTAGONIST(S):

_____
_____
_____
_____

NOTES: _____

_____
_____
_____
_____
_____

ABDUCTOR DIGITI MINIMI

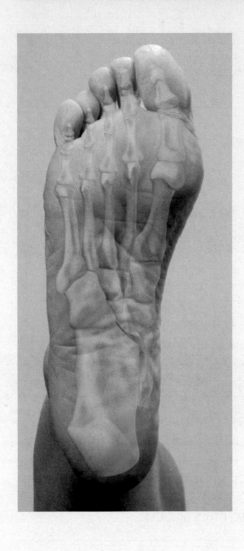

ORIGIN: _____

INSERTION: _____

ACTION(S): _____

NERVE: _____

ARTERIAL SUPPLY: _____

LOCATION AND/OR HOW TO PALPATE:
_____
_____
_____
_____
_____

WHEN MUSCLE IS SHORTENED:
_____
_____
_____
_____
_____

WHEN MUSCLE IS LENGTHENED:
_____
_____
_____
_____
_____

HOW TO STRETCH THIS MUSCLE:
_____
_____
_____

SYNERGIST(S):
_____
_____

ANTAGONIST(S):
_____
_____
_____
_____

NOTES: _____
_____
_____
_____
_____
_____

Palpation Exercises

Palpation of the muscles is important to reinforce their locations and to prepare for the application of muscle knowledge to massage therapy settings.

Palpation Exercise #1

This palpation exercise will require you to palpate the six deep lateral rotators of the hip and the hip adductors.

1. **Piriformis:** Have your partner lie prone, and find the greater sciatic notch. You can get a close idea of where the greater sciatic notch is located by bringing your partner's heel to his or her buttocks. The area where the heel contacts the buttocks will be the general location. To locate piriformis very specifically, find the PSIS, move about 2 inches inferiorly, and begin to press in through the thick gluteus maximus muscle, working your way laterally toward the greater trochanter. Piriformis lies between the greater sciatic notch and the greater trochanter. You can tell that you have found piriformis when you feel a thin strip of dense tissue, deep to gluteus maximus. What does this muscle have to do with sciatica?

2. The other lateral rotators in the group of the six all run from the ischium and obturator foramen toward the greater trochanter. Their names are the gemellus inferior and superior, obturator internus and externus, and quadratus femoris. Palpate this general area. The individual muscles are difficult to isolate.

3. **Adductors of the thigh:** Have your partner lie supine. Ask your partner to adduct the thigh against resistance by placing your hand on the medial thigh just proximal to the knee and asking your partner to press his or her thigh into your hand. Can you feel the adductors tighten? Remind yourself of the names of all five adductors, and note their basic locations, beginning with adductor magnus, the deepest and largest thigh adductor, which inserts quite distally on the linea aspera of the femur. Recall adductor longus and brevis, which lie more proximal in the medial thigh. Recall that pectineus is located within the femoral triangle and that this is an endangerment site. Finally, end by reviewing gracilis, the slender, most medial and superficial muscle of the thigh. The proximal attachments of the hip adductor muscles are in a sensitive area, as they are so close to the genitals. It is possible to instruct your client to perform friction to the tendons of origin of the adductors (near the pubis) as homework, rather than working in that area yourself, as it may not be appropriate for you to address this area.

    Recall the insertion of gracilis? What actions, other than adduction, can pectineus and gracilis perform?

Review

List three everyday actions you do that involve adduction of the femur:

1. _____
2. _____
3. _____

List three everyday actions you do that involve lateral rotation of the hip:

1. _____
2. _____
3. _____

Palpation Exercise #2

This palpation exercise will require you to palpate the gluteus muscles and tensor fascia latae.

1. **Gluteus medius and gluteus minimus:** Palpate gluteus medius. Have your partner in a supine position. Palpate just inferior to the iliac crest from just posterior to the ASIS over to the PSIS. Find the greater trochanter. Gluteus medius is a triangular-shaped muscle that lies between the iliac crest and the greater trochanter. Pressing right into the external surface of the ilium allows us to apply friction and direct pressure to these muscles with ease. All of gluteus minimus is deep to gluteus medius, and much of gluteus medius is deep to gluteus maximus. Find the small section of gluteus medius (just inferior to the anterior iliac crest) that is superficial. You can ask your partner to abduct his or her thigh to feel for contraction of gluteus medius and gluteus minimis.

2. **Gluteus maximus:** Have your partner lie prone. Find the lateral border of the sacrum and the posterior iliac crest. You have found most of the origin of gluteus maximus. Gluteus maximus inserts into the IT band and the gluteal tuberosity on the proximal, posterior femur. Gluteus maximus is entirely superficial and thus easy to palpate and massage. It is a thick, strong muscle and other than the quadriceps group, is the largest muscle in the body.

3. **Tensor fascia latae:** Have your partner lie supine. Find the iliac crest just posterior to the ASIS. TFL is located between this portion of the iliac crest and the IT band. If your partner has a tight TFL, it is probably a good idea to massage the IT band.

Palpation Exercise #3

This palpation exercise will require you to palpate the hamstrings and their related bone markings.

Bones/Bony Landmarks

1. **Ischial tuberosity:** Find this bone marking on the inferior ischium. It is sometimes called the "sits" bone, as we sit on our ischial tuberosities.

2. **Pes anserinus:** Revisit this flat area on the proximal, anterior, medial tibia.

3. **Head of fibula:** Find this rounded bone marking on the most proximal aspect of the fibula.

4. **Proximal, posterior, medial tibia:** Look for the insertion spot of semimembranosus. Can you feel the tendon of insertion, deep and just medial to the tendon of semitendinosus in the medial posterior knee area? Can you trace the tendon as it approaches its spot of insertion on the tibia?

Muscles

1. **Semimembranosus and semitendinosus:** Palpate the medial posterior thigh. Offer these muscles a nice pétrissage massage. Remember that semimembranosus is deep to semitendinosus. Semitendinosus inserts at pes anserinus.

2. **Biceps femoris:** Palpate the lateral aspect of the posterior thigh. This muscle runs from the ischial tuberosity to the head of the fibula.

3. After you have massaged your partner's hamstrings, have him or her turn over into a supine position and stretch the hamstrings. Why must the knee be extended (at least somewhat) to stretch the hamstrings? Make sure you check in with your partner, so you do not stretch the muscles too far.

Palpation Exercise #4

This palpation exercise will require you to palpate the iliopsoas, the quads, and related bone markings.

Bones/Bony Landmarks

1. **Lesser trochanter:** Note the location of the lesser trochanter on the proximal, medial femur. Why is this bone marking not palpable?

2. **ASIS and AIIS:** Once again, palpate the ASIS. Recall that the AIIS is inferior to the ASIS, but not easily palpable due to the inward curve of the ilium between the ASIS and AIIS, as well as the soft tissue in this area. But note the location of this bone marking, even though you cannot actually feel it.

3. **Linea aspera:** Recall the rough line that runs almost the entire length of the posterior femur. This bone marking is impossible to palpate, as it is covered by the hamstring muscles, most notably biceps femoris.

4. **Tibial tuberosity:** Find the patella and move directly distal about an inch or an inch and a half. Feel for the rough bump that is the tibial tuberosity. The quadriceps muscles insert here.

5. **Pes anserinus:** Revisit this flat area on the proximal, anterior, medial tibia once more. Look at the colored illustration of origin and insertion sites earlier in this chapter. Find the area indicating insertions of gracilis, semitendinosus, and sartorius. Palpate this relatively flat area on the medial, proximal anterior tibia.

Muscles

1. **Psoas major:** Work with your partner in a supine position. The psoas major originates on the transverse processes and bodies of the lumbar vertebrae and T12. It inserts on the lesser trochanter. Psoas major is deep to abdominal muscles and organs. Find the navel and ASIS, and slowly press with your fingertips along the line between these two landmarks. You may have to adjust the angle of your pressure or direction of your fingers to move through digestive organs as you work your way to the psoas major muscle. Press in on your partner's exhalations. When you feel you have reached the depth required to contact psoas major, ask your partner to flex his or her hip to see if you can feel fibers contract. *Note:* Palpation/massage of psoas major must be done with great care and clear communication with the client. If the client feels pain, stop your work.

2. **Iliacus:** Have your partner lie supine. Iliacus fills the iliac fossa on the anterior aspect of the ilium and inserts at the lesser trochanter. Find the anterior iliac spine between the ASIS and AIIS. Curl your fingers around the anterior iliac spine, pressing gently and medially into the iliac fossa. Ask your partner to flex his or her hip and try to feel the fibers contract.

3. **Quadriceps: Rectus Femoris:** Have your partner lie supine. The rectus femoris originates on the AIIS and just superior to the acetabulum. Rectus femoris inserts on the tibial tuberosity. The muscle is located superficially in the anterior thigh. Trace the AIIS to the tibial tuberosity, and you have traced rectus femoris. Again, ask your partner to flex his or her hip and feel for the contracting fibers, distal to the AIIS and in the anterior thigh.

4. **Quadriceps: Vastus Medialis:** Have your partner lie supine. The lateral portion of **vastus medialis** is deep to rectus femoris. Palpate just medially to rectus femoris. The origin of this muscle is the linea aspera on the posterior femur. The muscle wraps around the medial side of the femur, anterior to the adductors.

   It is possible to distinguish vastus medialis from the hip adductor muscles by isometrically contracting the quadriceps group. Have your partner flex his or her knee a bit. Then, position your hand on the anterior distal leg and have your partner press his or her anterior leg into your hand. This will cause the quadriceps to tighten, but will not affect the adductors. You should be able to feel the distinction between the contracted quadriceps and relaxed adductor muscles.

5. **Quadriceps: Vastus Lateralis:** Have your partner lie supine. The medial portion of vastus lateralis is deep to rectus femoris, but the lateral aspect is easily palpable. Remember that this muscle makes up the anterolateral aspect of the thigh.

Palpation Exercise #5

This palpation exercise will require you to palpate the posterior leg muscles and relevant bone markings that are attachment sites.

Bones/Bony Landmarks

Palpate the following bone markings:

1. Posterior aspect of the epicondyles of the femur. Feel for the rounded distal ends on the medial and lateral sides of the femur. Palpate posteriorly, noting the tendons of insertion of the hamstrings. Continue to move posteriorly, and palpate gently into the edges of the popliteal fossa to feel for the attachment sites of gastrocnemius.

2. Calcaneus and Achilles tendon: Find the thick Achilles tendon on the posterior, distal leg. Trace the tendon to its attachment point on the posterior calcaneus.

3. Posterior head and shaft of the fibula: Find the head of the fibula at the bone's most proximal aspect. Palpate just distal to the posterior aspect of the head of the fibula.

4. Proximal, posterior tibia (review the location of the soleal line)

Muscles

Gastrocnemius is the most superficial muscle in the posterior leg. It is a fleshy muscle with two heads. It is easy to pétrissage. Deep to gastrocnemius is soleus, a flat muscle whose inferior aspect is more distal than gastrocnemius. Plantaris, a variably present muscle is located in the posterior knee area. The tendon of insertion of plantaris lies between gastrocnemius and soleus. This tendon is long and extends distally to join the Achilles tendon and attach to the calcaneus. Deep to soleus are the muscles of the deep, posterior leg compartment.

1. **Gastrocnemius and soleus:** Have your partner lie prone with feet hanging off the end of the table. Palpate gently in the posterior knee area to find the most proximal portion of gastrocnemius between the hamstring's tendons of insertion. Trace the muscle distally toward the Achilles tendon. Ask your partner to plantarflex while you provide resistance. (You can lean gently into the bottom of the foot.) Palpate the central part of the posterior leg, feeling for both bellies of the gastrocnemius and the point at which they join. This point can be extremely tender. Feel distal to gastrocnemius to find soleus, which creates the contour of the distal leg. Palpate the Achilles tendon, the insertion of both muscles. Friction to the Achilles tendon can be helpful to clients who walk, run, or play sports. Make sure you hold the tendon in a taut position before providing friction to it.

2. **Soleus:** Test for flexibility of the soleus. Have your partner lie prone with knee flexed to 90 degrees. Ask your partner to dorsiflex the foot as much as possible. How is the range of motion? Why is restriction of dorsiflexion in this position likely to be caused by a shortened soleus muscle?

3. **Plantaris:** Palpate the plantaris, if your partner has one. Have your partner lie prone with knee flexed. *Gently* press into the popliteal space, between the two heads of the gastrocnemius muscle. Feel for muscle fibers running from the lateral epicondyle of the femur distally and medially. Remember that this muscle also inserts into the calcaneus via the Achilles tendon.

4. **Tibialis posterior, flexor digitorum longus, and flexor hallucis longus:** These muscles make up the deep, posterior leg compartment. They are difficult to isolate, but can be addressed by massaging the posterior leg, with the intention of affecting the deepest muscles.

Palpation Exercise #6

This palpation exercise will require you to palpate the peroneal muscles, anterior leg muscles, and relevant bone markings.

Bones/Bony Landmarks

1. Find the origin and insertion sites of all six muscles listed below in the illustration provided earlier in the chapter.

2. Note the location on the fibula of each of the peroneal's origins. Find the insertions of the peroneals on the foot.

3. Find the origin of extensor hallucis longus on the fibula and the interosseus membrane. Find the origin of extensor digitorum longus on the anterior fibula, tibia, and interosseus membrane. Find the origin of tibialis anterior on the anterior tibia and interosseus membrane. Find the insertion spots of these three muscles on the foot.

Muscles

1. **Peroneus longus and brevis:** Have your partner lie supine. The peroneus longus runs from the head of the fibula distally. The tendon of insertion passes posterior to the lateral malleolus and across the plantar surface of the foot to the base of the first metatarsal and medial cuneiform. The bulk of the muscle is between the head of the fibula and the lateral malleolus. As you palpate this region, have your partner evert against resistance, so that you can feel the muscle fibers tighten. The peroneus brevis is deep to the peroneus longus, running from the lateral shaft of the fibula to the fifth metatarsal. It is difficult to distinguish the fibers of these two muscles. Try to feel where both tendons pass behind the lateral malleolus.

2. **Peroneus tertius:** The peroneus tertius arises from the distal, anterior fibula and passes in front of the lateral malleolus to insert right near the brevis on the fifth metatarsal. Try to palpate the tendon of this muscle on the dorsal surface of the fifth metatarsal while everting and dorsiflexing.

3. **Extensor hallucis longus:** Have your partner lie supine. Look at the dorsal surface of the foot and note the tendon that heads for the big toe. This muscle is deep in the anterior leg compartment, which is located between the lateral tibia and the fibula. It is difficult to distinguish the muscles within the anterior leg compartment.

4. **Extensor digitorum longus:** Have your partner lie supine. Look at the dorsal surface of the foot and note the four tendons heading for the four lateral toes. This muscle is palpable in the most lateral aspect of the anterior leg compartment. However, it can be difficult to isolate.

5. **Tibialis anterior:** Have your partner lie supine. Palpate the medial side of the tibia, where there is little muscle. Move to the lateral aspect of the tibia and sink into the belly of the muscle. Tibialis anterior is the most superficial muscle in the anterior leg compartment. The tendon passes medially and inserts at the base of the first metatarsal and medial cuneiform.

Palpation Exercise #7

This palpation exercise will require you to palpate the intrinsic foot muscles. These all support longitudinal arches.

1. **Abductor hallucis:** Have your partner lie supine. Press into the tissue from the medial side of the heel to the medial side of the big toe.

2. **Flexor digitorum brevis:** Have your partner lie supine. Press into the plantar surface of the heel and move distally to the four lateral toes.

3. **Abductor digiti minimi:** Have your partner lie supine. Press into the tissue from the middle of the calcaneus to the lateral aspect of the fifth digit.

As you further palpate/massage your partner's foot, please review the following:

Deep to layer one lies layer two:

1. Lumbricals arise from the tendon of flexor digitorum longus and insert into the bases of the proximal phalanges and the extensor expansion. Lumbricals flex the MP joints and extend the PIP and DIP joints.

2. Quadratus plantae runs from the calcaneus to the tendon of flexor digitorum longus. This muscle helps flex the toes by adjusting the angle of pull on its tendon of insertion.

Deep to layer two is layer three:

1. Adductor hallucis adducts the big toe and supports the transverse arch of the foot.

2. Flexor hallucis brevis flexes the big toe.

3. Flexor digiti minimi (brevis) flexes the fifth digit.

Deep to layer three is layer four (deepest layer):

1. Plantar interossei lie deep between the metatarsals on the plantar surface of the foot and adduct the toes.

2. Dorsal interossei lie between the metatarsals on the dorsal side of the foot and abduct the toes.

Review

1. Palpate the iliac crest. What bone contains this crest? What three bones comprise the hip bones? What muscles attach to the iliac crest? Find the ASIS and PSIS.

2. Palpate/massage the adductors of the hip. What are their names? What is their collective origin and insertion? What is different about gracilis?

3. Palpate/massage your partner's hamstrings. What are the three names of the hamstrings? Where is their common origin spot? Where does each insert? How do you stretch them?

4. Palpate/massage the gastrocnemius and soleus. Review their actions. Can you stretch them independently of each other?

Clay Work Exercises

These exercises help reinforce names and locations of muscles. They require the use of small plastic skeletons and clay. In each exercise below, create each of the listed muscles out of clay, one at a time, and attach it to the plastic skeleton where appropriate. Also, list the origin, insertion, and action of each muscle in the spaces provided. Share your understanding of the muscles with your partner as you build them.

Clay Work Exercise #1: Piriformis and Hip Adductors

Muscle Name	Origin	Insertion	Action(s)	Location
1. Piriformis				
2. Adductor Magnus				
3. Adductor Longus				
4. Adductor Brevis				
5. Pectineus				
6. Gracilis				

Clay Work Exercise #2: Gluteal Region

Muscle Name	Origin	Insertion	Action(s)	Location
1. Gluteus Minimus				
2. Gluteus Medius				
3. Tensor Fascia Latae				
4. Gluteus Maximus				

Clay Work Exercise #3: Hamstrings, Quadriceps, Iliopsoas, and Sartorius

Muscle Name	Origin	Insertion	Action(s)	Location
1. Semimembranosus				
2. Semitendinosus				
3. Biceps Femoris				
5. Iliopsoas				
6. Vastus Intermedius				
7. Vastus Medialis				
8. Vastus Lateralis				
9. Rectus Femoris				
10. Sartorius				

Clay Work Exercise #4: Muscles of the Leg

Muscle Name	Origin	Insertion	Action(s)	Location
1. Popliteus				
2. Soleus				
3. Plantaris				
4. Gastrocnemius				
5. Tibialis Posterior				
6. Flexor Digitorum Longus				
7. Flexor Hallucis Longus				
8. Peroneus Tertius				
9. Peroneus Brevis				
10. Peroneus Longus				
11. Extensor Digitorum Longus				
12. Extensor Hallucis Longus				
13. Tibialis Anterior				

Clay Work Exercise #5: Intrinsic Foot Muscles

Muscle Name	Origin	Insertion	Action(s)	Location
1. Dorsal Interossei				
2. Palmar Interossei				
3. Adductor Hallucis				
4. Flexor Hallucis Brevis				
5. Flexor Digiti Minimi Brevis				
6. Lumbricals				
7. Quadratus Plantae				
8. Abductor Hallucis				
9. Flexor Digitorum Brevis				
10. Abductor Digiti Minimi				

Case Study Exercises

Case Study #1

A client comes into your office, and you notice that she has an anterior pelvic tilt.

What muscles might be shortened and contributing to this issue?

_____
_____
_____

What muscles might be lengthened and contributing to this problem?

_____
_____
_____

Case Study #2

A client comes in to your office. As you observe his standing posture, you notice that his feet are not pointing forward, but rather they point to the sides (hip lateral rotation).

What muscles might be shortened and contributing to this issue?

_____
_____
_____

What muscles might be lengthened and contributing to this problem?

_____
_____
_____

Case Study #3

Your client lets you know that she cannot fully flex her knee.

What muscles might be shortened and contributing to this issue?

_____
_____
_____

What muscles might be lengthened and contributing to this problem?

_____
_____
_____

Case Study #4

The outsides of your clients' shoes are noticeably more worn than the medial or inner sides. What muscles might be shortened and contributing to this phenomenon?

_____
_____
_____

What muscles might be lengthened and contributing to this phenomenon?

_____
_____
_____

Case Study #5

Your client has limited ability to fully abduct his thighs.

What muscles might be shortened and contributing to this issue?

_____
_____
_____

What muscles might be lengthened and contributing to this problem?

_____
_____
_____

Case Study #6

Your client has limited ability to dorsiflex her ankle.

What muscles might be shortened and contributing to this issue?

_____
_____
_____

What muscles might be lengthened and contributing to this problem?

_____
_____
_____

Review Exercises

These review exercises help you to recall what you have learned in this chapter and reinforce your learning.

Review Charts to Study

Piriformis and Adductors of Thigh

Muscle Name	Origin	Insertion	Action(s)	Location
Piriformis	Anterior sacrum	Greater trochanter	Lateral rotation of hip	Deep buttock region
Adductor Magnus	Inferior pubic ramus and ischial tuberosity	Linea aspera of femur	Adduction of hip	Medial thigh
Adductor Longus	Anterior pubis	Linea aspera	Adduction of hip	Medial thigh
Adductor Brevis	Anterior pubis	Linea aspera	Adduction of hip	Medial thigh
Pectineus	Anterior pubic ramus	Linea aspera	Flexion and adduction of hip	Medial thigh
Gracilis	Anterior pubis	Pes anserinus	Adduction of hip, flexion of knee, and medial rotation of knee	Medial thigh (most superficial, medial thigh muscle)

Gluteal Region

Muscle Name	Origin	Insertion	Action(s)	Location
Gluteus Minimus	Posterior or external ilium	Greater trochanter	Abduction and medial rotation of the hip	Lateral hip
Gluteus Medius	Posterior or external ilium	Greater trochanter	Abduction and medial rotation of the hip	Lateral hip
Tensor Fascia Latae	ASIS and anterior iliac crest	Iliotibial band	Abduction, medial rotation, and flexion of the hip; helps stabilize knee	Anterolateral hip
Gluteus Maximus	Posterior ilium and sacrum	Gluteal tuberosity and iliotibial band	Extension and lateral rotation of the hip	Superficial buttock region

Hamstrings, Quadriceps, Iliopsoas, and Sartorius

Muscle Name	Origin	Insertion	Action(s)	Location
Semimembranosus	Ischial tuberosity	Proximal, posterior, medial tibia	Extend hip and flex knee	Deep, medial posterior thigh
Semitendinosus	Ischial tuberosity	Pes anserinus	Extend hip and flex knee	Superficial, medial posterior thigh
Biceps Femoris	Ischial tuberosity and linea aspera	Head of the fibula	Extend hip and flex knee	Posterior lateral thigh
Iliopsoas	Transverse processes and bodies of T12–L5 and iliac fossa	Lesser trochanter	Flexion of hip (strongest) and lateral rotation of hip	Deep abdomen
Vastus Intermedius	Anterior femur	Tibial tuberosity via the patellar tendon	Extend knee	Deep anterior thigh
Vastus Medialis	Linea aspera	Tibial tuberosity via the patellar tendon	Extend knee	Anteromedial thigh
Vastus Lateralis	Linea aspera	Tibial tuberosity via the patellar tendon	Extend knee	Anterolateral thigh
Rectus Femoris	AIIS and close to ac-etabulum	Tibial tuberosity via the patellar tendon	Extend knee and flex hip	Superficial anterior thigh
Sartorius	ASIS	Pes anserinus	Flex, laterally rotate, and abduct hip and flex knee	Superficial anterior thigh

Muscles of the Leg

Muscle Name	Origin	Insertion	Action(s)	Location
Popliteus	Lateral epicondyle of the femur	Proximal, medial, posterior tibia	Medial rotation of tibia and flexion of knee	Deep, posterior knee
Soleus	Soleal line of tibia and posterior head of fibula	Calcaneus via Achilles tendon	Plantarflexion of the ankle	Deep to gastrocnemius in superficial posterior leg compartment
Plantaris	Lateral epicondyle of femur	Calcaneus via Achilles tendon	Flexion of knee and plantarflexion of ankle	Posterior knee
Gastrocnemius	Lateral and medial condyles of femur	Calcaneus via Achilles tendon	Flexion of knee and plantarflexion of ankle	Superficial, posterior leg
Tibialis Posterior	Posterior tibia, fibula, and interosseus membrane	Navicular, cuneiform bones, cuboid, and metatarsals 2, 3, and 4	Inversion of foot and plantarflexion of ankle	Deep posterior leg compartment
Flexor Digitorum Longus	Posterior tibia	Distal phalanges of four lateral toes, plantar surface	Flexion of four lateral toes and plantarflexion of ankle	Deep posterior leg compartment
Flexor Hallucis Longus	Posterior fibula	Distal phalanx of digit 1, plantar surface	Flexion of big toe and plantarflexion of ankle	Deep posterior leg compartment
Peroneus Tertius	Distal, anterior fibula	Base of the fifth metacarpal	Eversion of foot and dorsiflexion of ankle	Anterior leg compartment
Peroneus Brevis	Inferior two thirds of lateral fibula	Base of the fifth metacarpal	Eversion of foot and plantarflexion of ankle	Lateral leg compartment
Peroneus Longus	Lateral fibula including head of fibula	Base of first metacarpal and medial cuneiform	Eversion of foot and plantarflexion of ankle	Lateral leg compartment
Extensor Digitorum Longus	Lateral condyle of tibia and entire anterior fibula	Distal phalanges of four lateral toes, dorsal side	Extension of four lateral toes and dorsiflexion of ankle	Anterior leg compartment
Extensor Hallucis Longus	Anterior fibula and interosseus membrane	Distal phalanx of digit 1, dorsal surface	Extension of big toe and dorsiflexion of ankle	Anterior leg compartment
Tibialis Anterior	Lateral condyle and proximal half of anterior tibia	Base of first metatarsal and medial cuneiform	Inversion of foot and dorsiflexion of ankle	Anterior leg compartment

Intrinsic Foot Muscles

Muscle Name	Origin	Insertion	Action(s)	Location
Dorsal Interossei	Adjacent sides of metatarsals 1–5	Medial side of base of proximal phalanx of digit 1 and lateral sides of bases of proximal phalanges of digits 2–4	Abduct toes (digits 2–4)	Layer four (deepest) dorsal side of foot
Palmar Interossei	Medial sides of metatarsals 3, 4, and 5	Medial sides of bases of proximal phalanges of digits 3, 4, and 5	Adduct toes (digits 3–5)	Layer four (deepest) plantar side of foot
Adductor Hallucis	Oblique head: base of metatarsals 2–4; Transverse head: metatarsophalangeal joint capsules	Lateral side of base of proximal phalanx of digit 1	Adduct digit 1 (big toe)	Layer three plantar side of foot
Flexor Hallucis Brevis	Cuboid and lateral cuneiform, plantar surfaces	Base of proximal phalanx of digit 1	Flex digit 1 (big toe)	Layer three plantar side of foot
Flexor Digiti Minimi Brevis	Base of fifth metatarsal	Base of proximal phalanx of fifth digit	Flex fifth digit (little toe)	Layer three plantar side of foot
Lumbricals	Tendon of insertion of flexor digitorum longus	Bases of proximal phalanges of digits 2–5 and extensor expansion	Flex MP joints and extend DIP joints and PIP joints of the foot	Layer two plantar side of foot
Quadratus Plantae	Calcaneus	Tendon of insertion of flexor digitorum longus	Flex four lateral toes	Layer two plantar side of foot
Abductor Hallucis	Calcaneus	Medial side of proximal phalanx of digit 1	Adduct digit 1 (big toe)	Layer one (most superficial) plantar side of foot
Flexor Digitorum Brevis	Calcaneus	Medial and lateral sides of the middle phalanges of digits 2–5	Flex four lateral toes	Layer one (most superficial) plantar side of foot
Abductor Digiti Minimi	Calcaneus	Lateral side of the base of the proximal phalanx of the fifth digit	Abduct fifth digit (little toe)	Layer one (most superficial) plantar side of foot

Action Charts of Hip, Knee, Ankle, and Foot Movers

Please fill in the muscles that perform the hip, knee, ankle, and foot movements indicated:

HIP FLEXORS	HIP EXTENSORS
1.	1.
2.	2.
3.	3.
4.	4.
5.	

HIP LATERAL ROTATORS	HIP MEDIAL ROTATORS
1.	1.
2.	2.
3.	3.
4.	
5.	
6.	
7.	
8.	
9.	

HIP ADDUCTORS	HIP ABDUCTORS
1.	1.
2.	2.
3.	3.
4.	4.
5.	

KNEE FLEXORS	KNEE EXTENSORS
1.	1.
2.	2.
3.	3.
4.	4.
5.	
6.	
7.	
8.	

ANKLE PLANTARFLEXORS	ANKLE DORSIFLEXORS
1.	1.
2.	2.
3.	3.
4.	4.
5.	
6.	
7.	
8.	

FOOT EVERTORS	FOOT INVERTERS
1.	1.
2.	2.
3.	

TOE FLEXORS	TOE EXTENSORS
1.	1.
2.	2.
3.	3.
4.	4.
5.	5.

TOE ABDUCTORS	TOE ADDUCTORS
1.	1.
2.	2.
3.	

Review Exercise for Muscles Located in the Hip and Thigh Region

Fill in the appropriate muscle or bone marking in the space provided.

1. _____ is a deep buttock region muscle and laterally rotates the hip. It can cause sciatica when short.

2. _____ is the largest, deepest medial thigh muscle and adducts the thigh.

3. _____ is the larger of the two lateral hip muscles and performs abduction and medial rotation of the hip. It pulls the hip down when the weight is on the limb, so the other hip rises and the other limb can swing through when walking.

4. _____ is the largest muscle in the body (by volume). It performs lateral rotation and forceful extension of the hip.

5. _____ is the small lateral hip muscle that flexes, abducts, and medially rotates the hip, and it plays a role in stabilization of the knee. It inserts into the IT band.

6. _____ is the anterolateral quadriceps group muscle; it originates on the linea aspera.

7. _____ is the anteromedial quadriceps group muscle; it originates on the linea aspera.

8. _____ is the superficial quadriceps group muscle; it flexes the hip as well as extends the knee.

9. The insertion of all four quadriceps group muscles is on the _____.

10. The action of all four quadriceps group muscles is _____.

11. _____ is the lateral hamstring muscle, which inserts on the head of the fibula.

12. _____ is the deeper of the two medial hamstring muscles, which inserts on the proximal, medial posterior tibia.

13. _____ is the superficial of the two medial hamstring muscles, which inserts at pes anserinus.

14. The origin of the three hamstrings is _____ _____.

15. The actions of all three hamstrings are _____ and _____.

16. _____ is the *tailor muscle,* the longest muscle in the body. It performs lateral rotation, abduction and flexion of the hip, and knee flexion.

Review Exercise for Muscles Located in the Knee Area and Leg

Fill in the appropriate muscle in the space provided.

1. _____ is the small, deep muscle in the posterior knee region that performs medial rotation of the tibia.

2. _____ is the small muscle in the posterior knee region that is variably present. This muscle has a long tendon of insertion, which joins the calcaneus via the Achilles tendon.

3. _____ is the most superficial muscle in the posterior leg and performs knee flexion and plantarflexion of the ankle.

4. _____ is the ankle plantarflexor and is located directly deep to gastrocnemius.

5. _____ is the deep posterior leg compartment muscle that inverts the foot and plantarflexes the ankle.

6. _____ is the deep posterior leg compartment muscle that flexes the four lateral toes and plantarflexes the ankle.

7. _____ is the deep posterior leg compartment muscle that flexes the big toe and plantarflexes the ankle.

8. _____ is the lateral leg compartment muscle that everts the foot and plantarflexes the ankle. It is the shorter of a pair.

9. _____ is the lateral leg compartment muscle that everts the foot and plantarflexes the ankle. It is the longer of a pair.

10. _____ is the anterior leg compartment muscle that everts the foot and dorsiflexes the ankle.

11. _____ is the anterior leg compartment muscle that extends the four lateral toes and dorsiflexes the ankle.

12. _____ is the anterior leg compartment muscle that extends the big toe and dorsiflexes the ankle.

13. _____ is the anterior leg compartment muscle that inverts the foot and dorsiflexes the ankle.

Review Exercise for the Intrinsic Foot Muscles

Fill in the appropriate muscle in the space provided.

1. _____ is the muscle located in the fourth layer, deep between the metatarsals on the dorsal side of the foot; it abducts the toes.

2. _____ is the muscle located in the fourth layer, deep between the metatarsals on the plantar side of the foot; it adducts the toes.

3. _____ is the muscle located in the third layer on the plantar side of the foot; it flexes the big toe.

4. _____ is the muscle located in the third layer on the plantar side of the foot; it adducts the big toe.

5. _____ is the muscle located in the third layer on the plantar side of the foot; it flexes the fifth digit.

6. _____ is the muscle located in the second layer on the plantar side of the foot; it flexes the MP joints and extends the PIP and DIP joints of the four lateral toes.

7. _____ is the muscle located in the second layer on the plantar side of the foot; it helps flex the four lateral toes.

8. _____ is the muscle located in the first layer on the plantar side of the foot; it abducts the big toe.

9. _____ is the muscle located in the first layer on the plantar side of the foot; it flexes the four lateral toes.

10. _____ is the muscle located in the first layer on the plantar side of the foot; it abducts the fifth digit.

Appendix A
Answers to Chapter Review Questions

CHAPTER 1

1. List four characteristics of anatomical position:
   a. **Standing erect/upright**
   b. **Arms at sides**
   c. **Head and feet face forward**
   d. **Palms face forward**

2. Which plane divides the body into right and left sections?
   Sagittal

3. Which plane divides the body into anterior and posterior sections? **Transverse**

4. The chin is inferior to: **mouth, nose, eyes, forehead (anybody part above the chin)**

5. Name a body part superior to the navel: **sternum, chin, mouth (any body part above the navel)**

6. Name a structure medial to the shoulders: **sternum, spine (any body part closer to the midline than the shoulders)**

7. Name a structure on the anterior aspect of the body: **nose, mouth, navel, pubic symphysis, (any body part on the front of the body)**

8. Name something distal to your knees: **foot, ankle (anybody part lower than the knee)**

9. What side of your head is covered when you wear a hood? **Posterior and superior**

10. Which joint is directly proximal to the hand? **The wrist joint.**

CHAPTER 2

1. What are bones?
   Bones are a rigid form of connective tissue that provide an overall structure or framework for the body.

2. List five functions of bones:
   a. **provide an overall structure or framework for the body.**
   b. **protect organs**
   c. **serve as levers in movement-(movement is due to muscular contraction)**
   d. **produce blood cells (red cells, white cells and platelets)**
   e. **store minerals and fats**

3. Two main types of bone tissue are:
   a. **compact, which forms the outer layer of bones**
   b. **spongy, which is formed of thin "beams" of bone called trabeculae. Spongy bone houses red marrow, which produces blood cells.**

4. List the five shapes of bones: shapes of bones are a single word, so would only need one line for an answer.
   a. **long, such as the humerus**
   b. **short, such as the carpals and tarsals**
   c. **flat such as the sternum, ilium, and many bones of the skull**
   d. **irregular, such as the vertebrae**
   e. **sesamoid, such as the patella**

5. Skeleton is divided into axial and appendicular segments.
   a. The axial skeleton consists of:
      the bones of the skull, the vertebrae including the sacrum and coccyx, the sternum, the ribs and the hyoid.
   b. The appendicular skeleton consists of:
      all of the bones of the upper and lower extremities, and the bones which hold the extremities to the axial

skeleton. More specifically, the clavicle, scapula, humerus, radius, ulna, carpals, metacarpals and phalanges of the hand, the ilium, ischium, pubis, femur, patella, tibia, fibula, tarsals, metatarsals and phalanges of the foot.

6. Name and locate all the bone marking examples in the illustration below:

Items for students to label:
Head of the radius
Head of the fibula
Medial and lateral condyles of the femur
Medial and lateral epicondyles of the humerus
Greater and lesser tubercles of the humerus
Deltoid tuberosity and tibial tuberosity
Greater and lesser trochanters
Iliac crest
Spine of the scapula
Iliac fossa, infraspinous fossa
Bicipital groove
Obturator foramen

7. Define fascia, and give four examples of connective tissue structures that are called fascia?

Fascia is connective tissue that forms a continuous, three-dimensional web around and within every structure of the human body. Fascia surrounds and connects each cell. Examples include areolar tissue, reticular tissue, dense irregular tissue such as epimysium, and aponeuroses.

Joints

1. Fill in the appropriate functional classifications of joints:
   a. **synarthrotic** = "immovable" joint
   b. **amphiarthrotic** = slightly movable joint
   c. **diarthrotic** = freely movable joint

2. Structural classifications of joint use the following terms:
   a. **fibrous** joints are held together by fiber.
   b. **cartilaginous** joints are held together by cartilage.
   c. **synovial** joints contain all the components of synovial joints.

3. List the four components of a synovial joint:
   a. **articular cartilage on the ends of bones, which meet to form a joint**
   b. **synovial fluid within a synovial cavity**
   c. **joint sleeve or joint capsule**
   d. **reinforcing ligaments**

4. For each type of synovial joint listed below, please fill in the following: a., the movement permitted at this joint; b., the shape of the articulating surfaces; and c., an example of where this joint is in the body.

1. Plane or gliding
   a. side-to-side movement or back-and-forth movement, small gliding movements
   b. flat surfaces
   c. intercarpal, acromioclavicular, sternoclavicular, proximal tibiofibular joints
2. Condyloid or ellipsoidal
   a. flexion, extension, abduction, and adduction only
   b. oval indentation/ellipse and corresponding oval or egg-shaped structure
   c. wrist and atlanto-occipital joints
3. Saddle
   a. main actions are flexion, extension, abduction, and adduction
   b. saddle and legs of a rider
   c. joint between trapezium and first metacarpal
4. Pivot
   a. rotation only
   b. ring and axis or convex and concave surfaces
   c. radioulnar joints and atlantoaxial joint
5. Hinge
   a. flexion and extension only
   b. convex and concave surfaces
   c. elbow, knee, ankle, interphalangeal joints
6. Ball-and-socket
   a. ball and round socket
   b. flexion, extension, abduction, adduction, and rotation
   c. shoulder and hip

Muscles

1. What are muscles?

   Muscles are organs composed of fiber-like cells that are specialized for contraction

2. Three types of muscle tissue include:
   a. **skeletal,** which is **voluntary, striated,** and **attaches to bones, and contracts to allow movement of bones**
   b. **smooth,** which is **involuntary, nonstriated,** and **lines the walls of tubes and hollow organs, and contracts to move fluids and other substances**
   c. cardiac, which is **involuntary, striated,** and **is the muscle of the heart, which contracts to pump blood through the body**

3. Functions of muscles include:
   a. **movement of bones**
   b. **movement of fluids such as blood and lymph, and movement of other substances**
   c. **generation of heat**
   d. **maintenance of posture**
   e. **stabilization of joints**

4. Structure of a skeletal muscle:
   a. Each individual muscle cell is enclosed in a connective tissue sheath called an **endomysium.**
   b. Each fascicle, or group of muscle cells, is wrapped in a connective tissue sheath called a **perimysium.**
   c. Many fascicles, bound together to form a muscle, are wrapped in a covering called a **epimysium**
   d. The epimysium blends into a tendon or aponeurosis, attaching muscles to bone.

5. List and define the components of a skeletal muscle cell:

   Sarcolemma: a skeletal muscle cell membrane.
   Myofibrils: the structural components of a skeletal muscle cell that are made of myofilaments.
   Myosin: the primary protein of thick myofilaments that contain cross bridges to pull the actin toward the center of each sarcomere.
   Actin: the primary protein of the thin myofilaments. Actin myofilaments are pulled by myosin toward the center of each sarcomere.
   Sarcoplasmic reticulum: a specialized network of smooth tubes and sacs that surrounds each and every mibromybril of a skeletal muscle, and stores calcium.

6. Write out the steps involved in the sliding filament mechanism:

   Sliding filament mechanism is the process of skeletal muscle contraction. This process begins with a nerve impulse traveling down the spinal cord or cranial nerve toward a muscle. The impulse travels down the motor axon of a motor neuron and continues down the axon terminals until it reaches the synaptic end bulbs. Acetylcholine is released from the synaptic end bulbs to carry the nerve impulse across the synaptic cleft and attach to the sarcolemma. The sarcolemma becomes permeable to sodium, which moves from the interstitial space into the cell, increasing the positive charge of the cell. In response to this change in charge, the sarcolemma releases calcium. Calcium removes the troponin-tropomyosin from the actin, revealing myosin binding sites. Myosin's cross bridges can thus attach to the actin and pull it toward the center of the sarcomere, thus shortening the muscle.

7. Define a motor unit, and explain the relationship between motor units and the all-or-nothing principle.

   A motor unit is the combination of a single motor axon and all of the skeletal muscle cells innervated by this axon.

8. What is the difference between origin and insertion?

   The origin of a muscle is the more stable muscle attachment site (typically to bone) and insertion is the more movable muscle attachment site.

9. Give an example of a concentric contraction and an example of an eccentric contraction.

   An example of a concentric contraction is lifting a book by flexing the elbow. An example of eccentric contraction is slowly lowering the book, utilizing the muscles of elbow flexion as they lengthen.

CHAPTER 3

Case Study #1

A client comes to your office for a massage therapy session. As you observe her posture, you notice that her right shoulder is raised (right acromion is higher than the left) and the backs (dorsal side) of both hands face forward. Your task is to determine which muscles are out of balance to cause these postural issues.

The client is performing two actions. Which action is indicated by a raised shoulder/acromion on the right side?
Elevation of the *scapula* on the right side.

Which muscles perform the action your client is performing?
Levator scapula and upper trapezius

These muscles are likely to be shortened and should be massaged to assist in bettering the client's posture.

Which action is indicated by the fact that the back of both hands face forward?
bilateral medial (internal) rotation of *the arm/shoulder.*

Which muscles perform the action your client is performing?
Subscapularis, anterior deltoid, pectoralis major, latissimus dorsi, teres major

These muscles are likely to be shortened and should be massaged to assist in bettering the client's posture.

Where would you focus your massage to address these shortened muscles?
Subscapularis is located on the anterior scapula, anterior deltoid is the anterior shoulder, pectoralis major is located superficially in the chest, latissimus dorsi is a superficial low to mid back muscle and teres major along with latissimus dorsi makes up the posterior axilla.

Case Study #2

A client comes to see you and tells you that he is having difficulty raising his arm fully in front of him.

What action is the client having trouble performing?

Flexion of the *shoulder/arm*

What muscle would be shortened and limit the ability of the client to perform the above action?

Latissimus dorsi, teres major, infraspinatus, teres minor, and posterior deltoid

Remember that limits on performing an action are often caused by shortening of antagonists. The shortened muscles should be massaged to assist the client's range of motion. Where would you focus your massage to address these shortened muscles?

Latissimus dorsi is a superficial low to mid back muscle, teres major is located in the posterior axilla, infraspinatus is located inferior to the spine of the scapula, teres minor lies along the axillary border of the scapula, and posterior deltoid is located in the superficial shoulder.

Case Study #3
Your client has difficulty bringing her arm from a position in which it is abducted to 90 degrees, further out to the side of her body. She cannot raise her arm to a position where her arm is resting against the side of her head.

What action is the client having trouble performing?

Upward rotation of the *scapula*

What muscle would be shortened and limit the ability of the client to perform the above action?

Rhomboids, levator scapula, and pectoralis minor

Remember that limits on performing an action are often caused by shortening of antagonists. The shortened muscles should be massaged to assist the client's range of motion.

Where would you focus your massage to address these shortened muscles?

Rhomboids is a midlayer upper back muscle located between the scapula and the spine, levator scapula is located in the posterolateral neck, and pectoralis minor is deep in the anterolateral chest.

Case Study #4
As you observe your client's posture, you notice that her shoulders are more anterior than her ear lobes and her shoulders appear rounded. In addition, you notice that her scapulae seem far away from the spine.

Which action is the client performing?

Protraction of the *scapula*

Which muscles perform this action?

Pectoralis minor and serratus anterior

These muscles are likely to be shortened and should be massaged to assist in bettering the client's posture.

Where would you focus your massage to address these shortened muscles?

Pectoralis minor is deep in the anterolateral chest and serratus anterioris located in the lateral thorax.

Case Study #5
As you observe your client's posture, you notice that his elbows appear bent. As you ask your client about his daily activities you learn that he is a bodybuilder who lifts substantial weight as part of his workout.

Which action is the client performing through his posture?

Flexion of the *elbow/forearm*

Which muscles perform this action?

Brachialis, biceps brachii and brachioradialis

These muscles are likely to be shortened and should be massaged to assist in bettering the client's posture.

Where would you focus your massage to address these shortened muscles?

Brachialis is located deep in the anterior arm, biceps brachii is superficial in the anterior arm and brachioradialis is a superficial, lateral forearm muscle.

Case Study #6
As you interview your client, she informs you that she cannot fully extend her wrists. She is a massage therapist and uses the muscles in her hands and forearms on a daily basis.

When a client is unable to fully extend her wrist due to shortened muscles, which muscles are likely to be shortened?

Wrist flexors: flexor carpi radialis, flexor carpi ulnaris, and palmaris longus

Where would you focus your massage to address these shortened muscles?

The superficial, anterior forearm

Review Charts to Study

Origin, Insertion, Location, and Action Chart of the Muscles That Move the Arm				
Name of Muscle	Origin	Insertion	Basic Location	Action(s)
Coracobrachialis	Coracoid process of the scapula	Medial humerus	Medial arm (blends with short head of biceps brachii)	Adduction and flexion of the arm
Pectoralis Major	Medial clavicle, sternum, and costal cartilage of ribs 1–6	Bicipital groove of the humerus	Superficial chest	Medial rotation, flexion, extension from a flexed position, adduction, and horizontal adduction of the arm
Deltoid: Anterior	Lateral third of clavicle	Deltoid tuberosity	Anterior shoulder cap	Flexion, medial rotation, and horizontal adduction of the arm
Middle	Acromion	Deltoid tuberosity	Lateral shoulder	Abduction of the arm
Posterior	Spine of the scapula	Deltoid tuberosity	Posterior shoulder cap	Extension, lateral rotation, and horizontal abduction of the arm
Supraspinatus	Supraspinous fossa	Greater tubercle of the humerus	Superior to the spine of the scapula	Initiation of arm abduction
Infraspinatus	Infraspinous fossa	Greater tubercle of the humerus	Inferior to the spine of the scapula	Lateral rotation and extension of the arm
Teres minor	Axillary border of the scapula	Greater tubercle of the humerus	Along axillary border of the scapula	Lateral rotation and extension of the arm
Subscapularis	Subscapular fossa	Lesser tubercle of the humerus	Anterior scapula	Medial rotation of the arm
Latissimus Dorsi	Thoracolumbar aponeurosis, sacrum, posterior iliac crest, spinous processes of T7-L5, inferior 2–3 ribs, inferior angle of scapula	Bicipital groove of the humerus	Superficial low to mid back and posterior axilla	Extension, medial rotation, and adduction of the arm
Teres Major	Inferior angle of the scapula	Bicipital groove of the humerus	Posterior axilla	Extension, medial rotation, and adduction of the arm

Origin, Insertion, Location, and Action Chart of the Muscles That Move the Scapula

Name of Muscle	Origin	Insertion	Basic Location	Action(s)
Serratus Anterior	Lateral ribs 1–8	Anterior, vertebral border of the scapula	Lateral ribs	Protraction and upward rotation of the scapula
Pectoralis Minor	Ribs 3, 4, 5 close to costal cartilage	Coracoid process of the scapula	Deep anterolateral chest	Protraction, depression, and downward rotation of the scapula
Levator Scapula	Transverse processes of C1–C4	Superior angle of the scapula	Posterolateral neck	Elevation and downward rotation of the scapula
Rhomboids	Spinous processes of C7–T5	Vertebral border of the scapula	Between the scapula and the spine, midlayer	Retraction and downward rotation of the scapula
Trapezius: Upper fibers	External occipital protuberance and ligamentum nuchae	Lateral clavicle and acromion	Superficial, posterolateral neck and between neck and acromion	Elevation and upward rotation of the scapula
Middle fibers	Spinous processes of C7–T6	Spine of the scapula	Superficial upper and middle back	Retraction of the scapula
Lower fibers	Spinous Processes of T7–T12	Root of the spine of the scapula	Superficial middle back	Depression and upward rotation of the scapula

Origin, Insertion, Location, and Action Chart of the Muscles That Move the Elbow

Muscle Name	Origin	Insertion	Location	Action(s)
Brachialis	Distal half of anterior arm	Proximal anterior ulna including coronoid process and ulnar tuberosity	Deep anterior arm	Flexion of the elbow (strongest)
Biceps Brachii	Coracoid process and supraglenoid tubercle of the scapula	Radial tuberosity	Superficial anterior arm	Flexion of the elbow, supination of the forearm, and flexion of the arm
Brachioradialis	Lateral supracondylar ridge of the humerus	Styloid process of the radius	Superficial, lateral forearm	Flexion of the elbow (when the forearm is in neutral position)
Anconeus	Lateral epicondyle of the humerus	Olecranon process and proximal posterior ulna	Posterior elbow	Extension of the elbow
Triceps Brachii	Infraglenoid tubercle of the scapula and posterior humerus	Olecranon process	Posterior arm	Extension of the elbow and extension of the arm

Origin, Insertion, Location, and Action Chart of the Muscles That Rotate the Forearm

Name of Muscle	Origin	Insertion	Basic Location	Action(s)
Supinator	Lateral epicondyle of the humerus, supinator crest of the ulna, and ligaments of the elbow	Proximal, anterior radius	Wraps around the lateral aspect of the proximal forearm	Supination of the forearm
Biceps Brachii	Coracoid process and supraglenoid tubercle of the scapula	Radial tuberosity	Superficial anterior arm	Supination of the forearm, flexion of the elbow, and flexion of the arm
Pronator Quadratus	Distal ¼ of the anterior ulna	Distal ¼ of the anterior radius	Deep, distal, anterior forearm	Pronation of the forearm
Pronator teres	Medial epicondyle of the humerus and coronoid process of the ulna	Mid lateral shaft of the radius	Superficial, proximal, anterior forearm	Pronation of the forearm

Origin, Insertion, Location, and Action Chart of the Muscles That Move the Wrist

Muscle Name	Origin	Insertion	Location	Action(s)
Extensor Carpi Radialis Longus	Lateral supracondylar ridge of the humerus	Base of the second metacarpal	Superficial, posterior forearm	Extension and radial deviation of the wrist
Extensor Carpi Radialis Brevis	Lateral epicondyle of the humerus	Base of the third metacarpal	Superficial, posterior forearm	Extension and radial deviation of the wrist
Extensor Carpi Ulnaris	Lateral epicondyle of the humerus	Base of the fifth metacarpal	Superficial, posterior forearm	Extension and ulnar deviation of the wrist
Flexor Carpi Radialis	Lateral epicondyle of the humerus	Bases of the second and third metacarpals	Superficial, anterior forearm	Flexion and radial deviation of the wrist
Palmaris Longus	Medial epicondyle of the humerus	Palmar aponeurosis	Superficial, anterior forearm	Flexion of the wrist
Flexor Carpi Ulnaris	Medial epicondyle of the humerus and proximal ulna	Pisiform, hamate, and base of the fifth metacarpal	Superficial, anterior forearm, though most proximal aspect is posterior	Flexion and ulnar deviation of the wrist

Origin, Insertion, Location, and Action Chart of the Forearm Muscles That Move the Fingers and Thumb

Muscle Name	Origin	Insertion	Location	Action(s)
Abductor Pollicis Longus	Posterior radius, ulna, and interosseus membrane	Base of the first metacarpal	Deep posterior forearm	Abduction of the thumb at the CMC joint
Extensor Pollicis Brevis	Posterior radius and interosseus membrane	Base of the proximal phalanx of the thumb	Deep posterior forearm	Extension of the thumb at the MP joint
Extensor Pollicis Longus	Posterior ulna and interosseus membrane	Base of the distal phalanx of the thumb	Deep posterior forearm	Extension of the thumb at the IP joint
Extensor Indicis	Posterior ulna and interosseus membrane	Extensor expansion of the second digit	Deep posterior forearm	Extension of the second digit
Extensor Digitorum	Lateral epicondyle of the humerus	Base of middle phalanges and extensor expansion of digits 2–5	Superficial posterior forearm	Extension of digits 2–5
Extensor Digiti Minimi	Lateral epicondyle of the humerus	Extensor expansion over the 5th digit	Superficial posterior forearm	Extension of the fifth digit
Flexor Pollicis Longus	Anterior radius and interosseus membrane	Distal phalanx of the thumb	Deep anterior forearm	Flexion of the thumb at the IP joint
Flexor Digitorum Profundus	Anterior ulna and interosseus membrane	Distal phalanges of digits 2–5	Deep anterior forearm	Flexion of digits 2–5 at MP, PIP, and DIP joints
Flexor Digitorum Superficialis	Medial epicondyle of the humerus, coronoid process of the ulna, and anterior radius	Middle phalanges of digits 2–5	Midlayer anterior forearm	Flexion of digits 2–5 at MP and PIP joints

CMC, carpometacarpal; IP, interphalangeal; MP, metacarpophalangeal; PIP, proximal interphalangeal.

Origin, Insertion, Location, and Action Chart of the Intrinsic Hand Muscles

Muscle Name	Origin	Insertion	Location	Action(s)
Dorsal Interossei	Adjacent sides of metacarpals	Proximal phalanges of digits 2, 3, and 4	Dorsal side of hand, between the metacarpals	Abduction of digits 2, 3, and 4 at the MP joints
Palmar Interossei	Shafts of second, fourth, and fifth metacarpals	Proximal phalanges of digits 2, 4, and 5	Deep, palmar side of the hand, between the metacarpals	Adduction of digits 2, 4, and 5 at the MP joints
Lumbricals	Tendon of insertion of flexor digitorum profundus	Bases of the proximal phalanges of digits 2–5 and extensor expansion	Palmar side of the hand	Flexion of the MP joints and extension of the PIP and DIP joints
Adductor Pollicis	Transverse head: shaft of the third metacarpal. Oblique head: bases of the second and third metacarpals, capitate and adjacent carpals	Base of the proximal phalanx of the thumb	Webbing between the first and second digits	Adduction of the thumb at the CMC joint
Opponens Pollicis	Flexor retinaculum and trapezium	Lateral shaft of the first metacarpal	Thenar eminence (deepest)	Opposition of the thumb: combination of abduction and flexion at the CMC joint
Flexor Pollicis Brevis	Flexor retinaculum and trapezium	Base of the proximal phalanx of the thumb	Thenar eminence	Flexion of the thumb at the MP joint
Abductor Pollicis Brevis	Flexor retinaculum, trapezium, and scaphoid	Base of the proximal phalanx of the thumb	Thenar eminence	Abduction of the thumb at the MP joint
Opponens Digiti Minimi	Hook of hamate and flexor retinaculum	Medial border of the fifth metacarpal	Hypothenar eminence (deepest)	Opposition of the fifth digit: combination of flexion and adduction
Flexor Digiti Minimi	Hook of hamate and flexor retinaculum	Base of the proximal phalanx of the fifth digit	Hypothenar eminence	Flexion of the fifth digit
Abductor Digiti Minimi	Pisiform	Base of the proximal phalanx of the fifth digit	Hypothenar eminence	Abduction of the fifth digit

Review List of Arm and Scapula Movers to Fill in

Please list muscles that move the arm or scapula.

ARM MOVERS	SCAPULA MOVERS
1. **Coracobrachialis**	1. **Serratus anterior**
2. **Pectoralis major**	2. **Pectoralis minor**
3. Anterior **Deltoid**	3. **Levator scapula**
Middle **Deltoid**	
Posterior **Deltoid**	
4. **Supraspinatus**	4. **Rhomboids**
5. **Infraspinatus**	5. Upper fibers of **Trapezius**
	Middle fibers of **Trapezius**
	Lower fibers of **Trapezius**
6. **Teres minor**	
7. **Subscapularis**	
8. **Latissimus dorsi**	
9. **Teres major**	
10. Biceps brachii (additional arm flexor)	
11. Triceps brachii (additional arm extensor)	

Review Chart to Fill in

	LATISSIMUS DORSI AND TERES MAJOR	LEVATOR SCAPULA AND UPPER TRAPEZIUS	RHOMBOIDS AND MIDDLE TRAPEZIUS	SERRATUS ANTERIOR AND PECTORALIS MINOR
List some uses of these muscles in daily life.	**Wood chopping**	**Shrugging shoulders**	**Reach behind**	**Reach forward**
If these muscles are SHORTENED, what posture might you notice?	**Back of hands face forward**	**Raised shoulders**	**Shoulders pulled back**	**Shoulders pulled forward**
What would be the effect of LENGTHENED or dysfunctional muscles?	**Inability to perform forceful extension of the arm**	**Inability to raise shoulders fully**	**Inability to squeeze scapulae together**	**A lengthened serratus muscle can cause winged scapula**
How would you massage these muscles?	**Effleurage. Friction to the superficial mid to low back region and pétrissage to the posterior axilla**	**Pétrissage to area between neck and shoulder. Friction and direct pressure to the muscle attachment at the superior angle of the scapula**	**Effleurage and friction to the upper back, between the spine and scapulae.**	**Friction and/or direct pressure to the deep anterolateral chest and to the lateral rib area**

Action Charts of Arm and Scapula Movers

ARM EXTENORS	ARM FLEXORS
1. *Latissimus dorsi*	1. *Coracobrachialis*
2. *Teres major*	2. *Pectoralis major*
3. *Posterior fibers of deltoid*	3. *Anterior fibers of deltoid*
4. *Infraspinatus*	4. *Biceps brachii (weak arm flexor)*
5. *Teres minor*	
6. *Triceps brachii (weak arm extensor)*	
7. *Pectoralis major (from a flexed position only)*	

ARM MEDIAL ROTATORS	ARM LATERAL ROTATORS
1. *Subscapularis*	1. *Posterior fibers of deltoid*
2. *Anterior fibers of deltoid*	2. *Infraspinatus*
3. *Pectoralis major*	3. *Teres minor*
4. *Latissimus dorsi*	
5. *Teres major*	

ARM ADDUCTORS	ARM ABDUCTORS
1. *Coracobrachialis*	1. *Supraspinatus*
2. *Pectoralis major*	2. *Middle fibers of deltoid*
3. *Latissimus dorsi*	
4. *Teres major*	

ARM HORIZONTAL ADDUCTORS	ARM HORIZONTAL ABDUCTORS
1. *Pectoralis major*	1. *Posterior fibers of deltoid*
2. *Anterior fibers of deltoid*	

SCAPULA ELEVATORS	SCAPULA DEPRESSORS
1. *Levator scapula*	1. *Pectoralis minor*
2. *Upper fibers of trapezius*	2. *Lower fibers of trapezius*

SCAPULA PROTRACTORS	SCAPULA RETRACTORS
1. *Pectoralis minor*	1. *Rhomboids*
2. *Serratus anterior*	2. *Trapezius*

SCAPULA UPWARD ROTATORS	SCAPULA DOWNWARD ROTATORS
1. *Serratus anterior*	1. *Levator scapula*
2. *Upper fibers of trapezius*	2. *Rhomboid*
3. *Lower fibers of trapezius*	3. *Pectoralis minor*

Action Charts of Elbow, Forearm, and Wrist Movers

ELBOW FLEXORS	ELBOW EXTENSORS
1. *Brachialis*	1. *Triceps brachii*
2. *Biceps brachii*	2. *Anconeus*
3. *Brachioradialis*	

FOREARM SUPINATORS	FOREARM PRONATORS
1. *Supinator*	1. *Pronator teres*
2. *Biceps brachii*	2. *Pronator quadratus*

WRIST EXTENSORS	WRIST FLEXORS
1. *Extensor capri radialis longus*	1. *Flexor carpi radialis*
2. *Extensor capri radialis brevis*	2. *Flexor carpi ulnaris*
3. *Extensor capri ulnaris*	3. *Palmaris longus*

Review of Muscles Located in the Hand and Forearm That Move the Fingers and Thumb

Deep posterior forearm muscles:

1. *Abductor pollicis longus:* deep posterior forearm muscle that abducts the thumb

2. *Extensor pollicis brevis:* shorter deep posterior forearm muscle that extends the thumb

3. *Extensor pollicis longus:* longer deep posterior forearm muscle that extends the thumb

4. *Extensor indicis:* deep posterior forearm muscle that extends the second digit

Superficial posterior forearm muscles:

5. *Extensor digitorum:* superficial posterior forearm muscle that extends four fingers (digits 25); the origin is the lateral epicondyle of the humerus, and the tendon of origin is part of the common extensor tendon

6. *Extensor digiti minimi:* superficial, posterior forearm muscle that extends the fifth digit; the origin is the lateral epicondyle of the humerus, and the tendon of origin is part of the common extensor tendon

Deep anterior forearm muscles:

7. *Flexor pollicis longus*: deep anterior forearm muscle that flexes the thumb

8. *Flexor digitorum profundus:* deep anterior forearm muscle that flexes 12 phalanges

Midlayer, anterior forearm muscle:

9. *Flexor digitorum superficialis:* midlayer anterior forearm muscle that flexes four fingers

Review of Ten Intrinsic Hand Muscles

Three muscles that move the fingers: (Muscles that move the fingers must insert on the phalanges.)

1. *Dorsal Interossei:* DAB, dorsal side, deep between metacarpals, spreads or abducts the fingers

2. *Palmar Interossei:* PAD, palmar side, deep between metacarpals, adducts the fingers

3. *Lumbricals:* located on the palmar side of the hand, flexes MP joints, and extends the PIPs and DIPs; this muscle is located in both hands and feet

Four muscles that move the thumb: (All thumb movers insert on the thumb!)

1. *Adductor pollicis:* deep to the lumbricals, webbing between the first and second digits (thumb), adducts the thumb

2. *Opponens pollicis:* part of the thenar eminence, performs opposition of the thumb

3. *Flexor pollicis brevis:* part of the thenar eminence, performs flexion of the thumb

4. *Abductor pollicis brevis:* part of the thenar eminence, performs abduction of the thumb

Three muscles that move the little finger: (have digiti minimi in name, insert on the fifth digit)

1. *Opponens digiti minimi:* hypothenar eminence, performs opposition of the fifth digit

2. *Flexor digiti minimi:* hypothenar eminence, performs flexion of the fifth digit

3. *Abductor digiti minimi:* hypothenar eminence, performs abduction of the fifth digit

CHAPTER 4

Case Study #1

A client cannot fully open her jaw.

List three muscles that would likely be shortened and contributing to this problem:

Masseter, temporalis, and medial pterygoid

List two muscles that would likely be lengthened:

Platysma and digastric

Case Study #2

A client comes to your office, and you notice that her head is turned to the right.

List five muscles that could be shortened and contributing to this problem.

Left SCM, left scalenes, right suboccipitals, right splenius capitis, right splenius cervicis

Please note if the muscles are shortened on the right or left side:

List five muscles that could be lengthened and contributing to this problem.

Please note if the muscles are lengthened on the right or left side:

Right SCM, right scalenes, left suboccipitals, left splenius capitis, left splenius cervicis

Describe where you would focus your massage to assist this client in improving her posture.

Left anterolateral neck and right posterior neck.

Case Study #3

Your client cannot fully extend his neck.

List two muscles that could be shortened (bilaterally) and contributing to this problem.

Please note if the muscles are lengthened on the right or left side:

SCM and scalenes (bilaterally)

List three muscles that could be lengthened (bilaterally) and contributing to this problem:

Please note if the muscles are lengthened on the right or left side:

Splenius capitis, splenius cervicis and suboccipitals (bilaterally)

Describe where you would focus your massage to assist this client in improving the range of motion in his neck.

Anterolateral neck (bilaterally)

Case Study #4

A client comes in who cannot fully tilt his head to the left.

List five muscles that could be shortened (unilaterally) and contributing to this problem. Please note if the muscle is short on the right or left side:

Right SCM, right scalenes, right suboccipitals, right splenius capitis, and right splenius cervicis

List five muscles that could be lengthened (unilaterally) and contributing to this problem.

Please note if the muscles are lengthened on the right or left side:

Left SCM, left scalenes, left suboccipitals, left splenius capitis, and left splenius cervicis

Describe where you would focus your massage to assist this client in improving the range of motion in his neck.

Both anterolateral and posterior portions of the right side of the neck

Case Study #5

A client's trunk is turned to the left.

List five muscles that could be shortened and contributing to this problem.

Please note if the muscles are shortened on the right or left side:

Right rotators, right multifidus, right semispinalis, right external obliques, and left internal obliques.

List five muscles that could be lengthened and contributing to this problem.

Please note if the muscles are lengthened on the right or left side:

Left rotators, left multifidus, left semispinalis, left external obliques, and right internal obliques.

Case Study #6

A client is unable to turn his trunk to the left.

List five muscles that could be shortened and contributing to this problem.

Please note if the muscles are shortened on the right or left side:

Left rotators, left multifidus, left semispinalis, left external obliques, and right internal obliques.

List five muscles that could be lengthened and contributing to this problem.

Please note if the muscles are lengthened on the right or left side:

Right rotators, right multifidus, right semispinalis, right external obliques, and left internal obliques.

Case Study #7

A client is unable to fully flex her spine.

List five muscles that could be shortened and contributing to this problem.

Please note if the muscles are shortened on the right or left side:

Iliocostalis, longissimus spinalis, rotators, multifidus, semispinalis, interspinalis, and intertransversarii (all bilaterally)

List five muscles that could be lengthened and contributing to this problem.

Please note if the muscles are lengthened on the right or left side:

Rectus abdominis, external obliques, internal obliques (all bilaterally)

Case Study #8

A client is unable to inhale fully.

List three muscles that could be shortened and contributing to this problem.

Transverse abdominis, internal intercostals, serratus posterior inferior

List three muscles that could be lengthened and contributing to this problem.

Diaphragm (a single muscle) and external intercostals and serratus posterior inferior bilaterally

Review Charts to Study

Origin, Insertion, Location, and Action Chart of Jaw-Moving Muscles

Muscle Name	Origin	Insertion	Location	Action(s)
Medial Pterygoid	Medial pterygoid plate of the sphenoid bone	Mandible	Deep, lateral cheek	Elevate and protract mandible
Lateral Pterygoid	Lateral pterygoid plate of the sphenoid bone	Mandible	Deep, lateral cheek	Protract mandible
Temporalis	Lateral temporal bone	Mandible	Covers lateral temporal bone	Elevate mandible
Masseter	Zygomatic arch	Ramus of mandible	Superficial cheek	Elevate mandible
Platysma	Fascia over pectoralis major and anterior deltoid	Mandible and lower lip	Superficial, anterior neck and upper chest	Depress mandible

Origin, Insertion, Location, and Action Chart of Neck-Moving Muscles

Muscle Name	Origin	Insertion	Location	Action(s)
Scalenes	Transverse processes of C2–C7	Ribs 1 and 2	Anterolateral neck	Unilateral actions: lateral flexion and opposite-side rotation of the neck; Bilateral action: flexion of the neck
Sternocleidomastoid	Sternum and medial clavicle	Mastoid process of the temporal bone	Anterolateral neck	Unilateral actions: lateral flexion and opposite-side rotation of the neck Bilateral action: flexion of the neck
Suboccipitals	C1 and C2	C1 and the occiput	Deep, posterior neck, just below occiput	Unilateral actions: lateral flexion and same-side rotation of the neck Bilateral action: extension of the neck (between C1 and the occiput)
Splenius Capitis	Ligamentum nuchae and spinous processes of T1–T3	Occiput and mastoid process	Midlayer, posterior neck	Unilateral actions: lateral flexion and same-side rotation of the neck; Bilateral action: extension of the neck

(continued)

Origin, Insertion, Location, and Action Chart of Neck-Moving Muscles (*Continued*)

Muscle Name	Origin	Insertion	Location	Action(s)
Splenius Cervicis	Spinous processes of T3–T6	Transverse processes of T1–T3	Midlayer, posterior neck	Unilateral actions: lateral flexion and same-side rotation of the neck Bilateral action: extension of the neck

Origin, Insertion, Location, and Action Chart of Intrinsic Back Muscles

Muscle Name	Origin	Insertion	Location	Action
Segmentals: Interspinalis	Spinous process of C3–T1 and T12–L5	Spinous process of vertebra directly above origin	Between spinous process in cervical and lumbar regions	Extend spine (cervical and lumbar regions only)
Segmentals: Intertransversarii	Transverse process of C3–T1 and T11–L5 and the sacrum	Transverse process of vertebra directly above origin	Between transverse process in cervical and lumbar regions	Extend spine and laterally flex spine (cervical and lumbar regions only)
Transversospinalis: Rotatores	Transverse process of T2–L5	Spinous process of vertebra above	Lamina groove	Extend spine and rotate spine to the opposite side
Transversospinalis: Multifidus	Transverse processes of C2–L5 and the sacrum	Spinous processes of vertebrae 2–4 vertebrae above origin	Lamina groove	Extend spine and rotate spine to the opposite side
Transversospinalis: Semispinalis	Transverse processes of vertebrae T2–L5	Spinous processes of vertebra 3–6 vertebrae above origin	Lamina groove	Extend spine and rotate spine to the opposite side
Erector Spinae Group: Iliocostalis	Sacrum posterior iliac crest, posterior ribs 3–12	Ribs and transverse processes of C4–C7	Lateral band, ilium to ribs	All three extend and laterally flex spine
Erector Spinae Group: Longissimus	Transverse processes of C4–L5 and the sacrum	Transverse processes of cervical and thoracic vertebrae, ribs and the mastoid process	Middle band, lateral to transverse processes	All 3 extend and laterally flex spine
Erector Spinae Group: Spinalis	Ligamentum nuchae, spinous processes of C7–T2 and T11–L3	Spinous processes of cervical and thoracic vertebrae and occiput	Medial band, in lamina groove	All three extend and laterally flex spine

Origin, Insertion, Location, and Action Chart of Abdominal Wall Muscles

Muscle Name	Origin	Insertion	Location	Action(s)
Transverse Abdominis	Lateral inguinal ligament, iliac crest, thoracolumbar aponeurosis, internal costal cartilages, and ribs 7–12	Abdominal aponeurosis and linea alba	Deep anterolateral trunk	Compress contents of abdomen
Internal Oblique	Thoracolumbar aponeurosis, iliac crest, and inguinal ligament	Ribs and costal cartilage of ribs 9–12, linea alba	Midlayer, anterolateral trunk	Unilateral actions: lateral flexion and same-side rotation of trunk; Bilateral action: flex trunk
External Oblique	Ribs 5–12	Linea alba and anterior iliac crest	Superficial anterolateral trunk	Unilateral actions: lateral flexion and opposite-side rotation of trunk; Bilateral action: flex trunk
Rectus Abdominis	Pubic crest and pubic symphysis	Xiphoid process and costal cartilage of ribs 5–7	Superficial anterior trunk	Flexion of trunk
Quadratus Lumborum	Posterior iliac crest	Transverse processes of lumbar vertebrae and 12th rib	Deep, low back	Unilateral actions: lateral flexion of lumbar spine and hip hiking; Bilateral action: extension of lumbar spine

Origin, Insertion, Location, and Action Chart of Respiration Muscles

Muscle Name	Origin	Insertion	Location	Action(s)
Diaphragm	Lumbar vertebrae, inferior 6 ribs and their costal cartilage, posterior xiphoid process	Central tendon	Between thoracic and abdominopelvic cavities	Chief muscle of inspiration
Internal Intercostals	Superior border of rib below	Inferior border of rib above	Between ribs	Depress ribs in forced exhalation
External Intercostals	Inferior border of rib above	Superior border of rib below	Between ribs	Elevate ribs in inhalation
Serratus Posterior Superior	Inferior portion of ligamentum nuchae, spinous processes of C7–T3	Ribs 2–5	Midlayer mid to upper back	Elevate ribs in inhalation
Serratus Posterior Inferior	Spinous processes of T11–L3	Ribs 9–12	Midlayer low back	Depress ribs in forced exhalation

Jaw/mandible elevators:

1. *Medial pterygoid* is a lateral cheek muscle, deep to ramus of mandible.

2. *Masseter* is a superficial lateral cheek muscle and a "chewing muscle."

3. *Temporalis:* muscle that is located on the lateral temporal bone.

Jaw/mandible depressors:

1. *Platysma* is a superficial anterior neck and upper chest muscle.

2. *Digastric (suprahyoid)* joins the hyoid bone to the mandible.

Muscles that perform flexion, lateral flexion, and opposite-side rotation of the neck:

1. *Scalenes* is a lateral neck muscle, has anterior, middle, and posterior sections, can cause thoracic outlet syndrome when shortened.

2. *Sternocleidomastoid* is a superficial, anterolateral neck muscle, named for its attachments.

Muscles that perform extension, lateral flexion, and same-side rotation of the neck:

1. *Suboccipitals* consists of four pairs of deep muscles, located inferior to the occiput.

2. *Splenius capitis* is a midlayer posterior neck muscle that attaches to the ligamentum nuchae and the occiput.

3. *Splenius cervicis* is a midlayer, posterior neck muscle that attaches to transverse processes and spinous processes.

Spine Extensors:

1. *Interspinalis* is a segmental group member, joins spinous process to spinous process, located primarily in the cervical and lumbar regions, and extends neck and low back.

2. *Intertransversarii* is a segmental group member, joins transverse process to transverse process, is located primarily in the cervical and lumbar regions, extends and laterally flexes neck and low back.

3. *Rotatores* is a transversospinalis member that joins transverse processes to spinous processes one vertebrae above, extends and rotates the spine to opposite side, and is located in the lamina groove.

4. *Multifidus* is a transversospinalis member that joins transverse processes to spinous processes two to four vertebrae above, extends and rotates the spine to opposite side, and is located in the lamina groove.

5. *Semispinalis* is a transversospinalis member that joins transverse processes to spinous processes three to six vertebrae above, extends and rotates the spine to opposite side, and is located in the lamina groove.

6. *Iliocostalis* is an erector spinae group member that is located most laterally of the three erectors and performs lateral flexion and extension of the spine.

7. *Longissimus* is an erector spinae group member that is the central band of the three erectors and performs lateral flexion and extension of the spine.

8. *Spinalis* is an erector spinae group member that is located most medially of the three erectors and performs lateral flexion and extension of the spine.

Muscles of the Abdominal Wall:

1. *Transverse abdominis* is the deepest lateral abdominal wall muscle and performs compression of the contents of the abdomen.

2. *Internal obliques* is a midlayer lateral abdominal wall muscle that performs flexion, lateral flexion, and same-side rotation of the trunk.

3. *External obliques* is a superficial lateral abdominal wall muscle that performs flexion, lateral flexion, and opposite-side rotation of the trunk.

4. *Rectus abdominis* is an anterior abdominal wall muscle that is divided into segments and performs flexion of the trunk.

5. *Quadratus lumborum* is the deepest posterior abdominal wall muscle, attaches to the posterior iliac crest, the lumbar vertebrae, and the twelfth rib, and performs lateral flexion and extension of the lumbar spine.

Muscles of Respiration:

1. *Diaphragm* is the chief muscle of respiration and pulls the central tendon down to enlarge the volume of the thoracic cavity, causing pressure reduction on the thoracic cavity and causing air to enter the lungs.

2. *External intercostals* is a muscle located between the ribs and is generally said to assist in inhalation.

3. *Internal intercostals* is a muscle located between the ribs and is generally said to assist in exhalation.

4. *Serratus posterior superior* is a muscle located in the midlayer upper back, elevates ribs 25, and is generally thought to assist in inhalation.

5. *Serratus posterior inferior* is a muscle located in the midlayer of the low back and is generally said to assist in exhalation, although it may have a role in stabilizing the lower ribs, which can help the diaphragm function more efficiently.

CHAPTER 5

Case Study Exercises
Case Study #1

A client comes into your office and you notice that she has an anterior pelvic tilt.

What muscles might be shortened and contributing to this issue?

Iliopsoas, rectus femoris, QL, lumbar erectors, sartorius, TFL, pectineus

What muscles might be lengthened and contributing to this problem?

Gluteus maximus, the hamstrings, and rectus abdominis

Case Study #2

A client comes in to your office. As you observe his standing posture, you notice that his feet are not pointing forward, but rather they point to the sides (hip lateral rotation).

What muscles might be shortened and contributing to this issue?

Gluteus maximus, sartorius, piriformis, gemellus inferior and superior, obturator internus and externus, quadrates femoris, and iliopsoas.

What muscles might be lengthened and contributing to this problem?

Gluteus medius, gluteus minimus and TFL

Case Study #3

Your client lets you know that she cannot fully flex her knee.

What muscles might be shortened and contributing to this issue?

The four quadriceps group muscles: vastus intermedius, vastus medialis, vastus lateralis, and rectus femoris.

What muscles might be lengthened and contributing to this problem?

The hamstring and gastrocnemius

Case Study #4

The outsides of your clients' shoes are noticeably more worn than the medial or inner sides.

What muscles might be shortened and contributing to this phenomenon?

Tibialis anterior and tibialis posterior

What muscles might be lengthened and contributing to this phenomenon?

Peroneus longus, peroneus brevis, and peroneus tertius

Case Study #5

Your client has limited ability to fully abduct his thighs.

What muscles might be shortened and contributing to this issue?

Adductor magnus, adductor longus, adductor brevis, pectineus, and gracilis

What muscles might be lengthened and contributing to this problem?

Gluteus medius, gluteus minimus, TFL, and sartorius

Case Study #6

Your client has limited ability to dorsiflex her ankle.

What muscles might be shortened and contributing to this issue?

Gastrocnemius, soleus, tibialis posterior, flexor digitorum longus, flexor hallucis longus, peroneus longus, and peroneus brevis

What muscles might be lengthened and contributing to this problem?

Tibialis anterior, extensor digitorum longus, extensor hallucis longus, and peroneus tertius

Review Charts to Study

Piriformis and Adductors of Thigh

Muscle Name	Origin	Insertion	Action(s)	Location
Piriformis	Anterior sacrum	Greater trochanter	Lateral rotation of hip	Deep buttock region
Adductor Magnus	Inferior pubic ramus and ischial tuberosity	Linea aspera of femur	Adduction of hip	Medial thigh
Adductor Longus	Anterior pubis	Linea aspera	Adduction of hip	Medial thigh
Adductor Brevis	Anterior pubis	Linea aspera	Adduction of hip	Medial thigh
Pectineus	Anterior pubic ramus	Linea aspera	Flexion and adduction of hip	Medial thigh
Gracilis	Anterior pubis	Pes anserinus	Adduction of hip, flexion of knee, and medial rotation of knee	Medial thigh (most superficial, medial thigh muscle)

Gluteal Region

Muscle Name	Origin	Insertion	Action(s)	Location
Gluteus Minimus	Posterior or external ilium	Greater trochanter	Abduction and medial rotation of the hip	Lateral hip
Gluteus Medius	Posterior or external ilium	Greater trochanter	Abduction and medial rotation of the hip	Lateral hip
Tensor Fascia Latae	ASIS and anterior iliac crest	Iliotibial band	Abduction, medial rotation, and flexion of the hip; helps stabilize knee	Anterolateral hip
Gluteus Maximus	Posterior ilium and sacrum	Gluteal tuberosity and iliotibial band	Extension and lateral rotation of the hip	Superficial buttock region

Hamstrings, Quadriceps, Iliopsoas, and Sartorius

Muscle Name	Origin	Insertion	Action(s)	Location
Semimembranosus	Ischial tuberosity	Proximal, posterior, medial tibia	Extend hip and flex knee	Deep, medial posterior thigh
Semitendinosus	Ischial tuberosity	Pes anserinus	Extend hip and flex knee	Superficial, medial posterior thigh
Biceps Femoris	Ischial tuberosity and linea aspera	Head of the fibula	Extend hip and flex knee	Posterior lateral thigh
Iliopsoas	Transverse processes and bodies of T12–L5 and iliac fossa	Lesser trochanter	Flexion of hip (strongest) and lateral rotation of hip	Deep abdomen
Vastus Intermedius	Anterior femur	Tibial tuberosity via the patellar tendon	Extend knee	Deep anterior thigh
Vastus Medialis	Linea aspera	Tibial tuberosity via the patellar tendon	Extend knee	Anteromedial thigh
Vastus Lateralis	Linea aspera	Tibial tuberosity via the patellar tendon	Extend knee	Anterolateral thigh
Rectus Femoris	AIIS and close to acetabulum	Tibial tuberosity via the patellar tendon	Extend knee and flex hip	Superficial anterior thigh
Sartorius	ASIS	Pes anserinus	Flex, laterally rotate, and abduct hip and flex knee	Superficial anterior thigh

Muscles of the Leg

Muscle Name	Origin	Insertion	Action(s)	Location
Popliteus	Lateral epicondyle of the femur	Proximal, medial, posterior tibia	Medial rotation of tibia and flexion of knee	Deep, posterior knee
Soleus	Soleal line of tibia and posterior head of fibula	Calcaneus via Achilles tendon	Plantarflexion of the ankle	Deep to gastrocnemius in superficial posterior leg compartment
Plantaris	Lateral epicondyle of femur	Calcaneus via Achilles tendon	Flexion of knee and plantarflexion of ankle	Posterior knee
Gastrocnemius	Lateral and medial condyles of femur	Calcaneus via Achilles tendon	Flexion of knee and plantarflexion of ankle	Superficial, posterior leg
Tibialis Posterior	Posterior tibia, fibula, and interosseus membrane	Navicular, cuneiform bones, cuboid, and metatarsals 2, 2, and 4	Inversion of foot and plantarflexion of ankle	Deep posterior leg compartment
Flexor Digitorum Longus	Posterior tibia	Distal phalanges of four lateral toes, plantar surface	Flexion of four lateral toes and plantarflexion of ankle	Deep posterior leg compartment
Flexor Hallucis Longus	Posterior fibula	Distal phalanx of digit 1, plantar surface	Flexion of big toe and plantarflexion of ankle	Deep posterior leg compartment
Peroneus Tertius	Distal, anterior fibula	Base of the fifth metacarpal	Eversion of foot and dorsiflexion of ankle	Distal in the anterior leg compartment
Peroneus Brevis	Inferior two thirds of lateral fibula	Base of the fifth metacarpal	Eversion of foot and plantarflexion of ankle	Lateral leg compartment
Peroneus Longus	Lateral fibula including head of fibula	Base of first metacarpal and medial cuneiform	Eversion of foot and plantarflexion of ankle	Lateral leg compartment
Extensor Digitorum Longus	Lateral condyle of tibia and entire anterior fibula	Distal phalanges of four lateral toes, dorsal side	Extension of four lateral toes and dorsiflexion of ankle	Anterior leg compartment
Extensor Hallucis Longus	Anterior fibula and interosseus membrane	Distal phalanx of digit 1, dorsal surface	Extension of big toe and dorsiflexion of ankle	Anterior leg compartment
Tibialis Anterior	Lateral condyle and proximal half of anterior tibia	Base of first metatarsal and medial cuneiform	Inversion of foot and dorsiflexion of ankle	Anterior leg compartment

Intrinsic Foot Muscles

Muscle Name	Origin	Insertion	Action(s)	Location
Dorsal Interossei	Adjacent sides of metatarsals 1–5	Medial side of base of proximal phalanx of digit 1 and lateral sides of bases of proximal phalanges of digits 2–4	Abduct toes (digits 2–4)	Layer four (deepest) dorsal side of foot
Palmar Interossei	Medial sides of metatarsals 3, 4, and 5	Medial sides of bases of proximal phalanges of digits 3, 4, and 5	Adduct toes (digits 3–5)	Layer four (deepest) plantar side of foot
Adductor Hallucis	Oblique head: base of metatarsals 2–4; Transverse head: metatarsophalangeal joint capsules	Lateral side of base of proximal phalanx of digit 1	Adduct digit I (big toe)	Layer three plantar side of foot
Flexor Hallucis Brevis	Cuboid and lateral cuneiform, plantar surfaces	Base of proximal phalanx of digit 1	Flex digit I (big toe)	Layer three plantar side of foot
Flexor Digiti Minimi Brevis	Base of fifth metatarsal	Base of proximal phalanx of fifth digit	Flex fifth digit (little toe)	Layer three plantar side of foot
Lumbricals	Tendon of insertion of flexor digitorum longus	Bases of proximal phalanges of digits 2–5 and extensor expansion	Flex MP joints and extend DIP joints and PIP joints of the foot	Layer two plantar side of foot
Quadratus Plantae	Calcaneus	Tendon of insertion of flexor digitorum longus	Flex four lateral toes	Layer two plantar side of foot
Abductor Hallucis	Calcaneus	Medial side of proximal phalanx of digit 1	Adduct digit 1 (big toe)	Layer one (most superficial) plantar side of foot
Flexor Digitorum Brevis	Calcaneus	Medial and lateral sides of the middle phalanges of digits 2–5	Flex four lateral toes	Layer one (most superficial) plantar side of foot
Abductor Digiti Minimi	Calcaneus	Lateral side of the base of the proximal phalanx of the fifth digit	Abduct fifth digit (little toe)	Layer one (most superficial) plantar side of foot

Action Charts of Hip, Knee, Ankle, and Foot Movers

HIP FLEXORS	HIP EXTENSORS
1. *Iliopsoas*	1. *Gluteus maximus*
2. *Rectus femoris*	2. *Semimembranosus*
3. *Pectineus*	3. *Semitendinosus*
4. *Sartorius*	4. *Biceps femoris*
5. *TFL*	

HIP LATERAL ROTATORS	HIP MEDIAL ROTATORS
1. *Gluteus maximus*	1. *Gluteus medius*
2. *Piriformis*	2. *Gluteus minimus*
3. *Obturator internus*	3. *TFL*
4. *Obturator externus*	
5. *Gemellus superior*	
6. *Gemellus inferior*	
7. *Quadrates femoris*	
8. *Sartorius*	
9. *Iliopsoas*	

HIP ADDUCTORS	HIP ABDUCTORS
1. *Adductor magnus*	1. *Gluteus medius*
2. *Adductor longus*	2. *Gluteus minimus*
3. *Adductor brevis*	3. *TFL*
4. *Pectineus*	4. *Sartorius*
5. *Gracilis*	

KNEE FLEXORS	KNEE EXTENSORS
1. *Semimembranosus*	1. *Vastus interomedialis*
2. *Semitendinosus*	2. *Vastus medialis*
3. *Biceps femoris*	3. *Vastus lateralis*
4. *Gastrocnemius*	4. *Rectus femoris*
5. *Popliteus*	
6. *Plantaris*	
7. *Sartorius*	
8. *Gracilis*	

ANKLE PLANTARFLEXORS	ANKLE DORSIFLEXORS
1. *Gastrocnemius*	1. *Tibialis anterior*
2. *Soleus*	2. *Extensor digitorum longus*
3. *Plantaris*	3. *Extensor hallucis longus*
4. *Tibialis posterior*	4. *Peroneus tertius*
5. *Flexor digitorum longus*	
6. *Flexor hallucis longus*	
7. *Peroneus longus*	
8. *Peroneus brevis*	

FOOT EVERTORS	FOOT INVERTERS
1. *Peroneus longus*	1. *Tibialis anterior*
2. *Peroneus brevis*	2. *Tibialis posterior*
3. *Peroneus tertius*	

TOE FLEXORS	TOE EXTENSORS
1. **Flexor digitorum longus**	1. **Extensor digitorum longus**
2. **Flexor hallucis longus**	2. **Extensor hallucis longus**
3. **Flexor digitorum brevis**	3. **Extensor digitorum brevis**
4. **Flexor hallucis brevis**	4. **Extensor hallucis brevis**
5. **Flexor digiti minimi brevis**	5. **Lumbricals (IP joints)**
6. **Quadratus plantae**	
7. **Lumbricals (MP joints)**	

TOE ABDUCTORS	TOE ADDUCTORS
1. **Dorsal interossei**	1. **Plantar interossei**
2. **Abductor hallucis**	2. **Adductor hallucis**
3. **Abductor digiti minimi**	

Muscles Located in the Hip and Thigh Region

1. **Piriformis** is a deep buttock region muscle and laterally rotates the hip. It can cause sciatica when short.

2. **Adductor magnus** is the largest, deepest medial thigh muscle and adducts the thigh.

3. **Gluteus medius** is the larger of the two lateral hip muscles and performs abduction and medial rotation of the hip. It pulls the hip down when the weight is on the limb, so the other hip rises and the other limb can swing through when walking.

4. **Gluteus maximus** is the largest muscle in the body (by volume). It performs lateral rotation and forceful extension of the hip.

5. **TFL** is the small lateral hip muscle that flexes, abducts, and medially rotates the hip, and it plays a role in stabilization of the knee. It inserts into the IT band.

6. **Vastus lateralis** is the anterolateral quadriceps group muscle; it originates on the linea aspera.

7. **Vastus medialis** is the anteromedial quadriceps group muscle; it originates on the linea aspera.

8. **Rectus femoris** is the superficial quadriceps group muscle; it flexes the hip as well as extends the knee.

9. The insertion of all four quadriceps group muscles is on the **tibial tuberosity.**

10. The action of all four quadriceps group muscles is **knee extension.**

11. **Biceps femoris** is the lateral hamstring muscle, which inserts on the head of the fibula.

12. **Semimembranosus** is the deeper of the two medial hamstring muscles, which inserts on the proximal, medial posterior tibia.

13. **Semitendinosus** is the superficial of the two medial hamstring muscles, which inserts at pes anserinus.

14. The origin of the three hamstrings is the **ischial tuberosity**.

15. The actions of all three hamstrings are **flexion of the knee** and **extension of the hip**.

16. **Sartorius** is the **tailor muscle**, the longest muscle in the body. It performs lateral rotation, abduction and flexion of the hip, and knee flexion.

Muscles Located in the Knee Area and Leg

1. *Popliteus* is the small, deep muscle in the posterior knee region that performs medial rotation of the tibia.

2. *Plantaris* is the small muscle in the posterior knee region that is variably present. This muscle has a long tendon of insertion, which joins the calcaneus via the Achilles tendon.

3. *Gastrocnemius* is the most superficial muscle in the posterior leg and performs knee flexion and plantarflexion of the ankle.

4. *Soleus* is the ankle plantarflexor that is located directly deep to gastrocnemius.

5. *Tibialis posterior* is the deep posterior leg compartment muscle that inverts the foot and plantarflexes the ankle.

6. *Flexor digitorum longus* is the deep posterior leg compartment muscle that flexes the four lateral toes and plantarflexes the ankle.

7. *Flexor hallucis longus* is the deep posterior leg compartment muscle that flexes the big toe and plantarflexes the ankle.

8. *Peroneus (or fibularis) brevis* is the lateral leg compartment muscle that everts the foot and plantarflexes the ankle. It is the shorter of a pair.

9. *Peroneus (or fibularis) longus* is the lateral leg compartment muscle that everts the foot and plantarflexes the ankle. It is the longer of a pair.

10. *Tibialis anterior* is the anterior leg compartment muscle that everts the foot and dorsiflexes the ankle.

11. *Extensor digitorum longus* is the anterior leg compartment muscle that extends the four lateral toes and dorsiflexes the ankle.

12. *Extensor hallucis longus* is the anterior leg compartment muscle that extends the big toe and dorsiflexes the ankle.

13. *Peroneus tertius* is the anterior leg compartment muscle that inverts the foot and dorsiflexes the ankle.

Intrinsic Foot Muscles

1. *Dorsal interossei* is the muscle located in the fourth layer, deep between the metatarsals on the dorsal side of the foot; it abducts the toes.

2. *Plantar interossei* is the muscle located in the fourth layer, deep between the metatarsals on the plantar side of the foot; it adducts the toes.

3. *Flexor hallucis brevis* is the muscle located in the third layer on the plantar side of the foot; it flexes the big toe.

4. *Adductor hallucis* is the muscle located in the third layer on the plantar side of the foot; it adducts the big toe.

5. *Flexor digiti minimi brevis* is the muscle located in the third layer on the plantar side of the foot; it flexes the fifth digit.

6. *Lumbricals* is the muscle located in the second layer on the plantar side of the foot; it flexes the MP joints and extends the PIP and DIP joints of the four lateral toes.

7. *Quadratus plantae* is the muscle located in the second layer on the plantar side of the foot; it helps flex the four lateral toes.

8. *Abductor hallucis* is the muscle located in the first layer on the plantar side of the foot; it abducts the big toe.

9. *Flexor digitorum brevis* is the muscle located in the first layer on the plantar side of the foot; it flexes the four lateral toes.

10. *Abductor digiti minimi* is the muscle located in the first layer on the plantar side of the foot; it abducts the fifth digit.

Glossary

Abdominal aponeurosis: A bilayered sheet of connective tissue which serves as the insertion of three abdominal muscles. The right and left abdominal aponeuroses converge at the linea alba.

Abduction: A movement of a limb or body part away from the midline in the frontal plane. Abduction also refers to the movement of digits away from the midline of the hand (3rd digit) or away from the midline of the foot (2nd digit).

Actin: The thinner myofilament that contains myosin binding sites, where the myosin can attach and pull the actin toward the center of the sarcomere.

Action: The movement that a muscle creates when insertion moves toward origin.

Adduction: A movement of a limb or body part toward the midline in the frontal plane. Abduction also refers to the movement of digits toward the midline of the hand (3rd digit) or toward the midline of the foot (2nd digit)

Amphiarthrotic joint: "Slightly moveable joints, typically joined by fiber and/or cartilage.

Anatomical position: a position of reference from which directions are determined. Anatomical position includes standing upright, face and feet face forward, arms are at the sides, and palms face forward.

Antagonist: The muscle that performs an opposite action

Anterior: Front or toward the front.

Appendicular skeleton: Bones of the upper limbs, lower limbs, the clavicle, sternum, ilium, ischium, and pubis.

Atlantoaxial joint: The joint between the upper two cervical vertebrae, C1 and C2. C1 is called the atlas, after the Greek god Altas, who held up the world, and C2 is called the axis due to the projection it contains that points upward and fills the space in C1, due to the lack of a body.

Atlanto-occipital joint: The joint between the occiput and C1. C1 is called the atlas, as it "holds up, the head or the Greek god atlas.

Axial skeleton: Bones of the skull, spine, sternum, ribs, and hyoid bone.

Bone markings: Notable shapes, projections, and grooves on bones. Bone markings are often muscle attachment sites.

Caudal: Inferior, lower, pertaining to a tail.

Cephalad: Above or closer to the top of the head.

Circumduction: A combination of flexion, extension, adduction, and adduction.

Compact bone tissue: The superficial, dense layer of bone.

Concentric contraction: A muscle contraction that occurs when the muscle shortens and the distance between origin and insertion decreases.

Connective tissue: One of the four types of tissue on the body, connective tissue provides framework to the body and joins different structures together. Connective tissue contains cells, fibers, and ground substance in a manner that can create a liquid, gelatinous, or solid substance.

Coronal plane: The plane that divides the body into anterior and posterior sections. Also called the frontal plane.

Deep: Farther from the surface.

Depression: An inferior movement of a bone such as the scapula and mandible.

Diarthrotic joint: "Freely movable" joint. All synovial joints are classified as diarthrotic.

Distal: Farther (more distant) from the trunk. Distal is typically used to refer to a location on a limb, thus farther from the shoulder joint and closer to the finger tips/nails when referring to the upper limb, and farther from the hip joint and closer to the tips of the toes/toenails when referring to the lower limb.

Downward rotation: A turning movement of the scapula so that the glenoid fossa moves inferiorly, the inferior angle moves posteriorly, and the superior angle moves superiorly and anteriorly. Upward rotation of the scapula allows the arm to move from a positioning which it is pointed upward to a position in which it is abducted to 90 degrees. Downward rotation of the scapula also allows us to reach behind our bodies, toward and across the midline.

Eccentric contraction: A muscle contraction that occurs when the muscle lengthens while working and the distance between origin and insertion increases.

Elevation: A superior movement of a bone such as the scapula and mandible.

Endomysium: The connective tissue structure that wraps around an individual muscle cell.

Epimysium: The connective tissue structure that wraps around a muscle.

Eversion of the foot: A movement occurring at the intertarsal joints in which the sole of the foot is moved away from the mid sagittal plane. When eversion of both feet occurs simultaneously, the plantar surfaces of the foot are moved away from each other.

Extension: A straightening movement at a joint. Extension is often a posterior movement of a body part, with notable exception of the leg, foot, and toes.

Extensor mechanism: A complex connective tissue structure on the dorsal sides of the fingers, which contains loops or tunnels through which run the insertion tendons of finger extensor muscles. The extensor mechanism is also called the extensor expansion and the dorsal mechanism. This structure serves as a muscle insertion site for several muscles.

Fascia: A continuous, three-dimensional web of fibrous connective tissue that surrounds and connects tissues, organs, and cells of the body.

Fascicle: A group or bundle of muscle or nerve fibers wrapped together by connective tissue.

Flexion: A bending movement at a joint. Flexion is often a forward movement of a body part, with the notable exceptions of the leg, foot, and toes.

Flexor retinaculum: A connective tissue structure that forms the roof of the carpal tunnel. It attaches to the scaphoid and trapezium laterally and to the pisiform and hamate medially.

Frontal plane: The plane that divides the body into anterior and posterior sections. Also called the coronal plane.

Horizontal Abduction: A movement of a limb (usually the upper limb) in the transverse plane. The limb moves toward the mid sagittal plane.

Horizontal Adduction: A movement of a limb (usually the upper limb) in the transverse plane. The limb moves away from the mid sagittal plane.

Inferior: Below or closer to the feet.

Inguinal ligament: A ligament that runs from the ASIS to the pelvic tubercle.

Innominate bone: A hip bone, including the fused ilium, ischium, and pubis.

Insertion: The more movable attachment site of muscle to bone or connective tissue.

Inversion of the foot: A movement occurring at the intertarsal joints in which the sole of the foot is moved to face the mid sagittal plane. When inversion of both feet occurs simultaneously, the plantar surfaces of the foot are moved inward to face each other.

Isometric contraction: A muscle contraction that occurs when the tension in a muscle increases, but the length remains the same.

IT band: A thick band of connective tissue running along the lateral thigh from the ilium to the tibia. There is a band of fascia surrounding all the muscles of the thigh, and the IT band is a thickening of this fascia.

Lateral: Farther from the midline, closer to the sides. Lateral can also mean "side."

Lengthened muscle: The literal increase of the length of a muscle, while the muscle is at rest. Muscle lengthening often occurs with overuse and shortening of the opposing muscle(s).

Ligamentum nuchae: A thin ligament running from the external occipital protuberance to the spinous process of C7 and joining all the spinous processes between.

Linea alba: A "white line" of connective tissue that runs from the xiphoid process of the sternum to the pubic symphysis. The linea alba is located where the two abdominal aponeuroses converge in the center of the anterior abdomen. It darkens due to hormonal changes during pregnancy.

Medial: Closer to the midline or midsagittal plane.

Motor unit: The sum total of one motor neuron and all the skeletal muscle fibers the single neuron innervates.

Motor unit recruitment: The ability of a skeletal muscle cell to engage additional motor units to perform or maintain performance of an action.

Muscle fatigue: The inability of muscle cells to maintain contraction.

Muscle tone: The continuous contraction of a small number of motor units, giving the body firmness in the musculature.

Myofibril: The structural component of each skeletal muscle cell that runs the entire length of a muscle cell. Myofibrils contract and shorten. They are cylindrical in shape and contain thousands of threadlike protein structures beautifully positioned in organized rows and segments. There are hundreds of myofibrils within a muscle cell.

Myofilaments: Threadlike, protein structures organized in parallel rows, in a three-dimensional fashion within a myofibril. There are thousands of myofilaments within a myofibril.

Myosin: The thicker myofilament that contains cross bridges to pull the actin toward the center of the sarcomere.

Origin: The more stable attachment site of muscle to bone or connective tissue.

Pelvic girdle: The bowl-shaped skeletal structure housing lower digestive and reproductive organs. Made of ilium, ischium, pubis, and sacrum. The bones of the lower extremity connect to the pelvic girdle.

Perimysium: The connective tissue structure that wraps around a fascicle.

Plantar fascia: Thick connective tissue on the sole of the foot, which runs from the calcaneus to the toes.

Posterior: Back or closer to the back.

Protraction: An anterior movement of the scapula or mandible.

Proximal: Closer to the trunk. Proximal is typically used to refer to a location on a limb, thus proximal means closer to the shoulder joint when referring to the upper limb, and closer to the hip joint when referring to the lower limb.

Retraction: A posterior movement of the scapula or mandible.

Rotation: A turning movement at a joint. The shoulder and hip rotate both medially and laterally.

Sagittal plane: The plane that cuts the body into right and left sections.

Sarcolemma: A skeletal muscle cell membrane.

Sarcomere: A segment of a myofibril, from Z line to Z line. Sarcomeres are the functional unit of contraction for a skeletal muscle cell.

Sarcoplasmic reticulum: A network of tubes and sacs that wraps around each myofibril.

Shortened muscle: The literal reduction of the length of a muscle, while the muscle is at rest. Muscle shortening typically occurs with overuse and with maintaining the muscle's position in a shortened state.

Shoulder girdle: The clavicle and scapula.

Sliding filament mechanism: The process whereby myosin pulls actin toward the center of a sarcomere and muscle shortening occurs.

Spongy bone tissue: The internal portion of bone is comprised of thin, lattice-like structures called trabeculae. The spaces within the trabeculae contain red marrow, which produces blood cells.

Superficial: Closer to the surface.

Superior: Above or closer to the top of the head.

Synarthrotic joint: "Immovable" joint. While the sutures are classified as immovable joints, they do in fact permit minute movements. Synarthrotic joints are typically joined by fiber.

Synovial joint: Joints that contain a synovial capsule filled with synovial fluid. The articulating surfaces of the bones that come together to form synovial joints have a layer of hyaline cartilage. Most synovial joints are stabilized by ligaments either within the joint capsule or superficial to it.

Synergist: A muscle that performs as action in common with another muscle.

Temporal-mandibular joint: The jaw joint, between the head or condyle of the mandible and the mandibular fossa of the temporal bone.

Thoracolumbar aponeurosis: A sheet of connective tissue covering the sacrum and fanning laterally and superiorly. It attaches to the spinous processes of T7-L5 and serves as a portion of the origin of latissimus dorsi.

Transverse plane: Horizontally oriented plane that divides the body into upper and lower sections.

Upward rotation: A turning movement of the scapula so that the glenoid fossa moves superiorly, the inferior angle moves anteriorly, and the superior angle moves inferiorly and posteriorly. Upward rotation of the scapula allows the arm to move from a positioning that it is abducted to 90 degrees, to a position in which the arm points upward.

Ventral: Front or toward the front.

Volar: Anterior, primarily referring to the palmar side of the hand or plantar side of the foot.